Anatomical and Physiological Bases of Speech

Anatomical and Physiological Bases of Speech

David Ross Dickson, Ph.D.

Professor of Pediatrics
Director, Speech and Hearing
Mailman Center for Child Development
University of Miami School of Medicine
Miami, Florida

Wilma Maue-Dickson, Ph.D.

Manager, Physician Education Program
Cordis Corporation
Associate Professor of Surgery
University of Miami School of Medicine
Miami, Florida

Little, Brown and Company
Boston

Library of Congress Catalog Card No. 81-84195
ISBN 0-316-184314
Printed in the United States of America
HAL

Cover design by Betsy Hacker

Contents

Preface

This book is designed to be used by both the beginning and the advanced student. Students frequently enter their first course in anatomy and physiology with little or no background in the physical sciences. Therefore, the first two chapters present background information necessary to the study of the anatomy and physiology of respiration, phonation, articulation, and audition presented in the subsequent chapters. The final chapter deals with the structure and function of the nervous system.

In order for a text to be useful to the student beyond the confines of its specific content, it must stress principles. Thus a great deal of attention is given to basic principles of the structure and function of the neuromuscular mechanism as well as biomechanical potential, which is essential to an understanding of physiology. Mastering these fundamentals enables the student to organize and evaluate new information.

The authors wish to express their gratitude to a number of individuals who have contributed their energies, their thoughtful criticism, and their encouragement toward the completion of this text. Foremost among these have been Barbara Ward and her predecessor, Sarah Boardman, of the Allied Health Department at Little, Brown and Company. Their patience has been inexhaustible, and their thoughtful and constructive criticism has been insightful. We would also like to thank Noreen Frans and Roger Dalston for their assistance in reviewing specific parts of the text in its draft forms and Katherine Arnoldi, Book Editor at Little, Brown and Company, for her essential and exacting copyediting.

Support for research by the authors that led to the development of some of the information contained herein was provided by a number of agencies, including the National Institute of Dental Research, the Health, Research and Services Foundation of Pittsburgh, the Mailman Foundation, and the Hearing, Education and Research Foundation of Miami.

D. R. D.
W. M.-D.

1   Introduction

This volume is concerned with the biological processes involved in the production and reception of speech. The purpose of the present chapter is to provide the reader with a brief overview of the speech-hearing process and the acoustic events interposed between the biological processes of speech production and reception and to introduce the reader to the study of anatomy.

THE SPEECH-HEARING PROCESS

Figure 1-1 presents a simple schematic of the major events involved in the speech-hearing process. The organs of speech are activated by brain and spinal cord mechanisms (central processes) to produce an acoustic signal, which is received and processed by the listener. Sensory information from the energizing (motor) pathways, from the speech organs, and from the acoustic output are fed back into the central processor in order to control the function of the speech organs.

Figure 1-2 illustrates the major components of the speech organ system that produce the acoustic output we call speech. Air is taken into and is expelled from the lungs during **respiration.** As air is pumped from the lungs it passes through the larynx, where the air stream is periodically interrupted. This periodic interruption of the air stream results in **sound.** The nature of this sound is changed as it passes through the pharynx and the nasal and/or oral cavities. The nature of the change is a function of muscles that vary the shapes of the cavities and their entrances and exits. The process of **exhalation** is that part of respiration during which air is pumped out of the lungs. The action of the larynx in producing sound is called **phonation**. The process by which the nature of the sound is changed as it passes through the cavities above the larynx is called **resonance**. The movements of the structures above the larynx that serve to change the configuration of those cavities is called **articulation.**

1-1. *Schematic of the speech-hearing process.*

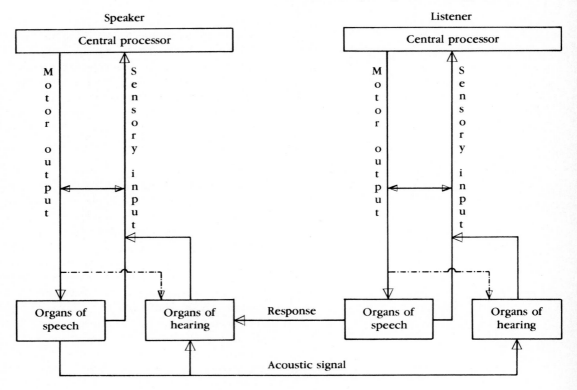

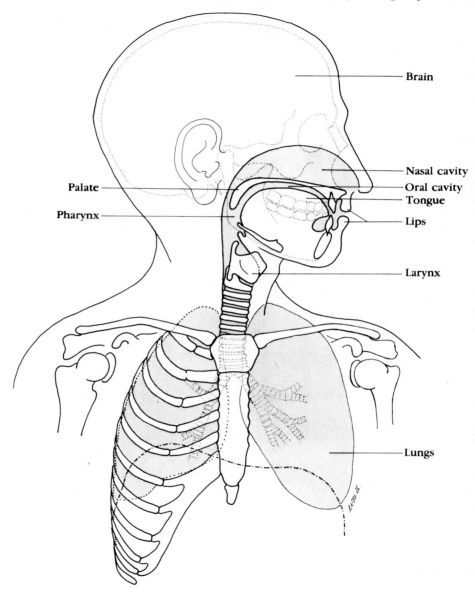

1-2. *Major components of the speech organ system.*

Brain

Nasal cavity

Oral cavity

Tongue

Palate

Lips

Pharynx

Larynx

Lungs

Figure 1-3 illustrates the major components of the hearing organ system, which receives and processes acoustic signals. Sound is received via the external ear and external ear canal and strikes the eardrum. This sets the eardrum into **vibration**. The resulting vibrations are transmitted through the middle ear cavity by a chain of three small bones called the ossicles. The ossicles transmit the vibrations to the inner ear, which is fluid-filled. The resulting vibrations in the fluid activate sensory nerve endings that translate the vibratory movements into **electrical signals**. These electrical signals are transmitted to the brain via the auditory nerve.

Each of these components of the speech-hearing system will be dealt with in detail in subsequent chapters. The following section provides a brief overview of the nature of sound. Although a comprehensive discussion of acoustics is beyond the scope of this volume, certain fundamentals are necessary to provide a context for study of the biological events that will be addressed.

1-3. *Major components of the hearing organ system.*

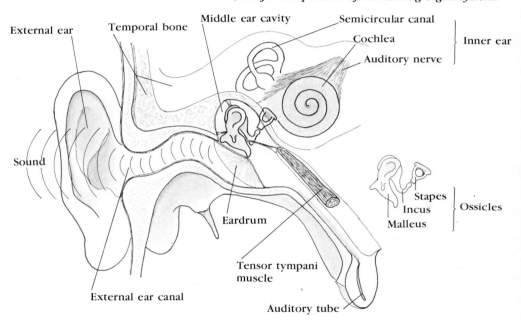

ACOUSTICS

Sound can be defined as vibrations occurring in some medium (such as air) that, when applied to the auditory mechanism, give rise to the sensation of hearing. A **vibration** is an oscillatory movement of any substance, whether it be an atom, a molecule, or some substance that they compose. In order to understand vibration we first need to examine the related principles of elasticity, inertia, and momentum.

Elasticity is the tendency of a substance to return to its original shape or size after being deformed. The greater that tendency, the greater the degree of elasticity. A rubber ball dropped to the floor will bounce because of its elasticity. The ball is deformed by striking the floor. Its tendency to return to its original shape provides the energy for the bounce. A steel ball has an even greater tendency to return to its original shape when deformed and so is more elastic and will bounce even higher if of the same weight as the rubber ball. Putty, if deformed, will remain so, and thus is not elastic. Thus elasticity has to do not with how easy the substance is to deform, but rather with how strong a tendency it has to return to its original shape. It is important to note that gases (such as air) demonstrate a high degree of elasticity when compressed (as demonstrated by compressing a filled balloon). Because the molecules of a gas such as air are elastic, they bounce off one another as they continually collide. This random activity of bumping and bouncing causes the molecules to maintain approximately equal separation from one another unless some external force intervenes. If an external force pushes some of the molecules of a gas closer together, they will push against their neighbors and rebound until all of the molecules are again evenly spaced.

Inertia is the property of any substance at rest to remain at rest and any substance in motion to remain in motion. Once thrown, a ball would continue to move forever were it not for the effects of gravity and the resistance encountered by the ball as it collides with air molecules.

Momentum is the property of a moving substance that determines the length of time before the substance ceases movement when the forces operating on it are constant. Momentum is a function of the mass and velocity of the substance and the resistance to which it is subjected. The greater the **mass** (weight per unit volume) and **velocity** and the less the **resistance,** the greater is the momentum.

Now let us examine the nature of **vibration.** If a violin string is pulled away from its rest position and released, it will move back toward rest position owing to its elasticity. However, when the string reaches rest position, its momentum, due to inertia, will carry it beyond rest position until its elasticity causes it to stop and return again toward rest position. This back and forth movement (vibration) will continue until the forces of elasticity and resistance bring it to a gradual halt. The back and forth motion of the string can be plotted over time (Figure 1-4) and is called **harmonic motion.** The motion of the string from rest position to one side, back through rest to the opposite side and back to rest position again is called one **cycle.** The rate (**frequency**) of vibration can then be referred to as the number of cycles that occur each second. The measure of cycles per second is called **hertz** (Hz). The maximum degree to which the string departs from rest position during any one cycle is called **amplitude.** The energy released per unit time by this motion is called the **intensity** of the vibration and is a direct function of its frequency and amplitude. If either the frequency or the amplitude of vibration is increased, the velocity of the string will increase.

The type of wave illustrated in Figure 1-4 is called harmonic because of its similarity to movement described by a rotating disk. If the motion of any point on the circumference of a uniformly revolving circle were plotted on a graph, its motion would describe a similar shape. Thus any distance along a harmonic wave can be measured in degrees of a circle. As vibration occurs, the number of degrees of a cycle which have occurred up to any given moment is called the **phase** of a cycle. The distance between any two points of the same phase on successive cycles is called the **wavelength** of the sound. Wavelength decreases with increased frequency since more cycles pass any given point each second. Wavelength increases as the speed of sound transmission increases. The speed (velocity) of sound is dependent upon the density and elasticity of the medium through which it passes.

When the string is pulled back and released, the rapid motion of the string causes air molecules to pile up ahead of the string. Thus a region of high molecular density is created (Figure 1-5). Because of the increased number of molecules undergoing random motion within a confined space, increased molecular density creates increased pressure. The high-pressure region (**condensation**) created by the motion of the string continues to move in the same direction owing to its own inertia. The string rebounds in the opposite direction creating an area of low molecular density or low pressure (**rarefaction**). As the string continues to vibrate, more condensations and rarefactions are created, which in turn create additional pressure variations by their own movement. Thus, while none of the air molecules moves very far, a pressure wave is generated that moves away from the string.

The **acoustic pressure wave** is similar to the wave produced in water by dropping a stone into it. The primary motion of the water molecules is up and down (analogous to the back and forth movement of the air molecules), with the wave peaks analogous to condensations and the valleys analogous to rarefactions. While the molecules move primarily up and down, the wave is propagated outward away from the stone.

Thus far we have seen how a simple pressure wave can be generated by a vibrating string. Such a pressure wave introduced to the human ear would be "heard," that is, create a sensation of hearing, if the frequency of vibration were at least 20 Hz but not more than 20,000 Hz and if it were of sufficient intensity. Changes in the frequency of vibration are perceived as changes in **pitch,** while changes in intensity are perceived as changes in **loudness.**

Loudness can be varied by changing the force of vibration. The harder we pluck the string, the greater the fluctuation in pressure. This is perceived as increased loudness. Pitch is altered by changing the frequency of vibration. The rate at which a string will vibrate (the number of cycles per second) is a function of the length, mass, and tension of the string.

1-4. *Phases of a harmonic wave.*

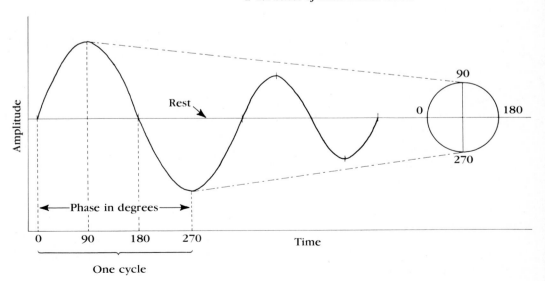

Tension is directly related to frequency, whereas length and mass are inversely related to frequency. We increase the frequency of a violin string by tightening (stretching) it. As tension increases, frequency increases. We also can increase the frequency with which the violin string vibrates by sliding our finger down the string, thus shortening the part of the string that is free to vibrate. Lower frequency strings on the violin are also heavier (have greater mass) than higher frequency strings.

Thus far we have examined **simple** harmonic vibration. Such vibration is called simple because it results in a single frequency and therefore a single pitch.

In the previous analogy of the string, a single frequency was produced. If we were to place a weight on the center of the string, the string as a whole would vibrate when plucked, but in addition, the upper and lower halves of the string would vibrate independently. The upper and lower halves of the string would vibrate at twice the frequency of the string as a whole, because of the relationships between length and frequency. Thus, two frequencies would be produced simultaneously. This would create a **complex** wave. In Figure 1-6 we see the result of combining two simple waves with different frequencies and intensities into a single complex wave. In nature, simple waves, also called pure tones, are extremely rare. Most objects when set into vibration produce multiple frequencies.

1-6. *Combination of two pure tones (A,B) into a complex tone (C). The frequency and also the intensity relationship of pure tones A and B is 2:1.*

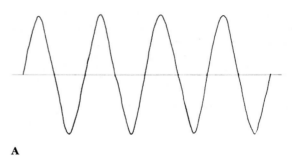

A

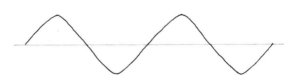

B

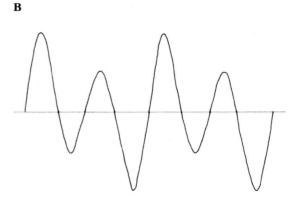

C

1-5. *Condensation, rarefaction, and propagation. Row 1 represents the uniform distribution of air molecules. Rows 2 through 5 trace successive stages in the movement of areas of condensation (ab, bc, cd, de), followed by areas of rarefaction.*

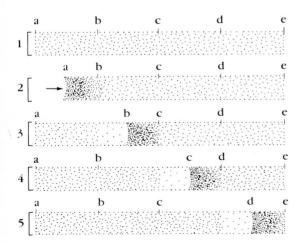

Complex sounds are of two types, called harmonic and inharmonic. **Harmonic** sounds are those in which all frequencies are simple multiples of the lowest frequency. In this case, the lowest frequency is called the **fundamental frequency** and all higher frequencies in the sequence are called **overtones.** Each of the frequencies, including the fundamental frequency, is called a **harmonic.** A note produced by a stringed instrument such as a piano is harmonic. If the frequencies that compose the complex tone do not have this relationship and are, therefore, **inharmonic,** they are heard as dissonant. One can produce a dissonant sound by simultaneously striking two adjacent keys on a piano or by hitting a drum. Most sounds in nature are inharmonic.

Thus far we have discussed the vibration that would occur if an object were set into vibration and then left alone to vibrate at a frequency or frequencies that is a function of its own internal characteristics. This is called **free vibration.** If the pressure wave generated by our string were to strike another object (such as another string or an eardrum) with sufficient intensity, it would cause that object to vibrate at the frequency imposed upon it by the pressure wave. That imposed vibration is called **forced vibration.** It is this type of vibration that makes all forms of acoustic communication possible.

Now we need to consider the interaction of two objects, one set into vibration by the vibration of the other. They are **coupled** together by the intervening pressure wave. The result is that each will affect the vibration of the other. Two strings, not enclosed and with some space between them, may interact only slightly, and their coupling is termed **loose.** However, let us take the case of a vibrating reed in the end of a clarinet, which sets the air column inside the clarinet into forced vibration. Here the coupling is **tight,** and the air column may have a greater effect on the way in which the reed vibrates than the reed has on the air column.

Forced vibration of a substance will attain the greatest amplitude when the frequency of the pressure wave causing the forced vibration is equal to the frequency at which the substance would vibrate freely (its **natural frequency**). Each of the two strings in our example has a frequency at which it will vibrate freely depending upon its length, mass, and tension. Regardless of these factors, the second string will vibrate in response to the first if there is sufficient intensity. However, if the natural frequency of the second string is not the same as the imposed frequency, it will offer some resistance to the vibration, thus reducing the intensity of its response. As the imposed frequency approaches the natural frequency, the intensity of response will increase until it reaches its maximum when the two frequencies are equal. This latter condition, when the applied frequency is equal to the natural frequency in forced vibration, is called **resonance.**

The principle of resonance can also be applied to forced vibration of an enclosed body of air. If a vibrating string is placed over an empty bottle, the air in the bottle will be set into vibration. The intensity of the sound generated by the vibrating air mass will be greatest at its **resonant frequency.** The resonant frequency of a contained body of air is a function of its size (volume), the size of the opening of the container, and the length of its neck. The larger the volume of air, the smaller the opening, and the longer the neck, the lower will be the resonant frequency. Air contained within a tube also has a resonant frequency that is a function of the length of the tube (because of the interaction of the tube length and the wavelength of the sound) and whether one or both ends of the tube are open.

Human Sound Production

In the human speech mechanism, air pumped from the lungs through the larynx, pharynx, and oral and/or nasal cavities provides the medium for propagation of sound. The larynx serves as the source of complex harmonic vibration. It does so by alternately interrupting the air stream from the lungs at a rapid rate. As the air column passing through the larynx is intermittently interrupted, a series of "puffs" or condensations separated by rarefactions are created. As this process continues, a pressure wave is propagated up through the cavities that lie above the larynx. Thus the larynx as a sound source is tightly coupled to a complex system of cavities.

The sound produced by the larynx consists of a fundamental frequency and a large number of overtones of decreasing intensity (Figure 1-7A). As the sound generated passes through the speech system cavities, it interacts with the multiple resonances of those cavities. In the resulting sound exiting from an open speech cavity system there are peaks and valleys in intensity across the spectrum of overtones due to the resonance factors (Figure 1-7B). The resonance peaks are called **formants.** Changes in the size and shape of the pharyngeal and oral cavities produced by muscular action alter the resonance factors and, therefore, alter the nature of the resulting sound.

Sounds produced with the oropharyngeal cavity system open are called **vowels.** Different vowels are produced by changing the resonance factors. **Consonants** are sounds that may or may not include a harmonic component generated at the

larynx but do contain noise elements generated (in the English language) in the mouth. This noise is produced either by stopping and releasing the air stream passing through the mouth or by forcing the air stream through a restricted space. Examples of the former are the initial consonants in the words "peat" and "ton." When a laryngeal sound component is added to these sounds, we have the words "beet" and "done." Examples of the latter are the initial consonants in the words "sue" (or "zoo") and "fat" (or "vat"). A third class of speech sounds is called **semivowels.** This includes such sounds as the initial sounds in the words "run" and "long." These sounds are called semivowels because they do not contain the noise element of consonants but are produced with a partially restricted airway.

INTRODUCTION TO ANATOMY

Speech production and reception cannot be fully comprehended without first understanding the dynamics of the structures that underlie these processes. In the human body, as in any mechanical system, knowledge of its construction is fundamental to an appreciation of how a system functions and, more particularly, how it may malfunction. Unfortunately, the underlying system mechanics in many areas of concern to speech and hearing physiology are still not completely understood.

There are several reasons for this. Historically, anatomical research has been stimulated by the search for information needed to either cure disease or make surgical intervention possible. Thus, organs such as the heart, kidneys, lungs, and liver have been subjected to thorough study. In contrast, areas of the body of less surgical or medical interest have received far less attention. For example, while the skeletal system as a whole has received its fair share of attention, the joints of the larynx have been carefully researched only during the past decade when surgical treatment of laryngeal diseases began to shift toward less than total removal of the larynx. Similarly, there was little interest in the study of the muscles of articula-

---

1-7. *Acoustic spectrum of sound (A) produced at the larynx and (B) after modification by the speech cavity system.*

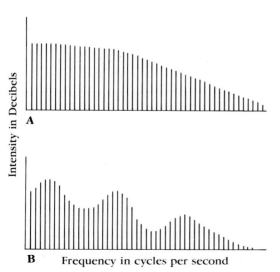

A

B   Frequency in cycles per second

Intensity in Decibels

tion until researchers and clinicians began to ask how speech is learned and why pathologies of speech take the forms they do. Major impetus for the study of the palate and pharynx accrued from the combined interest of speech scientists and surgeons in the problems associated with cleft palate. The area of greatest lack of information is the human central nervous system because of its great complexity. While some pathways have been described and functions hypothesized, this information is based almost entirely on studies of subhuman animals. Descriptions of human central nervous system function are largely hypothetical or theoretical. In terms of complex functions such as thought and memory, little is known.

The lack of definitive anatomical information basic to an understanding of the speech mechanism has made physiological study very difficult and has, at times, led to serious misevaluations of function. Some of the resulting misconceptions are still found in modern texts. Careful physiological studies based on adequate understanding of the anatomy of the structures involved in speech and hearing have been conducted only recently and are still ongoing.

Only by a thorough understanding of the structural mechanics that dictate the boundaries within which function must occur can we formulate reasonable hypotheses of function or read and interpret new research intelligently as it becomes available. These concerns regarding normal structure and function are even more imperative when we direct our attention to structural and functional pathologies, about which even less is known.

Anatomical Terminology

In order to communicate effectively about the structure and function of the human body it is necessary to become familiar with standard anatomical terminology. Three categories of anatomical terms are employed: those that denote parts, those that are used to refer to position and planes of the body, and those that indicate direction. Most of the terms in these categories are of Greek or Latin origin. Parts of the body are usually named for their shape, attachments, or function. For example, the trapezius muscle resembles a trapezoid in shape. The sternocleidomastoid muscle attaches to the sternum, the clavicle, and the mastoid process. The levator veli palatini muscle elevates the soft palate (velum). It can be seen that it will be to the student's advantage to learn the English equivalents of the terms used. These terms can be found in any standard medical dictionary.

Terms that describe positions and planes of the human body are all defined with reference to the body as it stands in the **anatomical position,** that is, with the body erect, arms at the side, and palms of the hands facing forward (Figure 1-8). The definitions of each of these terms is provided in Table 1-1.

It will avoid considerable confusion if these terms are examined in some detail. In the study of the human body, it is frequently helpful to show the body cut open, or to talk about it as if it were. Whenever possible, the three standard planes in space, each perpendicular to the other two, are used. Often the use of these planes, which correspond to the x, y, and z axes in mathematics, avoids confusion to the viewer. The three perpendicular planes separate the body into upper and lower parts, left and right parts, and front and back parts, respectively. The first of these planes, which divides the human body into upper and lower parts, is called the **horizontal plane.** It lies perpendicular to the other two planes and parallel to the floor. A horizontal plane through the human body standing in the anatomical position is also a **transverse plane** through the long axis of the body. However, a transverse plane is not always a horizontal plane, since the term transverse always denotes a section across the longitudinal axis of any object or any part of the body. For example, a transverse section through a rib would not lie in the horizontal plane.

1-8. *Illustration of anatomical terminology. A, Anatomical position; B, Transverse plane; C, Coronal plane; D, Sagittal plane; E, Sutures of the skull.* ▶

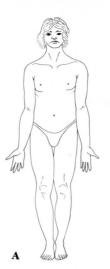

A

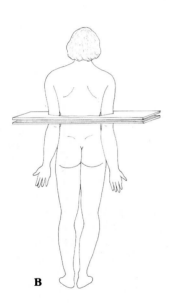

B

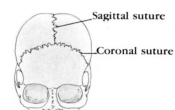

Sagittal suture

Coronal suture

E

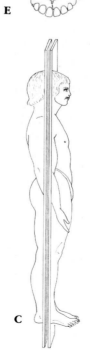

C

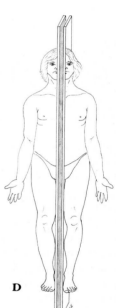

D

Table 1-1. Anatomical Terminology Applied to the Human Being in the Anatomical Position

Term	Meaning	Synonyms
Horizontal plane	Divides the body into upper and lower parts	
Transverse plane	Divides the body or any body part across its longitudinal axis	
Sagittal plane	Divides the body into right and left parts	
Coronal plane	Divides the body into front and back parts	Frontal plane
Superior	Above	Rostral, cephalad
Inferior	Below	Caudad
Anterior	Toward the front of the body	Ventral
Posterior	Toward the back of the body	Dorsal
Superficial	Toward the surface of the body	
Deep	Away from the surface of the body	
Lateral	Away from the midsagittal plane	
Medial	Toward the midsagittal plane	
Proximal	Closer to a given point of reference	
Distal	Farther from a given point of reference	

A vertical cut that separates the body into left and right parts is called a **sagittal plane,** since such a cut would pass through or parallel to the sagittal suture of the skull. A midsagittal plane passes exactly through the midline of the body and divides it into left and right halves. The third plane passes from side to side through the body and is perpendicular to the sagittal plane. It divides the body into front and back parts and is called a **coronal plane** since it passes through or parallel to the coronal suture of the skull. There is no "midcoronal" plane since the body is not symmetrical from front to back. In the human being the coronal plane is also called the **frontal plane.**

Another group of terms is used to denote relative position within the body. **Superior** means above; in the human being, this is the same as **rostral** or **cephalad,** both of which mean "toward the head." **Inferior** means below; in the human being, this is the same as **caudad,** which means "toward the tail." **Anterior** means toward the front of the body and, in the human being, is the same as **ventral,** which means "toward the belly." **Posterior** means toward the back of the body and, in the human being, is the same as **dorsal,** which means "toward the back."

Superficial means toward the surface of the body, while **deep** means away from the surface of the body. **Lateral** means toward the side, or, more specifically, away from the midsagittal plane, while **medial** means toward the midsagittal plane. **Proximal** means closer to any point of reference, and **distal** means farther from any point of reference. In general use the understood reference is the axis of the body. For example, with the arm extended, the elbow is proximal to the hand but distal to the shoulder.

It should be noted that many of the terms used to describe positions and planes within the body have specific definitions that are appropriate both for human beings standing erect, belly forward,

Table 1-2. Metric Equivalents (Values Rounded)

1 meter (m) = 39.37 inches

1 centimeter (cm) = 0.01 m = 0.3937 inch

1 millimeter (mm) = 0.10 cm

1 micrometer (μm) = 0.001 mm = 10^{-6} m (formerly called micron)

1 nanometer (nm) = 0.001 μm = 10^{-9} m (formerly called millimicron)

and for quadrupeds, that is, animals that stand on all fours, belly downward. For example, coronal, sagittal, transverse, ventral, dorsal, caudad, and cephalad all have definitions that allow their application without regard to the position of the body in space. Other terms can only be used appropriately when body position has already been defined. For example, we have already discussed the definition of the word ventral, which means "toward the belly." In human beings ventral is synonymous with anterior, but in quadrupeds, ventral is synonymous with inferior. Likewise, cephalad is synonymous with superior in human beings, but is synonymous with anterior in quadrupeds. In view of the purpose of the current text, terms denoting anatomical position and direction will hereafter be used only as they apply to the human being standing in the anatomical position.

Finally, the **metric system** will be used throughout this text when referring to the size of the structures. Since many of the structures that will be described measure less than 1 mm, the reader should be familiar with the terms listed in Table 1-2.

The structure and function of the organs involved in speech and hearing can best be understood against a background of our understanding of the constituents of those organs (cells and tissues), the functional interaction of tissues and organs, and the methods by which anatomical and physiological questions are answered. These topics will be discussed in this chapter.

CELLS AND TISSUES

The human body is composed of approximately 100 trillion individual cells. Each of these cells carries on basic life functions, including the ingestion of nutrients, the breakdown and utilization of those nutrients through metabolic activity, and the discharge of wastes. Most cells also reproduce themselves. Tissues are groups of cells whose structure has become modified during the embryological period to provide specialized functions. The four basic types of tissues are epithelium, connective tissue, nerve, and muscle.

Epithelium

Epithelium consists of sheets of cells that cover the external surfaces of the body and line its cavities. The cells that constitute epithelium have several distinguishing characteristics related to their functions. They contain very little intercellular substance, and adhere closely to one another. Epithelial cells are also avascular, that is, not directly supplied by the bloodstream. Epithelium serves the functions of protection and absorption. For example, the epithelium that forms the superficial layer of the skin protects the body from external forces and from loss of fluid. The epithelium that forms the lining of the intestines absorbs nutrients into the body. In addition to this **covering epithelium,** there are three types of specialized epithelium: glandular epithelium, myoepithelium, and neuroepithelium. **Glandular epithelium** forms glands that invaginate from the body surfaces. **Myoepithelium** forms smooth muscle cells of the glands. **Neuroepithelium** is composed of cells that have specialized into sensory nerve endings of the cochlea, vestibule, nasal cavities, and tongue and subserves the sensations of hearing, balance, smell, and taste. Thus the functions of epithelium are protection, synthesis and secretion, absorption, and sensation.

Epithelial cells can also be classified morphologically by their shape and by the number of cell layers that occur (Figure 2-1). Single-layered epithelium is called **simple epithelium.** Epithelium that consists of two or more layers is called **stratified epithelium.** Simple epithelium is found most often where there is transport of material across the cell layers, as in the lining of blood vessels. Three of the terms used to denote the shape of these cells are **squamous** (flat), **cuboidal,** and **columnar.** Thus, a single layer of flat epithelial cells is referred to as simple squamous epithelium. Similarly, a single layer of tall prismatic epithelial cells is referred to as simple columnar epithelium. Stratified squamous epithelium refers to multi-layered epithelium in which the cells are of a squamous configuration. Stratified columnar epithelium refers to multi-layered epithelium in which the superficial layers of cells are tall and prismatic in shape.

There are several other types of epithelium that cannot be completely described within these categories. Some simple columnar epithelium appears to be stratified rather than simple and is referred to as **pseudostratified epithelium.** There are also certain types of stratified epithelium that are somewhat atypical. Called **transitional epithelium** and **germinal epithelium,** they occur in the urinary tract and in the ovary, respectively.

In addition, some epithelial cells have **cilia.** Ciliated epithelium is found in the respiratory and digestive tracts, where the cilia provide a transport function for mucus.

Connective Tissue

The principal types of connective tissue are connective tissue with special properties, connective tissue proper, cartilage, and bone. **Connective tissue with special properties** includes such types as **adipose tissue,** which serves as a receptacle for fat deposits, and **hematopoietic tissue,** which is associated with blood cell formation, and will not be of concern to us here.

Connective tissue proper characteristically has few living cells and a large amount of nonliving intercellular material (Figure 2-2). Three types of fiber make up the major part of this tissue: collagen, elastic, and reticular. **Collagen fibers** are the predominant type. Although colorless, these fibers give a white appearance when found in dense bundles. They are not stretchable. **Elastic fibers** are very thin, threadlike, and yellow in color. When cut, they recoil as would a stretched rubber band. They can be stretched to $1\frac{1}{2}$ times their natural length when force is applied. **Reticular fibers** are extremely fine and delicate. They have many of the characteristics of collagen fibers and are often continuous with them.

Connective tissue proper is described as loose or dense. **Loose connective tissue** is also called **areolar tissue.** It contains all three types of fibers but is delicate and not resistant to stretch. It fills the spaces of the body (e.g., between muscle fibers and between organs) and so serves as the packing material of the body. In **dense connective tissue,** collagen fibers predominate, making it less flexible and more resistant to stress. Dense connective tissue is described as irregular or regular. **Irregular connective tissue** is composed of collagenous bundles which are arranged in a random pattern and resist stress from all directions equally. An example of this type of connective tissue is found in the skin. In **regular connective tissue,** the collagen fibers are arranged in a definite pattern, and the fibers are formed in response to prolonged stress in the same direction. This type affords the greatest resistance to traction forces. Tendons, aponeuroses, and most ligaments (Figure 2-3) are of this type. **Tendons** are composed of dense bundles of regular connective tissue separated by loose connective tissue and attach muscles to bones. Broad flat tendons are called **aponeuroses. Ligaments** consist entirely

2-1. *Epithelial tissue. A, Found in the kidney and lung; B, Found in skin, intestine, and vagina; C, Found in the kidney; D, Found in the gallbladder; E, Found in the male urethra; F, Found in the trachea; G, Found in the urinary tract; H, Found in the ovary.*

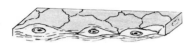

A. Simple squamous

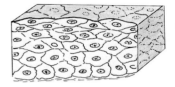

B. Stratified squamous

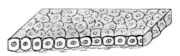

C. Cuboidal

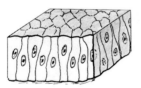

D. Simple columnar

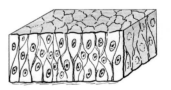

E. Stratified columnar

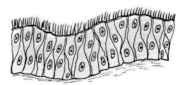

F. Pseudostratified columnar ciliated

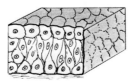

G. Transitional

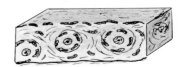

H. Germinal

2-2. *Connective tissue.*

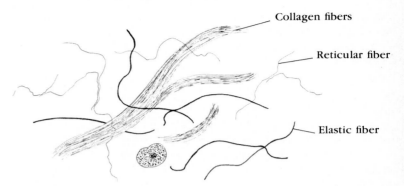

Collagen fibers

Reticular fiber

Elastic fiber

A. Loose (areolar) connective tissue

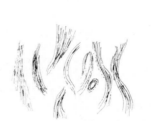

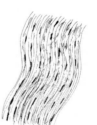

B. Dense irregular
connective tissue

C. Dense regular
connective tissue

2-3. *Ligaments (A), tendons (B), and aponeuroses (C).*

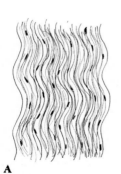

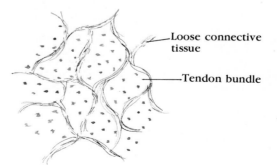

Loose connective
tissue

Tendon bundle

A   B   C

of regular connective tissue and connect bones and cartilages. Thus they limit motion at joints. Ligaments not of this type are the suspensory ligaments of the penis and the yellow ligaments of the vertebral column, which are composed of thick elastic fibers and are, therefore, stretchable. The various terms used to describe connective tissue proper are summarized in Table 2-1.

Cartilage (Figure 2-4) is characterized by its rigid consistency, flexibility, and slight elasticity. It is less rigid than bone. Unlike connective tissue proper, it has form that is resistant to pressure. It is composed principally of **matrix** within which are scattered cells that produce and maintain the matrix. Matrix is the principal component of cytoplasm. Little is known about the chemical composition of matrix, but it is thought to consist primarily of protein and carbohydrate molecules. Fibers are embedded within the matrix. Cartilage is classified by the types of fibers found in its matrix. The three types of cartilage are hyaline, elastic, and fibrous.

Hyaline cartilage contains an extremely fine network of collagen fibers. It is the most common type of cartilage and is also the most rigid form. Examples of hyaline cartilage can be found in the nose, in the larynx, and in the rib cage where it is interposed between the bony ribs and the sternum (breastbone). **Elastic cartilage** contains a dense network of elastic fibers as well as some collagen fibers. It is, therefore, less rigid. This is the type of cartilage that gives form to the external ear. **Fi-**

Table 2-1. Descriptive Terms for Connective Tissue

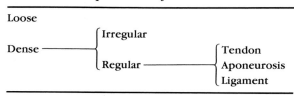

brous cartilage** (fibrocartilage) is characterized by cells that typically occur in rows and collagen fibers that occur in bundles. An example of fibrocartilage is found in the disks between the vertebrae.

Cartilage provides protection where some degree of flexibility is required and serves as a shock absorber, as in the case of intervertebral disks. In addition, it covers bony surfaces within certain types of joints and facilitates smooth gliding and lack of friction within the joint. Cartilage is typically surrounded by a layer of fibrous connective tissue called the **perichondrium.** An exception to this is found in the case of hyaline cartilage within joint cavities.

Bone (Figure 2-5) is similar to cartilage in that it is composed of cells distributed within a large body of matrix containing collagen fibers. However, in this case the matrix and the collagen fibers are impregnated with minerals that impart rigidity and hardness. The principal minerals found in bone are **calcium phosphate** and **calcium carbonate.** Bones are typically surrounded by a layer

2-4. *Types of cartilage.*

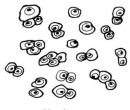

Hyaline

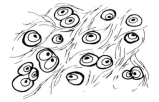

Elastic

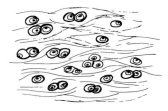

Fibrous

of fibrous connective tissue called the **perios-teum,** to which tendons and ligaments attach. Bone is classified according to its internal structure as spongy (also called cancellous) or compact. It is also classified according to its mode of development as either membranous or endochondral bone.

Spongy bone is characterized by the presence of internal interconnecting cavities, while **compact bone** is dense and devoid of such cavities. However, the bony tissue in each is similar in composition. Most bones of the body contain regions that are spongy and regions that are compact.

In **membranous bones,** cells that give rise to bone (called **osteoblasts**) differentiate within **membranes** (sheets of dense connective tissue) and form bony tissue. In **endochondral bones,** osteoblasts form bone on or around a preexisting cartilage, which serves as a model for the developing bone. As bones grow and develop, they both increase in size and are subject to remodelling (Figure 2-6). These changes are brought about by addition of bone and resorption of bone. Addition of bone is a function of the osteoblasts. Bone resorption is a function of cells called **osteoclasts.**

2-5. *Types of bone as seen in a section through the hip joint.*

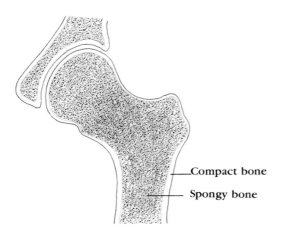

Compact bone
Spongy bone

Except for parts of the clavicle (collarbone), all membranous bones are part of the skull. All other bones of the body are endochondral. Bone, being rigid, forms the supporting skeleton of the body.

Nerve Tissue

Nerve tissue is composed of two types of cells: neurons, also called nerve cells, and neuroglia, also called glial cells. **Neurons** have the capacity to respond to changes in their environment by conduction and transmission of signals to other neurons, muscles, and glands. Thus the over 10 billion neurons in the human nervous system constitute a communication network that extends throughout the body. **Neuroglia** supports and takes part in the activity of neurons.

While neurons exist in a variety of forms, a typical neuron (Figure 2-7A) consists of a cell body, also called the **perikaryon,** one long cylindrical process called the **axon,** and a branching network of short processes called **dendrites.** The cell body is the trophic (nutritional) center of the cell. It manufactures nutrients, which are then transported throughout the cell processes. The perikaryon is also capable of receiving and conducting neural impulses. The dendrites are the principal sites for reception of neural impulses and transmit signals toward the cell body. Axons typically are long processes that conduct signals away from the cell body and in some neurons interconnect the dendrites and the cell body.

Functionally, neurons are classified as motor, sensory, or internuncial. **Motor neurons** (also called **motoneurons**) conduct signals from the central nervous system (CNS) to muscles and glands and are thus called **effector neurons.** **Sensory neurons** receive stimuli from the periphery of the body, from special sense organs, and from other organs of the body and conduct and transmit the resulting signals to the CNS. The majority of neurons are **internuncial;** that is, they serve to relay signals from one neuron to another. Internuncial neurons are found primarily within the CNS.

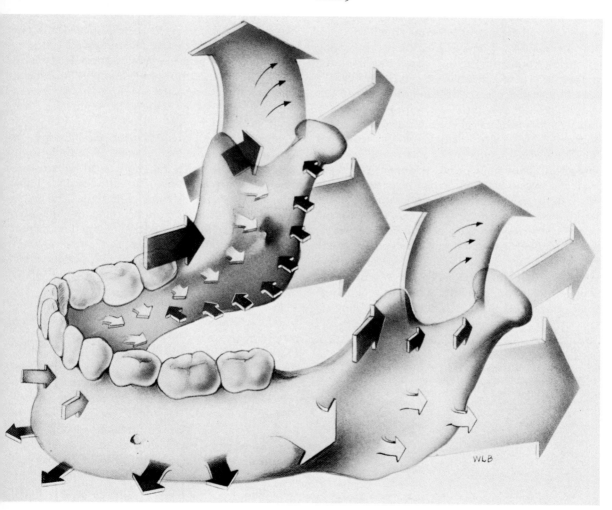

Neurons are also classified as multipolar, bipolar, or unipolar according to the number of processes that emanate from the perikaryon. Most neurons are **multipolar** (Figure 2-7A), possessing one relatively long axon and many branching dendrites. Motoneurons are of this type. Their perikaryon and dendrites are within the spinal cord, and their axon may be very long, extending from the spinal cord out to the fingers or toes. **Bipolar** neurons (Figure 2-7B) have two long processes, both called axons, extending from the perikaryon. The dendrites are located at the end of one of these processes. These neurons are sensory and are found only in the cochlear, vestibular, retinal, and olfactory nerves. **Unipolar** neurons (Figure 2-7C), also called **pseudounipolar** neurons, have a single process extending from the perikaryon. This single process contains two fused branches that join a long axonal process that extends both centrally and peripherally from the perikaryon. Unipolar neurons are sensory and form the sensory part of spinal and cranial nerves.

Sensory neurons, which receive signals from the body's periphery and organs, are typically unipolar. Motoneurons are typically multipolar and have a single long axon. A **nerve** is made up of a large number of axons (axis cylinders) all traveling together as a part of the **peripheral nervous system (PNS)**, that is, external to the CNS. Within the CNS, groups of axis cylinders are called **tracts** or **pathways** and constitute the **white matter** of the CNS. The cell bodies of neurons are located in clusters both outside of and within the CNS. Outside of the CNS these clusters are called **ganglia.** Within the CNS these clusters are called **nuclei.** Within the brain, neuronal cell bodies also occur in layers. The layers and clusters of cell bodies within the CNS form the **grey matter.** There is an exception to the above terminology: The term ganglia is sometimes used to refer to collections of neuronal cell bodies within the brain (e.g., the **basal ganglia**).

In order to understand how neurons function, it is helpful, as a frame of reference, to examine some of the characteristics common to all cells of the body. Cells are made up of an intracellular chemical gel surrounded by a cell membrane. The cell is immersed in the extracellular fluid of the body. The cell contains small organs (organelles), which serve its general cellular functions, and a nucleus. Several features of the cell and its environment are relevant to an understanding of both nerve and muscle function.

The intracellular and extracellular fluids are termed **electrolytes,** since the molecules which they contain carry electrical charges. Molecules that are electrically charged are called **ions.** Positively charged ions are called **cations,** while negatively charged ions are called **anions.** The cell membrane, which separates the intracellular and extracellular fluids, is made up of layers of molecules and is **semipermeable,** that is, it allows some substances to pass through and not others. Further, it has the capacity to vary its permeability. Thus we have the potential for intracellular and extracellular ions to be exchanged through the cell membrane. To put it differently, the cell membrane can exert a degree of control over the passage of those ions. The intracellular fluid contains a high concentration of protein anions (A^-) and potassium cations (K^+) and a low concentration of sodium cations (Na^+). The extracellular fluid contains a high concentration of

2-7. *Types of neurons. A, Typical (multipolar) neuron; B, Bipolar neuron; C, Unipolar (pseudounipolar) neuron.*

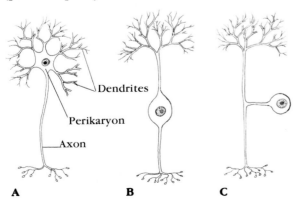

Dendrites

Perikaryon

Axon

A   **B**   **C**

Na$^+$ and chloride (Cl$^-$) and a low concentration of K$^+$. Figure 2-8 illustrates these relationships. In addition to considering the chemical concentrations, we must also examine the electrical concentrations. Most, if not all, cells of the body are negatively charged. That is, the intracellular fluid is electrically negative relative to the extracellular fluid. This difference ranges from about 9 to 100 millivolts (mV). In neurons it is −70 mV and in muscle cells it is −90 mV. This value is called the **resting membrane potential** and is a function of the ionic differences across the cell membrane, which are largely controlled by the membrane permeability. The cell membrane is practically impermeable to the large protein anions and to

other large organic anions that are found in high concentration within the cell. The cell membrane is moderately permeable to Cl$^-$ and Na$^+$, and quite freely permeable to K$^+$.

Now let us look at electrochemical forces acting on Cl$^-$, K$^+$, and Na$^+$. Cl$^-$ is found in higher concentration outside the cell and so would tend to diffuse into the cell to equalize its concentration. However, since Cl$^-$ carries a negative electrical charge, it is repelled by the intracellular negative charge. The magnitude of intracellular negative electrical charge necessary to counteract the tendency for chloride to flow into the cell is, in the case of the neuron, −70 mV. Since this is the charge found within the cell, the concentration of

2-8. Major electrochemical forces across a neuronal membrane. Large arrows indicate the direction of the chemical (concentration) gradient for each ion. The arrows in column A indicate the direction of the electrical gradient for each ion. Column B shows the net diffusion of each ion across the membrane. A$^-$ (large anions) do not cross the membrane. Chlorine (Cl$^-$) crosses the membrane but is in electrochemical equilibrium. Column C shows the action of the sodium pump for each of the ions.

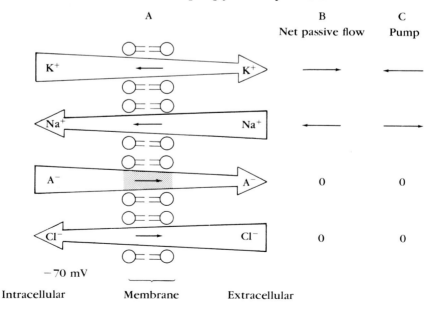

chloride can be completely explained by the known electrochemical factors. Potassium is concentrated inside of the cell and so, based on chemical concentration only, would tend to flow out of the cell. However, the negative charge within the cell would attract K^+ and resist its flow out of the cell. Equilibrium for K^+ exists at an intracellular charge of -90 mV. Thus the -70 mV charge within the neuron is not quite sufficient to account for the K^+ concentration. Thus we would expect K^+ to gradually flow out of the cell.

The case for sodium is quite different. Na^+ is concentrated outside the cell, therefore it would tend to flow into the cell. In this case the negative electrical charge inside the cell would attract sodium and increase that tendency. It would require a $^+60$ mV charge within the cell to prevent the influx of sodium. Thus, especially for sodium, but also for potassium, there must be some active metabolic process that pumps sodium out of the cell and, to a lesser extent, draws potassium into the cell. This metabolic process has been called the **sodium pump** and is the subject of intense research. Apparently, the energy for this process is provided by a chemical called **adenosine triphosphate(ATP)** located within the cell membrane, which facilitates transport of sodium out of the cell. Sodium transport is linked to movement of potassium into the cell. Further, the rate of extrusion of sodium from the cell is a function of the sodium level within the cell.

In any cell, stimulation of the cell membrane can cause a fluctuation in the resting electrical potential. This is accounted for by a built-in control mechanism. For example, stimulation to a cell causes its electrical potential to fall, which triggers movement of K^+ out of the cell and, to a lesser degree, Cl^- into the cell. This chemical flow restores the cell's electrical potential, which, in turn, leads to restoration of the chemical balance. In a neuron or muscle cell a drop in intracellular electrical potential triggers an increase in cell membrane permeability to sodium. The effect is small, and the cell is able to recover if the change in potential is below about 15 mV. If the change reaches 15 mV, however, a massive influx of sodium occurs, with an irreversible drop in membrane potential. The drop overshoots the zero point (Figure 2-9) and the intracellular fluid actually becomes positively charged for a brief instant. As this process occurs, the cell membrane begins to reduce its permeability to sodium. Also, the electri-

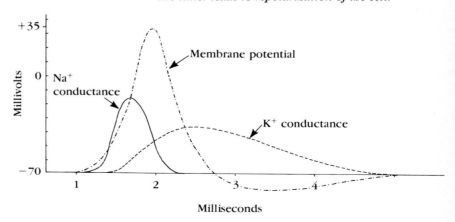

2-9. *Changes in membrane potential and permeability during an action potential. There is a massive influx of sodium (Na^+) and a slightly delayed and less dramatic efflux of potassium (K^+) from the cell. The latter leads to repolarization of the cell.*

cal balance of sodium reverses as the cell develops a positive charge. These factors lead to recovery, that is, to repolarization of the cell membrane. This electrical change from rest to overshoot and back is called an **action potential.**

As long as the drop in electrical potential does not exceed the critical 15 mV, the chemical response remains localized on the cell membrane. However, if the drop exceeds that value and thus triggers depolarization, adjoining parts of the membrane also undergo depolarization, which "travels" down the neuron like a wave propagated by a stone dropped into water, with repolarization following (Figure 2-10). If the stimulus to a neuron is of sufficient strength, it will produce an action potential. Further increase in the strength of the stimulus will have no effect on the nature or magnitude of the action potential. The action potential will occur or will not depending on the stimulus strength and so is said to be "all-or-none" in character.

From the point of stimulation, the action potential will travel without regard to direction. For example, if an axon received an adequate stimulus at the midpoint of its length, an action potential would be conducted both "down" the axon to its distal terminus and "up" the axon to the cell body. However, neurons normally receive stimuli on their dendrites, cell bodies, and on the "root" of

the axon where it joins the cell body (called the **axon hillock**). Therefore action potentials are normally conducted "down" the axon rather than "up."

The strength of the stimulus required to trigger an action potential is affected by the magnitude of the electrical potential of the cell membrane at any point in time. If stimulation occurs that causes a local response on the cell membrane but is insufficient to trigger an action potential, the cell membrane becomes hypersensitive to further stimulation, since its potential has become less than 70 mV. Then it may take less than a 15 mV change to trigger an action potential. However, when the cell membrane is undergoing rapid depolarization and for part of the recovery period, the neuron is refractory to further stimulation. The period from the onset of the action potential until repolarization is about one-third complete is called the **absolute refractory period,** meaning that the neuron will not respond to further stimulation of any strength. The time from that point in the recovery period until the recovery rate begins to slow (Figure 2-11) is called the **relative refractory period,** meaning that the neuron will respond to a stimulus only if that stimulus is stronger than would be required if the neuron were at rest. From Figure 2-11 it can be seen that during the period from initial stimulation to complete recovery, the neuron goes through several stages of excitability. First, during the period of local response, the threshold of excitability (the magnitude of stimulus required to induce a response) is lowered. Then comes the absolute refractory period followed by the relative refractory period. As recovery levels off, the threshold is again lower than normal. At this point, the repolarization process overshoots slightly resulting in a cell membrane potential greater than 70 mV, during which a greater than normal stimulus is required until the 70 mV resting potential is achieved. Since the absolute refractory period may only last for about one millisecond, many stimuli per second can activate the neuron.

Now we can examine what happens when the action potential reaches the distal end of the axon.

2-10. *Wave of depolarization travelling down an axon followed by repolarization.*

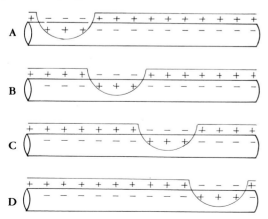

Axons typically terminate in a complex of branches called the **terminal arborization** or **telodendria** (Figure 2-12). Each branch of this terminal arborization ends in an **end bulb** (also called a **terminal bouton**). The end bulbs may be adjacent to another neuron, in which case the junction of the two is called a **synapse,** or to a muscle cell, in which case the junction is called a **myoneural junction.** Synapses will be considered here; neuromuscular junctions will be described later in the discussion of muscle tissue. At a synapse a small portion of the cell membrane of one neuron (the **presynaptic cell**) interfaces with a small portion of the cell membrane of a second neuron (the **postsynaptic cell**). Usually an axon adjoins a dendrite, cell body, or axon hillock. Most commonly, the terminal bouton of the axon interfaces with a small projection from a dendrite called a **dendritic spine.** However, in some cases the presynaptic cell may be a dendrite. The two cell membranes are separated by a **synaptic cleft,** which is approximately 20 nm wide. Typically, the end bulb of the axon contains small **vesicles,** which in turn contain a chemical agent. A number of different chemical agents may occur, but a single axon will apparently contain only one of them. If a single action potential reaches the presynaptic membrane, it causes some of these vesicles to be released into the synaptic cleft. The chemical they contain is then released onto the postsynaptic membrane. Some of these chemicals (such as **acetylcholine** and **epinephrine**) cause a local response depolarization of the postsynaptic membrane and so are called **ex-**

2-11. *The action potential and associated refractory periods.*

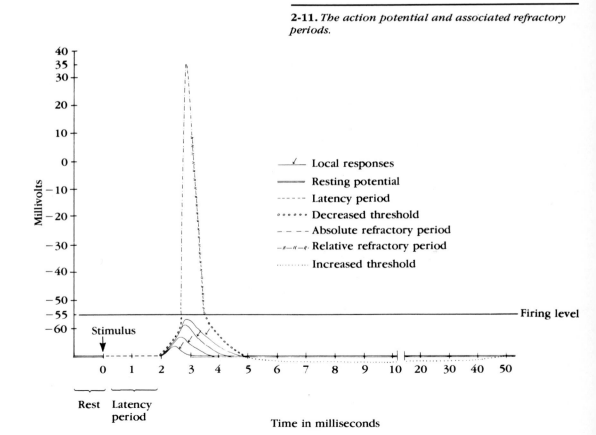

citatory mediators. This change in postsynaptic membrane potential is called the **excitatory postsynaptic membrane potential** (**EPSP**) since, while it is not sufficient to generate an action potential in the postsynaptic neuron, it does reduce the threshold of exitability. There are two ways in which the EPSP can be increased to the point where it will generate an action potential. **Spatial summation** can occur by the action of more than one synapse on the same postsynaptic cell. In this case the EPSPs summate (Figure 2-13) and may be sufficient to generate an action potential. **Temporal summation** of EPSPs will occur if repeated stimuli reach the postsynaptic membrane so that new EPSPs occur before previous ones have died out by the normal process of repolarization. The activity of the chemical mediator in the synaptic cleft is cancelled by a counteracting chemical that forms in the cell membranes. Rapid removal of the

mediator is essential in order for the postsynaptic membrane to repolarize.

Other chemicals (such as the amino acid called **glycine**) are found in the end bulbs of some axons. Release of these chemicals, called **inhibitory mediators,** reduces the threshold of excitability of the postsynaptic membrane, the reverse of the effect of the excitatory mediators. The response they generate is, therefore, called the **inhibitory postsynaptic membrane potential** (**IPSP**). Thus the summation of EPSPs and IPSPs controls the activity of the postsynaptic cell. The IPSP is very important functionally. Not only may it be a factor in learning and in the control of movement, but the inhibition of the IPSP by poisons such as strychnine can cause uncontrolled excitation seen clinically as hyperactivity of muscles and convulsions.

The complexity of the synaptic system of the

2-12. *Neurons and synapses. A, Multipolar neuron; B, Terminal bouton of one neuron may synapse with another neuron at any one of several points; C, Close-up view of the synapse.*

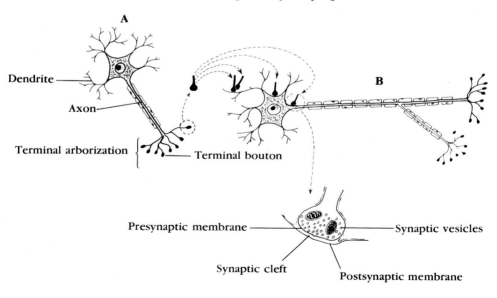

A

Dendrite

Axon

Terminal arborization

Terminal bouton

B

Presynaptic membrane

Synaptic cleft

Synaptic vesicles

Postsynaptic membrane

C

body is so great as to be beyond comprehension. Ganong has pointed out that in some motoneurons ". . . it has been calculated that if the cell body were the size of a tennis ball the dendrites of the cell would fill an average-sized living room . . ." and that functionally, ". . . there are approximately 10^{14} synapses in the human brain and that, on the average, each of the more than 10 billion neurons in the nervous system has 100 inputs converging on it while it in turn diverges to 100 other neurons" [6]. Synapses can be so numerous as to essentially cover the entire dendritic tree and cell body of a neuron. The ratio of neurons to synapses in some parts of the brain have been estimated at 1:40,000.

As indicated earlier, some peripheral sensory neurons receive their stimuli from the skin, muscles, tendons, joints, internal organs, and other body structures. Other sensory neurons are specialized for purposes of audition, taste, vision, olfaction, and motion. These stimuli are mediated through sensory receptors at the peripheral terminus of the sensory axis cylinder. For present purposes those receptors having to do with the sense of touch and pressure will be examined. Touch and pressure may be mediated simply by naked nerve endings in the epithelium where the stimulus of touch is sufficient to generate action potentials in those endings. Other nerve endings for touch and pressure are covered by a layered capsule of connective tissue and are called **pacinian corpuscles** (Figure 2-14). If sufficient mechanical stress is placed on the nerve endings, an action potential is generated. The rate at which action potentials are generated (up to the limit imposed by the absolute refractory period) is a function of the degree of mechanical stress. Therefore, we can interpret degrees of stress even though the action potential itself follows the all-or-none law. This same principle holds for the receptors having to do with body movement. The particular sensation received or interpreted has to do with the

2-13. *Neural summation. A, Spatial summation of simultaneous subthreshold synaptic impulses increases until the firing level is reached. B, Temporal summation occurs when the time interval between individual subthreshold synaptic impulses decreases until firing level is reached.*

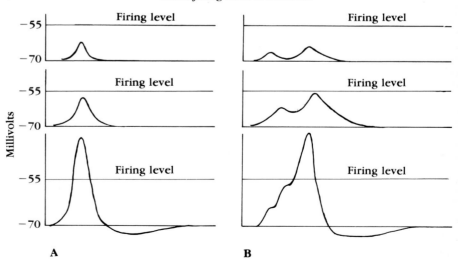

area of the brain to which those sensations are conducted. Thus if a sensory pathway is stimulated anywhere in its course, the sensation produced will be the same as though the sensory ending were stimulated; it is not the ending itself that determines what type of sensation (e.g., light, pain, touch) is interpreted by the brain. The structure and function of receptors having to do with movement will be discussed after consideration of muscles and joints. Receptors relating to audition will be examined in Chapter 6 (Audition).

Neuroglia is composed of specialized connective tissue cells that support neurons. There are five types, one in the peripheral nervous system and the other four in the central nervous system. That found in the PNS is the **Schwann cell.** Many of the axis cylinders of the PNS travel either singly or in groups within infoldings of the periphery of the Schwann cell (Figure 2-15). In most cases,

however, Schwann cells wrap themselves around the axis cylinder in multiple layers. In this case, the interfaces of the Schwann cell membranes within the wrapping produce a substance called **myelin.** The thicker the axis cylinder, the more layers of myelin are produced. These axis cylinders are said to be **myelinated.** A typical Schwann cell of a myelinated axis cylinder covers about 1 mm of the length of the axis cylinders. Thus it takes many Schwann cells to cover a long axis cylinder. Adjacent Schwann cells are separated by an extremely small space, and even here there is some interdigitation of adjacent Schwann cells (Figure 2-16). These spaces between successive lengths of myelin are called **nodes of Ranvier.** Myelin is an effective insulator of the axis cylinder and prevents depolarization of the neuronal cell membrane where it is covered. It is thought that the action potential in a myelinated axis cylinder essentially jumps from one node of Ranvier to the next. In other words, an action potential in one node is sufficient to trigger one in the next node in the direction of conduction. This is called **saltatory conduction.** Another way of viewing this is by analogy to propagation of a wave through water. As illustrated in Figure 2-17, a wave in an open tank will take a definable period of time to propagate from one point to another. However, if

2-14. *Pacinian corpuscle.*

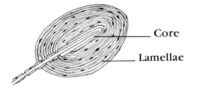

Core

Lamellae

2-15. *Relationship between axons and the cells of Schwann (diagrammatic). A, Unmyelinated axon; B, Myelinated axon. (Redrawn and reproduced, with permission, from Ganong WF:* Review of Medical Physiology, *9th ed. Copyright 1979 by Lange Medical Publications, Los Altos, California.)*

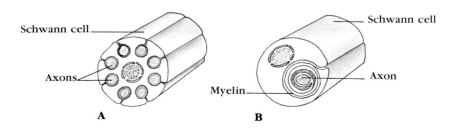

Schwann cell

Axons

Myelin

Schwann cell

Axon

A

B

the center of the tank is covered, the pressure response between those same two points is almost instantaneous. Saltatory conduction of an impulse is much more rapid than conduction along a nonmyelinated axis cylinder.

The four types of neuroglia in the CNS are astrocytes, oligodendrocytes, microglia, and ependymal cells. These cells are much smaller but far more numerous than neuronal cells. The function of the CNS glial cells is not completely understood. **Astrocytes** attach to blood vessels and neurons; they are thought to play a role in conduction of nutrients and also serve a function in maintenance of the ionic balance in the CNS. The **oligodendrocytes** produce the myelin sheath of axis cylinders within the CNS. The myelin, which is white, gives the characteristic appearance of the white matter of the CNS. However, the oligodendrocytes also

2-16. *Node of Ranvier. A, Longitudinal view; B, Longitudinal section.*

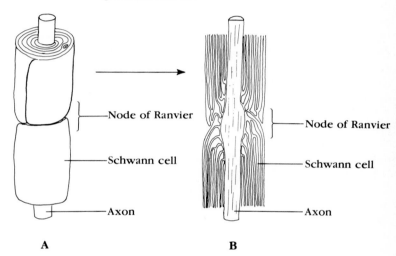

A   B

2-17. *Saltatory conduction in a myelinated neuron compared to a wave in a tank. If pressure is applied at point* a *in the uncovered tank at the left, a wave will be propagated across the surface of the water. If a lid partially covers the surface of the water as at the right, pressure applied at point* a *is instantaneously transferred to point* b *in a manner analogous to saltatory conduction in a myelinated neuron.*

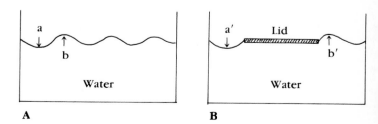

A   B

have a poorly understood metabolic interaction with the neurons. **Microglial cells** are thought by some to function as phagocytes (scavenger cells) of the CNS. **Ependymal cells** are columnar and line the cavities of the CNS.

As indicated previously, nerves in the PNS are made up of a large number of axis cylinders, usually some combination of long axons of sensory neurons and axons of motoneurons. As illustrated in Figure 2-18, the connective tissue covering of the nerve is called the **epineurium.** The axis cylinders are typically arranged in bundles, with each bundle surrounded by a second layer of connective tissue, the **perineurium.** Surrounding each of the myelinated or nonmyelinated axis cylinders is a third layer of connective tissue, the **endoneurium.**

Two types of postnatal growth and development occur within the nervous system that are particularly relevant to muscular function and learning in the child. The dendritic arborizations and number of synapses in the newborn are but few in comparison to what is found in the older child. Dendritic arborization and synaptic connections multiply at an extraordinary rate as the child develops, particularly during the first two years of life. In addition, the long axis cylinders of the PNS, which are largely unmyelinated at birth, become myelinated during the first year or so of postnatal life. These changes are related to the developing coordination and complexity of the child's motor activity and to the explosive rate at which language and other brain functions mature.

Muscle Tissue

Muscle cells are characteristically long and slender. Their unique functions in the body derive from their capacity to shorten their longitudinal length by as much as 50% in response to stimulation. Three basic types of muscle cells are found in the human body: cardiac, smooth, and skeletal. **Cardiac muscle** is found in the heart and has special properties that permit its lifelong regular and uninterrupted function. **Smooth muscle** is characterized by slow, steady contractions and is found around blood vessels, in the intestines, in the iris of the eye, and in some of the internal organs of the body. **Skeletal muscle,** also called **striated muscle** because of its microscopic appearance, controls skeletal movements and is the only type of muscle that is normally under conscious control. That is, while we may not be conscious of contracting individual skeletal muscles, we are aware of and can control the activity that results from those contractions. This is in contradistinction to activities resulting from the contraction of cardiac and smooth muscle. Under ordinary circumstances, we cannot consciously control heart rate, dilation of the pupils, or constriction of the blood vessels. We will be primarily concerned with skeletal muscle throughout the discussion of the speech and hearing mechanism.

A typical striated muscle, portrayed in Figure 2-19A, is cylindrical in form, tapers at each end, and terminates in a tendon that attaches to bone or cartilage. The muscle is encased in a connective tissue sheath called **epimysium.** Examination of a

2-18. *Connective tissue layers in a peripheral nerve.*

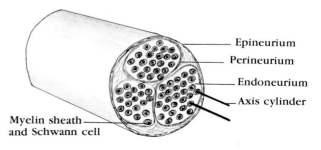

cross-section (Figure 2-19B) reveals that the muscle is compartmentalized into subsections called **fascicles,** each of which is surrounded by its own connective tissue sheath called the **perimysium.** Each fascicle is composed of a great many individual muscle **fibers.** The **endomysium,** another layer of connective tissue, surrounds each muscle fiber.

Close examination of the individual muscle fibers within the endomysium reveals that a muscle fiber is an individual specialized cell (Figure 2-19C). It contains many nuclei and is surrounded by a cell membrane called the **sarcolemma.** It contains the usual protoplasm characteristic of all cells, but in this case it is called **sarcoplasm.** The muscle cell or fiber is long and slender in appearance and typically does not extend the full length

of the muscle. The diameter of a typical muscle fiber ranges from approximately 10 to 100 μm in diameter. The tendons of the muscle insert into folds of the sarcolemma. It is important to remember that in no case do muscle fibers themselves attach directly to bone or cartilage.

Each muscle fiber is made up of several hundred to several thousand individual **myofibrils,** which lie parallel to one another and course the entire length of the muscle fiber. Each of these myofibrils is approximately 1 μm in diameter. Each myofibril is composed of short overlapping chains of protein molecules arranged longitudinally within the myofibril (Figure 2-19D). Each of these chains is called a **myofilament.** There are two types of myofilaments, one thicker than the other. The thick and thin filaments are interlocked in a three-dimensional alternating array as illustrated in Figure 2-19E. Comparison of a diagram of the myofibril and the photomicrograph of a myofibril (Figure 2-20) shows the reason for the striated or striped appearance of a skeletal muscle. The characteristic light and dark bands have been labeled for reference purposes. The **Z line** is the region where adjacent thin filaments are interconnected. The region between successive Z lines is called a **sarcomere.** The **A band** within each sarcomere is the region of the thick filaments. The darkest portions within the sarcomere are where the thick and thin filaments overlap. The dark **M line** in the center of the sarcomere is caused by a bulge in the thick filaments at that point. Also at the M line are interconnections among the thick filaments, which apparently serve to hold them in position.

The process of muscle contraction occurs within the sarcomere as the thin filaments slide over the thick filaments, shortening the sarcomere (Figure 2-21). In order to understand this sliding process, the thick and thin filaments need to be examined in greater detail.

The thick filaments are composed of chains of molecules called **myosin.** Each myosin molecule has an enlarged head at the end closest to the Z line. These heads extend into the space between the thick and thin filaments and, because of their function, are called **crossbridges.** The thin fila-

2-19. *Structure of striated muscle.*

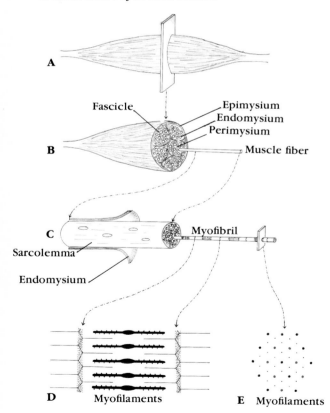

A

Fascicle
Epimysium
Endomysium
Perimysium

B
Muscle fiber

C
Myofibril

Sarcolemma

Endomysium

D   Myofilaments

E   Myofilaments

ments are composed of chains of three molecules: **actin, tropomyosin,** and **troponin** (Figure 2-22). These are called the actin filaments since over 80% of the molecules are actin. The long tropomyosin molecules wrap around the chains of globular actin molecules. The troponin molecules are attached at intervals along the length of the tropomyosin. The troponin contains three subunits. One of these (**troponin T**) binds to the tropomyosin. Another (**troponin I**) inhibits interaction between the myosin and actin filaments. The third (**troponin C**) is the site for binding calcium (Ca^{++}), which initiates the process of contraction.

When a muscle is at rest, troponin I is bound to the actin molecules and troponin T is bound to the tropomyosin molecules. The tropomyosin covers sites on the actin that, if exposed, would bind with the myosin molecules. Depolarization by an action potential causes calcium to be released into the myofibril. The calcium binds with the troponin C; causing the bond between troponin I and actin to weaken. This in turn permits the tropomyosin to move, exposing the sites on the actin that will bind with myosin. The result is actin-myosin binding. This bond causes a change in the shape of the myosin molecule such that the head of the myosin molecule swivels, pulling the actin molecule with

2-20. *Photomicrograph (A) and diagram (B) of a myofibril. (Photomicrograph reproduced, with permission, from Ganong WF:* Review of Medical Physiology, *10th ed. Copyright 1981 by Lange Medical Publications, Los Altos, California.)*

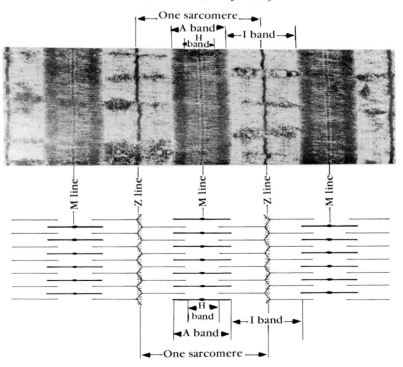

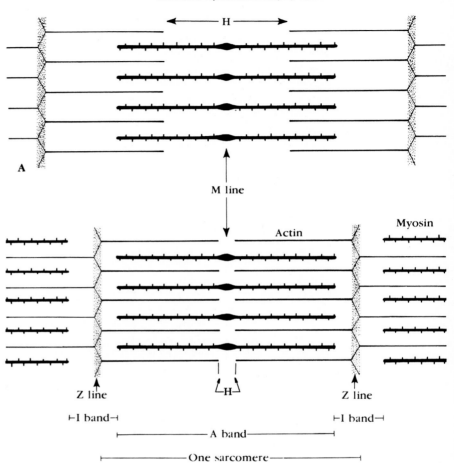

2-21. *Schematic of filament sliding in muscle contraction. A, Relaxation; B, Contraction.*

2-22. *Structure and function of thick and thin filaments in striated muscle. (Top figure reproduced, with permission, from Ganong WF:* Review of Medical Physiology, *10th ed. Copyright 1981 by Lange Medical Publications, Los Altos, California. Bottom figures reproduced, with permission, from Katz AM: Congestive heart failure.* N Engl J Med *293:1184, 1975.)*

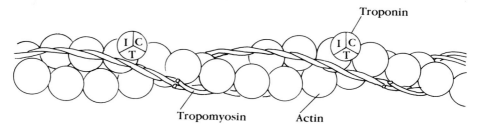

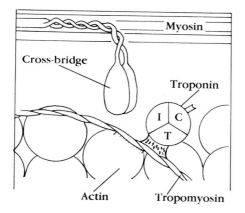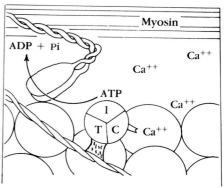

it. Thus the actin filaments slide toward the M line, shortening the sarcomere. At this point ATP, which is present in the sarcoplasm, provides the energy to pump the calcium out of the myofibril and the muscle returns to rest. Each cycle (Table 2-2) shortens the sarcomere by approximately 1%.

This contractile process does not have a refractory period. Thus if repeated stimuli are received before relaxation occurs, the sarcomere will continue to shorten up to a maximum of about 50% of its resting length. If the active transport of calcium out of the myofibril is inhibited for any reason, relaxation of the muscle cannot occur and sustained contraction called **contracture** results. It might seem paradoxical that hypocalcemia (low calcium level) will result in hyperactivity rather than reduced activity of muscle; however, reduction of calcium lowers the threshold of excitability at synapses and **motor end-plates** (myoneural junctions).

Next we need to examine how depolarization of the muscle cell membrane (sarcolemma) occurs

Table 2-2. Sequence of Events in Contraction and Relaxation of Skeletal Muscle

Steps in contraction

1. Discharge of motor neuron
2. Release of transmitter (acetylcholine) at motor end-plate
3. Generation of end-plate potential
4. Generation of action potential in muscle fibers
5. Inward spread of depolarization along T-tubules
6. Release of Ca^{++} from lateral sacs of sarcoplasmic reticulum and diffusion to thick and thin filaments
7. Binding of Ca^{++} to troponin C, uncovering myosin binding sites on actin
8. Formation of cross-linkages between actin and myosin and sliding of thin on thick filaments, producing shortening

Steps in relaxation

1. Ca^{++} pumped back into sarcoplasmic reticulum
2. Release of Ca^{++} from troponin
3. Cessation of interaction between actin and myosin

Source: Reproduced, with permission, from Ganong WF, *Review of Medical Physiology*. 10th ed. Copyright 1981 by Lange Medical Publications, Los Altos, California.

at the motor end-plate. The myoneural junction is similar in structure and function to the synapse (see Nerve Tissue). At the myoneural junctions, the terminal bouton of one motor axon fits into a folded depression within the sarcolemma. The gap between the nerve and muscle cell membranes is similar to the synaptic cleft. When an action potential reaches the terminal bouton, acetylcholine is released into the cleft. The acetylcholine increases the permeability of the sarcolemma to a degree normally sufficient to cause depolarization. Only in recent years have we understood how the action potential generated by depolarization of the sarcolemma at the myoneural junction reaches each of the myofibrils of the muscle. We are used to thinking of a cell membrane as simply surrounding a cell like the skin of an orange. However, imagine drilling multiple holes in the orange so that each hole passed among the small cells of the orange sections with each cell in contact with one of the holes. Now imagine that the skin of the orange lined each of those holes. This is analogous to the way in which each sarcomere of each myofibril within each muscle fiber is adjacent to the cell membrane. These lined holes are called **tubules,** and all of the tubules of a muscle fiber are called the **T-system.** The T-system is associated anatomically with the **sarcoplasmic reticulum,** a specialized form of the **endoplasmic reticulum,** which contributes to metabolic processes in cells throughout the body. In general, endoplasmic reticulum is a complex series of tubules with walls of membrane formed within the cytoplasm of the cells. Pairs of tubules of the sarcoplasmic reticulum lie adjacent to each of the myofibrils and interposed between members of these pairs is a tubule of the T-system. The combination of one branch of the T-system and two associated tubules of the sarcoplasmic reticulum has been termed a **triad** (Figure 2-23).

The action potential of an axon triggers the release of acetylcholine into the myoneural cleft. This triggers depolarization of the underlying sarcolemma, and an action potential is generated and conducted throughout the sarcolemma of that muscle fiber. As the action potential reaches any

2-23. *The T-system (A) and the sarcoplasmic reticulum (B) in skeletal muscle. (Figure A reproduced, with permission, from Peachey LD: The sarcoplasmic reticulum and transverse tubules of the frog's sartorius.* J Cell Biol *25:209, 1969, by copyright permission of the Rockefeller University Press, as modified in Bloom W, and Fawcett DW:* A Textbook of Histology, *9th ed. Copyright 1968 by W. B. Saunders Company, Philadelphia, Pennsylvania. Figure B reproduced, with permission, from Hoyle G: How is muscle turned on and off?* Sci Am *22:84, 1970. Copyright © by Scientific American, Inc., All rights reserved.)*

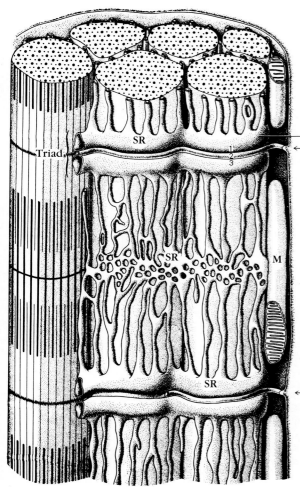

A

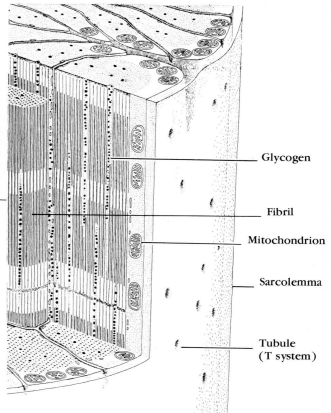

B

particular part of the T-system, it triggers the release of stored calcium from the sarcoplasmic reticulum into the adjacent sarcomere, and the process of contraction occurs.

The reaction to a single action potential would be a very brief contraction followed by relaxation. This brief contraction is called a **twitch.** Incomplete relaxation occurring between stimuli is called **incomplete tetanus. Complete tetanus** (Figure 2-24) occurs when action potentials are sufficiently close together to maintain maximal contraction.

Muscles contain elastic and viscous components in series with the muscle fibers. This means that a muscle (unlike a sarcomere) is capable of contracting without reducing its overall length. This normally occurs only when the muscle is prevented from shortening by the action of other muscles or other factors that inhibit joint movement, as in pushing against an immobile object. This is called **isometric** (equal length) contraction as opposed to contraction resulting in shortening of the muscle, called **isotonic** (equal tension) contraction. In isometric contraction, tension is produced by the contractile process. In the majority of muscles, maximum tension is produced when a muscle is at its resting length. Most common body movements require only minor shortening of muscles; thus, maximal tension can be produced. While muscles can contract up to 50% of their resting length, they do not do so under normal circumstances. More typically, muscles function within 10% of their resting length. This is one example of the efficiency with which the body operates. Another is seen in the velocity of contraction. Velocity is inversely proportional to load, and the highest velocity occurs at the muscle's resting length.

Muscles of the body vary greatly in size, and range from a few millimeters in length and approximately 1 mm in diameter to the very large muscles of the arms, legs, and torso which may be 30 or 40 cm or more in length and several centimeters in diameter.

Striated muscles occur in the body in a variety of forms. When we think of a muscle, we most commonly envision long cylindrical muscles such as those found in the arms and the legs. These muscles are called **fusiform muscles** (Figure 2-25). In some cases, however, such as in the abdominal wall, muscles occur in the form of broad flat sheets. In either case, the muscle fascicles all lie parallel to one another, and their potential range of motion is dictated by the length of the muscle. The longer the muscle, the greater its range of motion. The power of the muscle, as is true of all muscles, is dictated by the number of muscle fibers.

2-24. *Isometric tension as a function of time in a single muscle fiber during continuously increasing and decreasing stimulations. (Redrawn and reproduced, with permission, from Buchthal F:* Dan Biol Medd, *17:1, 1942.)*

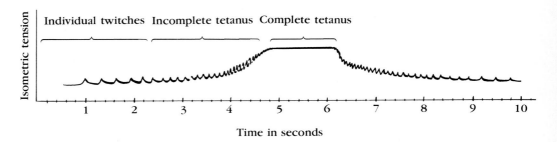

Time in seconds

Some muscles adopt a form that provides for many short muscle fibers, an advantage when great power over a short range of motion is required. One such type of muscle is called **penniform** (also called **pennate**) because it gives the appearance of one side of a feather. The tendon in such a muscle, instead of being found at the two ends of the muscle, runs the entire course of the muscle with the muscle fascicles branching off from it. In this case, the potential range of the muscle is determined by the length of any one of the fascicles, while the power of the muscle is a function of the sum of its fibers. Thus a penniform muscle will

typically have a shorter potential range of motion but greater power `han a fusiform muscle of the same size. Muscles are classified as **bipenniform** if they have muscle fascicles arising from both sides of a tendon that runs the full length of the muscle. **Multipenniform** muscles are characterized by fascicles that converge on multiple tendons.

In some cases, fascicles may converge from a broad area of attachment on one bone to a single point on another. These are called **radiate** muscles. In exceptional cases, the muscle fascicles originate from a central tendon and radiate

2-25. *Architecture of skeletal muscle.*

Fusiform

 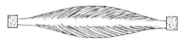

Penniform (unipenniform)   Bipenniform

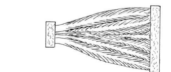

Multipenniform

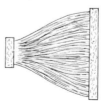 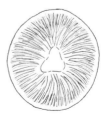

Radiate   Circumpennate

through 360 degrees to a circular insertion. These are called **circumpennate** muscles. An example of this type of muscle is the diaphragm. The majority of muscles discussed in this text are fusiform; exceptions will be noted as such.

NEUROMUSCULAR RELATIONSHIPS

Skeletal muscles receive their stimuli from motoneurons. A motoneuron typically has its cell body within the spinal cord or brain stem with a long axon extending to the muscle, where it branches to form myoneural junctions with a number of muscle fibers (Figure 2-26). The combination of a neuron and associated muscle fibers is termed a **motor unit.** The motor unit is the functional unit of a muscle, since if the neuron is stimulated and produces an action potential, it will stimulate all of the muscle fibers in the motor unit to contract. Motor units vary dramatically in size, with some containing only three or four muscle fibers and others containing over 150 muscle fibers. Another way of describing the nerve-muscle relationships for a particular muscle is in terms of the nerve-to-muscle fiber ratio. That is the ratio of the number of neurons (thus also the number of axons) to the number of muscle fibers.

Muscles concerned with fine, precise, controlled movement, such as those that produce movement of the fingers and eyes, have small motor units. Muscles concerned with gross movements and power, such as the large muscles of the back, arms, and legs, have large motor units. The degree to which a muscle contracts is due not only to the rate of stimulation of its fibers but also to the number of fibers stimulated. Thus, small motor units can provide for finer degrees of muscle function than can large motor units.

With minimal voluntary activity, a relatively small number of motor units will be active. As muscular effort increases, additional motor units discharge. This process is called **recruitment** of motor units. Active motor units during muscle function are spread throughout the muscle and fire asynchronously in order to provide for smooth function. If all neurons to a muscle fired in synchrony, movements would be jerky and tremulous.

During voluntary activity, motor units are not recruited at random, since not all motor units have the same properties. Motor units are classified as fast or slow depending upon the duration of the twitch contraction (Figure 2-24). **Fast muscles** have twitch durations as short as 7 or 8 msec, while in **slow muscles,** twitch duration can be as long as 100 msec. This difference has been related to the rate of metabolism of ATP in the muscles. Twitch duration is fairly constant within a motor unit but varies across motor units. The metabolic difference is associated with a difference in the color of the muscle fiber. Faster fibers are light in color, while slow fibers are darker and red in color; thus fast and slow muscle fibers are also called **white fibers** and **red fibers** respectively. In some animals, such as birds, whole muscles are either white or red, while red and white fibers are intermixed in human muscles. Ganong [6] reports that

The differences between types of muscle units are not inherent but are determined in part by their innervation. The nerves to fast and slow muscles have been crossed and allowed to regenerate. When regrowth was complete and the nerve that previously supplied the slow muscle innervated the fast one, the fast muscle became slow. The reverse change occurred in the previously slow muscle. There were also appropriate changes in ATPase content. There is evidence that substances can flow down neurons and enter muscle. However, the effect of the nerve on the chemistry of the muscle appears to be due to the pattern of discharge in the nerve rather than a trophic factor per se.

As expected, the axons associated with slow muscle fibers are smaller in diameter and thus conduct action potentials more slowly than axons associated with fast muscle fibers. The slower motor units are more resistant to fatigue, and in large muscles such as those of the arms, legs, and back, these are recruited first. Fast units are recruited when a higher level of activity is required. Thus large muscles have a large number of slow units. Muscles that perform fine skilled motion have a large number of fast units. Slow motor units are sometimes called **tonic units** since they are related to slow, steady contraction. Fast units are sometimes called **phasic units** since they respond and fatigue more rapidly.

Neuromuscular interaction requires more than the function of the motor unit. In addition to the activation of muscles to contract, sensory information must be fed back to the CNS to control movement. Feedback mechanisms in learning control of movement will be dealt with in greater de-

tail in Chapter 7 (Nervous System). However, an understanding of reflex activity in the control of muscle contraction is essential to an understanding of basic muscle function.

A simple **reflex arc,** illustrated in Figure 2-27, consists of a sensory receptor, its associated sensory neuron, one or more synapses in the CNS, a motoneuron, and its associated effector. A reflex arc is termed **monosynaptic** if the sensory

2-26. *Myoneural junction.*

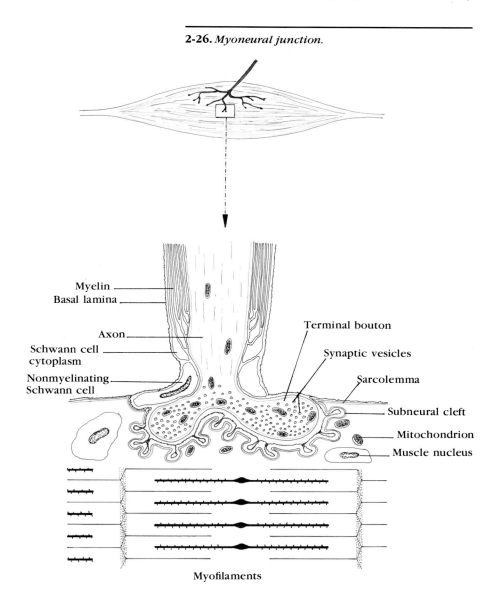

Myelin
Basal lamina

Axon

Schwann cell cytoplasm

Nonmyelinating Schwann cell

Terminal bouton

Synaptic vesicles

Sarcolemma

Subneural cleft

Mitochondrion

Muscle nucleus

Myofilaments

neuron stimulates the motoneuron directly or **polysynaptic** if one or more interneurons are interposed between the sensory neuron and one or more motoneurons. The preemptive reflex is the **withdrawal reflex.** In this case, a noxious stimulus such as pain to the skin results in flexion (bending) of the limbs on the side of the stimulus to pull them away and extension of the opposite limbs to support the body and prepare for flight. This is obviously a complex polysynaptic reflex arc. However, owing to a reflex arc, a stimulus can produce a direct response for protection at the spinal cord or brain stem level without the necessity for involvement of higher brain centers. The pathway is direct from the receptor to the effectors. This does not mean, however, that reflex arcs cannot be controlled by higher brain centers. For example, if you accidentally touch the edge of a knife, you may exhibit a withdrawal response that will be inhibited the next time you do so if you learn that the knife is not sharp.

Two types of receptors, one located within a muscle and the other on its tendon, provide direct input to reflex arcs for the control of muscle function. The receptor located within the muscle is called the **muscle spindle** and is the receptor for the **stretch reflex.** The stretch reflex may be monosynaptic or polysynaptic. All other known reflex arcs are polysynaptic.

The muscle spindle (Figure 2-28) contains up to ten small short muscle fibers arranged parallel to the other fibers of the muscle. The muscle fibers of the spindle are termed **intrafusal** in contradistinction to the regular fibers of the muscle, termed **extrafusal.** The intrafusal muscle fibers are of two types, nuclear bag and nuclear chain. The **nuclear bag fibers** are characterized by a swelling in their center that contains multiple nuclei. The **nuclear chain fibers** lack this swelling, and their nuclei are arranged in tandem. The nuclear chain fibers are attached to the nuclear bag fibers in parallel. The complex of intrafusal fibers is encapsulated in connective tissue. The ends of the intrafusal fibers are contractile, while their centers apparently are not.

Two types of sensory (afferent) nerve fibers are associated with the spindle. The **primary fibers** are rapidly conducting fibers wrapped around the centers of the intrafusal fibers in what are called **annulospiral endings. The secondary fibers** are

2-27. Monosynaptic and polysynaptic reflex arcs.

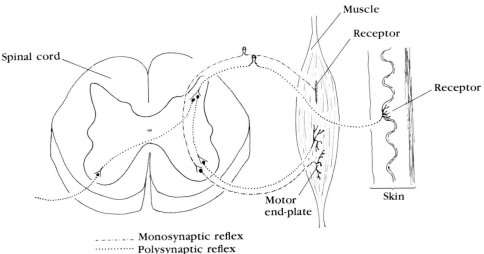

_ _ _ _ _ _ Monosynaptic reflex
·············· Polysynaptic reflex

more slowly conducting and terminate on the ends of the nuclear chain fibers (and perhaps the nuclear bag fibers) in what are called **flower spray endings.** Both types of endings are stimulated when the spindle is stretched during stretching of the muscle. The activation of these endings by stretching the muscle causes excitation of its motoneurons via the reflex arc, and the muscle contracts. This reflex is most apparent when the stretch is sudden. The knee-jerk response to tapping the tendon of the leg extensor at the knee is an example. However, the stretch reflex is essential to maintenance of posture and smooth, con-

trolled movement. The primary and secondary sensory endings respond differently to stretch. Both endings begin to fire when the intrafusal fibers are stretched and continue to fire so long as the muscle is in the stretched state. However, the primary endings increase their rate of firing as the velocity of stretch increases. Thus the primary fibers signal both the active process of stretching and the maintenance of stretch (Figure 2-29).

The intrafusal muscle fibers are also supplied with motoneurons known as **gamma efferents.** Although small, these fibers are abundant, making up about 30% of the motoneurons that exit from

2-28. *The muscle spindle and its relationships to extrafusal muscle fibers and to the spinal cord: a, Annulospiral ending; b, Nuclear bag intrafusal muscle fiber; c, Nuclear chain intrafusal muscle fiber; f, Flowerspray ending; g, Golgi tendon organ; m, Extrafusal muscle fibers; p, Motor end-plate. Afferent fibers are sensory while efferent fibers are motor.*

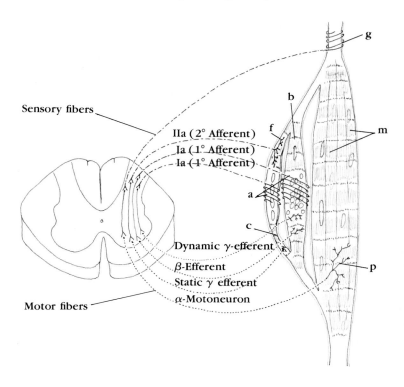

Sensory fibers

IIa (2° Afferent)
Ia (1° Afferent)
Ia (1° Afferent)

Dynamic γ-efferent
β-Efferent
Static γ efferent
α-Motoneuron

Motor fibers

the spinal cord. The motor supply to the intrafusal fibers permits contraction (shortening) of these fibers with a consequent increase in their sensitivity to stretch. In addition, when the extrafusal fibers contract, shortening the muscle, the intrafusal fibers contract also in order to maintain their length ratio to the muscle and, therefore, their sensitivity to stretch. It has been hypothesized that the nuclear bag fibers respond to dynamic (changing) length, while the nuclear chain fibers respond only to static (changed) length.

In skilled movement, muscle spindle discharge apparently is regulated by the CNS to assist in the discharge of the **alpha motoneurons** (motoneurons to the extrafusal muscle fibers) to develop initial speed of movement. When the gamma efferents are blocked, reduction in the initial acceleration and velocity of motion has been recorded [1, 17].

The sensory endings on the tendons of muscles are called **Golgi tendon organs.** They respond when adequate stress is placed on the tendon during both stretch and contraction of the muscle. They conduct impulses via rapidly conducting neurons, giving rise to an IPSP on the motoneuron of the same muscle but an EPSP on the muscles that would act in opposition. Thus the tendon organs serve to temper motor activity and inhibit activity in a muscle when high levels of stress occur at the tendon.

The motoneurons that supply both the intrafusal and extrafusal muscle fibers receive input within the spinal cord or the brain stem from many sources. The ratio of motoneurons to synapses in the spinal cord can be in excess of 1:5000. These relationships will be explored further in Chapter 7.

MUSCULOSKELETAL RELATIONSHIPS

Motion of the human body or of its parts is made possible by the presence of joints, which permit movement between skeletal components, and muscles, which serve as the motive force for these movements. The structure of a joint determines the range within which motion can occur. For all joints, motion is further restricted by associated ligaments. If one were to examine the body from an engineer's point of view, several types of joints would be recognized (Figure 2-30). A first level of differentiation might be between those joints that are not freely movable and those that are. Joints that are not freely movable are of two types: those in which no motion occurs, and those in which only slight motion can occur. Immovable joints are called **fibrous joints** (also called **synarthro-**

2-29. *Response patterns of primary afferent (Ia) and of secondary afferent (IIa) fibers to the contraction and stretch of the associated extrafusal muscle fibers (EM): 1, rest; 2, increasing contraction; 3, steady contraction; 4, decreasing contraction; 5, increasing stretch; 6, steady stretch; 7, recoil from stretch; 8, rest.*

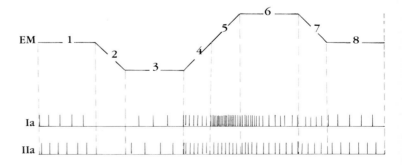

dial joints). Fibrous joints are exemplified by the **sutures** of the skull. In this instance, the bones have grown together and are joined by fibrous tissue. In some sutures fusion becomes so complete that the suture eventually becomes obliterated.

Joints in which only slight movement is permitted are called **cartilaginous joints** (also called **amphiarthrodial joints**). The most common type of cartilaginous joint is the **symphysis,** such as that which occurs between the two halves of the pelvis anteriorly.

Freely movable joints are called **synovial joints** (also called **diarthrodial joints**). Synovial joints have several characteristics important to their function. The joint itself is enclosed by a fibrous capsule lined by a membrane. This articular capsule secretes synovial fluid, which lubricates the joint. The opposing bony surfaces within the articular capsule are smooth and are covered by hyaline cartilage. The synovial fluid and cartilage serve to protect the joint from impact and friction.

The fibrous capsule limits motion of the joint.

There are six types of synovial joints, classified according to their structure and function (Figure 2-31). They will be described here in ascending order of the degree of movement permitted at each.

In a **plane joint** (**arthrodial joint**), the opposed surfaces are flat or slightly curved and permit sliding of one surface over the other. This is exemplified by some of the joints between successive vertebrae.

In a **hinge joint** (**ginglymus joint**), motion in only one plane is permitted. This is a back and forth or flexion-extension motion, as exemplified by the elbow and finger joints.

A **pivotal joint** (**trochoid joint**) consists of a rounded process inserted into a bony **fossa** (trench or channel) that has the appearance of a sleeve or a ring. This structure plus strong bands of ligaments permit only a rotational movement about the longitudinal axis of the rounded process.

2-30. *Examples of major types of joints. A, Coronal suture of the skull (fibrous joint); B, Pubic symphysis (cartilaginous joint); C, Hip joint (synovial ball and socket joint).*

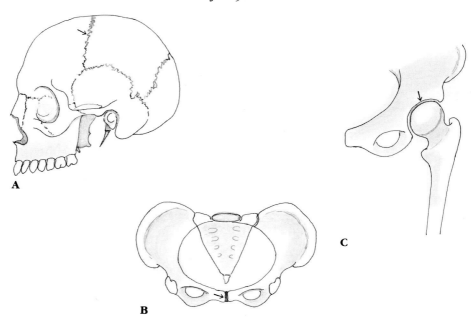

A

B

C

An additional ligament in this type of joint is called the **annular ligament,** which holds the rounded articular process in place and provides for its socket. This type of joint is exemplified by the joint between the first and second cervical (neck) vertebrae (the locus of much of the rotational movement of the head) and also within the complex joint of the elbow (the point of rotation for the forearm and hand).

A **condyloid joint** (**condylarthrodial joint**) consists of an ovoid process that fits into an elliptical-shaped cavity. It allows two types of motion at right angles to each other. Condyloid joints are exemplified by the wrist, which can be moved from side to side or from flexion to extension. However, since the two dimensions of the oval are unequal, rotation cannot occur at a condyloid joint. The joint between the lower jaw and the skull is another example of this type of joint.

A **saddle joint** (**articulatio sellaris**) permits

2-31. *Examples of different types of synovial joints. A, Intervertebral articulations (plane joints); B, Atlanto-axial joint (pivotal joint); C, Elbow joint (hinge joint); D, Hip joint (ball and socket joint); E, Third joint of the thumb (saddle joint); F, Temporomandibular joint (condyloid joint).*

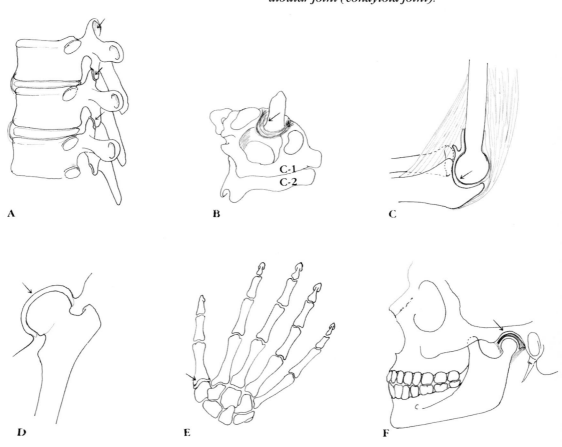

the same type of motion as a condyloid joint. However, the opposing surfaces in this joint consist of a concavity facing a convexity. The third joint of the thumb is an example of this type of joint.

A **ball and socket joint (enarthrodial joint)** is structured as its name implies and allows the greatest degree of freedom of motion in all directions. The hip and shoulder joints are of this type.

A joint can be thought of as the fulcrum of a lever. A common type of lever is a balance (Figure 2-32). Imagine a long board placed over a fulcrum with a load of bricks on one end and you pushing on the other end. By analogy, the board is the bone

to be moved, the fulcrum is the joint that permits the motion, the bricks (load) represent the resistance to the motion, and you represent the muscle that is going to perform the work. If the load is closer to the fulcrum than you are, you can move the load with less effort with the lever than you could without it. Thus the lever provides a mechanical advantage. If the load is more distant from the fulcrum than you are, it will take more effort on your part to move the load with the lever than it would take to move it without the lever. In this case you are working at a mechanical disadvantage. However, in this case you can move the load with great speed since a small movement on your

2-32. *Types of levers. a, Diagram; b, Function (mechanical disadvantage); c, Function (mechanical advantage).*

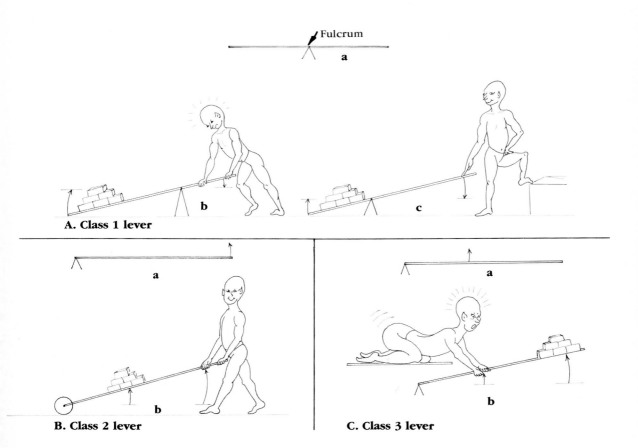

A. Class 1 lever

B. Class 2 lever

C. Class 3 lever

end results in extensive movement at the other end. This type of lever, in which the fulcrum (joint) is between the load to be moved and the muscle, is called a **class 1 lever.** It is very common in the human body and is used to provide stability, rapid movement, or mechanical advantage.

In a **class 2 lever** the fulcrum (joint) is at one end of the lever arm (bone), the force applied (muscle attachment) is at the other end and the load is in between. A wheelbarrow is an example of a class 2 lever. This type of lever always provides a mechanical advantage but is uncommon in the human body.

In a **class 3 lever** the fulcrum is at one end, the load at the other, and the force is applied between them. Such a lever always works at a mechanical disadvantage but provides a means of rapid extensive movement of the load with minimal shortening of the muscle. This is the most common type of lever in the body.

The angle between the direction of shortening of a muscle's fibers and the direction of motion required or permitted will also affect the efficiency with which a muscle can perform work. For example, examine Figure 2-33. The round object in the center represents a bone that can move only in the direction indicated by the arrow within the circle. Arrows a, b, c, and d represent muscles that pull in the direction indicated by their arrows.

Muscle *a* would be able to accomplish this motion most efficiently, while muscles *b* and *c* would have decreasing efficiency. Muscle *d,* pulling at a right angle to the direction of movement, would have no ability to move the object since, if the object moved, muscle *d* would actually be stretched. Proceeding from muscle *a* to muscle *d,* we move from a condition where contraction can be translated directly into motion to conditions where an increasing amount of muscle work will be expended to pull in a direction in which motion cannot occur. The term **vector** is used to indicate the combination of power and direction of pull of a muscle relative to the direction of movement. Figure 2-34 illustrates a class 3 lever with two muscles (*a* and *b*) having different directions of pull. Muscle *a* is more efficient because of its direction of pull relative to the motion allowed by the joint.

A muscle can serve one or more of several functions. When a muscle provides the major force for a motion, it is called the **prime mover.** A muscle that opposes a prime mover is called an **antagonist.** In some cases the pull of a prime mover results not only in the movement desired but in additional, undesired motion. For example, the thyrohyoid muscle lowers the small hyoid bone in the neck. However, contraction of that muscle also

2-33. *Relationship between vector of motion and work load. If the bone can move only in the direction of the arrow it contains, muscles* a *through* d *would have to contract with increasing degrees of force to provide the same amount of motion of the bone, given equal resistance to motion.*

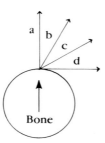

2-34. *Example of muscles acting on a class 3 lever. Muscle* a *is more efficient than muscle* b.

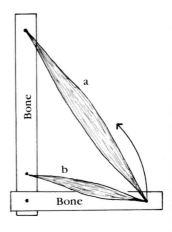

elevates the larynx. Thus another muscle, in this case the sternothyroid, acts to prevent motion of the larynx. A muscle that serves to prevent unwanted motion produced by a prime mover is called a **synergist.** In some functions, such as lifting, it is necessary to bring many muscles into play to stabilize the body as a whole so that required work can be accomplished efficiently. These muscles are called **postural muscles** or **fixators.**

By convention, attachments of muscles to bones or cartilages are termed origins and insertions. In the arms and legs, the proximal attachment is usually called the **origin** and the distal attachment is called the **insertion.** Frequently the term origin is used to denote the fixed end of the muscle and the term insertion denotes the end that moves when the muscle contracts. However, which of two or more bones undergoes movement when a muscle contracts frequently depends upon body position (the effect of gravity) and/or what other muscles may be functioning at the same time to stabilize one or the other of the bones involved. Therefore, use of the terms origin and insertion is frequently more confusing than helpful. The terms will be used for convenience in later chapters but only to indicate standard nomenclature and not necessarily the function of the muscles.

ANALYSIS OF MUSCLE FUNCTION

Thus far we have learned that a number of factors must be considered to ascertain the role of a muscle or group of muscles in any particular function. Among these are such factors as the nerve-to-muscle fiber ratio, which provides an index to the relative number of motor units; motor unit size; types of motor units, whether fast or slow; conduction rate of individual nerve fibers; and the distribution and function of sensory endings in the muscles and tendons. Unfortunately, little definitive information is available at present with regard to these factors for the muscles of speech. Thus, these areas cannot be systematically included in the analyses of the functional potential of speech musculature in the following chapters.

We have also learned that muscles can act as prime movers, assist prime movers, or act as antagonists, synergists, or fixators. Therefore, a muscle that contracts during a movement is not necessarily a prime mover for that activity. Also, two or more activities may occur simultaneously. In addition, muscle function can be affected by other activities and by body position and gravity. Analysis of joints and ligaments will indicate the range within which a given motion can occur. Evaluation of the nature of the lever involved and the vector of associated muscles will help in analyzing muscle potential for a motion. Now let us review other factors that will assist us in analyzing the role of muscles in motion patterns.

Muscles do not ordinarily do work that can be done by gravity. Muscles assist gravity only when force or speed in the direction of gravity is required. This means that in some cases muscle function depends upon body position. If the force of gravity causes a more rapid motion than is desired, a muscle will act to resist that motion and thereby provide a braking function.

Muscular energy is not used where the normal recoil of stretched tissues will suffice. For example, during inhalation in the upright posture, the rib cage is moved away from its rest position and against gravity. This requires the expenditure of energy for the contraction of muscles. During exhalation, however, unless there is some requirement that it be done rapidly or forcefully, the muscles of inhalation gradually "turn off," and the normal recoil of stretched nonmuscular tissue and gravity move the rib cage back to its resting position.

While several muscles frequently work together to provide a single function, two or more muscles do not normally serve a function that can be accomplished by a single muscle. In general it is well to keep in mind that the musculoskeletal system functions logically and with a minimum of effort to provide required motion.

Motion at joints is the principal function of most striated muscles. Muscles most commonly act on the joint that lies between the two ends of the muscle (Figure 2-35). While this is not invariably true, it gives the investigator or student a probable place to begin analysis of function of a particular muscle. If a muscle has a broad area of attachment at one end and a localized attachment at the other end, typically the principal function of the muscle is to move the bone that receives the more localized attachment.

In some cases the nature of a muscle's attachments gives one a reasonable probability of deducing its function. If we were to attach rope from a twenty-story building to a small metal box and then shorten the rope, it would be within reasonable probability that the box would move and the building would stay where it was. An example of such reasoning might apply to the sternohyoid muscle, which attaches at its lower end to the sternum and thereby to the entire rib cage, and attaches at its upper end to the very small and relatively free hyoid bone. It would be a reasonable hypothesis that this muscle's sole function would be to lower the hyoid bone and not to elevate the rib cage.

The contraction of a muscle fiber results in an increase in its **stiffness** when it is contracted against resistance. This increase in stiffness is of general importance in the maintenance of posture and of special importance, as we shall see later, in the function of the larynx.

Finally, the smallest functional unit of a muscle is the motor unit. The degree of activity of a muscle can be changed in two ways: by the recruitment of motor units, and by an increase in the rate of neural stimulation. Fine control of muscle activity can be achieved only when the strength required is low relative to maximum strength. The degree of control is a function of the size of the motor units and the range of neural stimulus rate available. When we are operating at maximum strength, all motor units are active at their maximum stimulus rates and tetanus results. The closer we come to this state, the less fine control we can exert over our movements. Fine motor skills are possible only when a small percentage of available strength is required.

METHODS OF INVESTIGATION

In order to understand and appraise new information as it becomes available, it is necessary to examine some of the most commonly used methods employed in research in anatomy and physiology, including the types of information that can be gained from these methods and their major shortcomings. We will mention here only those methods in common use with human subjects. Certain methods, while they are extremely valuable, can only be used on subhuman animals because they necessitate destructive processes on the living subject. A major example of this is the study of nerve function by induced degeneration of nerve fibers.

A word of caution should be voiced regarding animal experimentation. Even with regard to basic anatomy, there are important differences among animal species, particularly in those structures of the head and neck that concern us in this volume. Therefore, before results of experiments on subhuman species can be applied directly to human beings, equivalence between the two species in the area under investigation must be demonstrated.

2-35. *The biceps muscle as an example of a muscle that lies across a joint.*

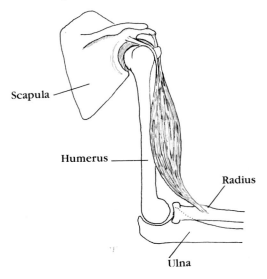

Scapula

Humerus

Radius

Ulna

Dissection

The primary study methods of the anatomist are gross dissection and histological sectioning. **Histology** refers to the study of tissues or to microscopic anatomy. Histological study necessitates infiltration of the tissues with a plastic medium such as celloidin or wax, which permits the tissue to be cut into very thin slices (**sections**). Section thickness for histological study ranges from 1 to 20 or 30 μm. Sections are then stained with a series of chemicals that, with the addition of a binding chemical, will each adhere to only one type of tissue. Thus muscle tissue may appear to be red, connective tissue blue or green, nerves black, and so forth. An example of a histological sagittal section through a human fetal head is shown in Figure 2-36.

Dissection and sectioning techniques cannot be undertaken on living tissue except in the case of very small tissue samples obtainable by biopsy. In the study of cadaveric materials, there are some problems of tissue shrinkage involved in fixation of

2-36. *Sagittal section through the head of a human fetus.*

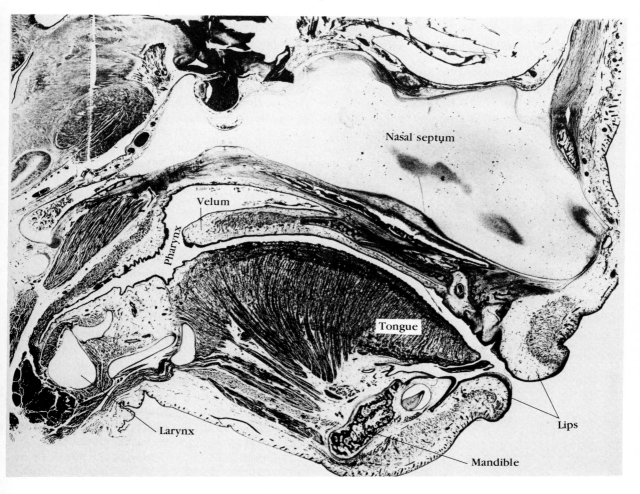

the tissue that may affect the outcome of the study unless they are carefully controlled. Obviously, only structure, not function, can be examined by these methods. The advantage of histological sectioning is that an entire organ can be cut into very thin sections so that anatomical relationships can be studied without the destruction of tissue that is unavoidable in gross dissection. Although some investigators, including the present authors, have developed techniques for histological study of specimens as large as the intact adult larynx and whole human fetal heads, the histological method is normally undertaken only on relatively small specimens. Currently it is not possible to obtain thin serial sections on any partially bony structure the size of the adult human head. However, large organs composed only of soft tissue, such as the brain and heart, can be studied successfully by histological methods.

Another disadvantage of the histological method is the difficulty of reestablishing valid three-dimensional relationships from the series of thin sections obtained. The shape of a three-dimensional object may be subject to extreme distortion unless stringent methods of control are employed. For example, imagine slicing a cylinder into extremely thin sections (Figure 2-37A) and then trying to put it back together again piece by piece. Without some built-in alignment system, it would be easy to end up with a cylinder whose surface and long axis were at a greatly altered angle (Figure 2-37B). Now imagine trying to re-

construct a human head, in which no single landmark lies in a straight line across or through the whole head. It is easy to see how the attempt to reconstruct hundreds of thin serial sections could result in a gross distortion of both form and interrelationships among structures.

Some tissue types present unique problems to the researcher. For example, nerve cells, because of their very high oxygen requirements, are the first cells to begin to disintegrate after death. This process begins immediately after death, and total destruction of the peripheral nerve endings may take less than an hour. Thus unless tissue is fixed chemically to stop the destructive process, misleading results can be obtained. For example, in studies of the presence of muscle spindles in the human larynx, some investigators have found these endings in the superficial musculature of the larynx [2, 3, 5, 7, 10, 11, 13–16, 18], while others have not [4, 8, 9]. Since it is unlikely that these endings occur in some human larynges and not in others, one reasonable hypothesis is that where spindles were not found, too much time had elapsed between death and fixation, allowing time for destruction of those endings.

Radiography

Some patterns of motion and certain anatomical details can be viewed in the living subject by means of x-rays. As in photography, x-rays can consist of "still" pictures or "motion" pictures. X-rays are photoelectron beams that pass through the tissues of the body. Some of the electrons are absorbed by the tissues through which they pass. Dense tissues absorb more electrons than less dense tissues. If a film sensitive to these electrons is placed on the opposite side of the body from the source of the photoelectron beam, a picture can be obtained that represents the relative densities of the different parts of the structure being viewed. Relatively soft tissues will be differentiated from relatively hard tissues, and air columns will stand out from surrounding tissues.

A number of x-ray methods are discussed briefly below. However, there is one problem common to

2-37. *Example of distortion possible in sectioning and reconstruction of anatomical specimens.*

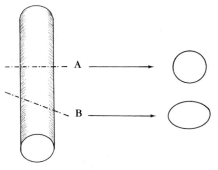

all of these methods. They all involve levels of radiation potentially hazardous to the subject. In large amounts, radiation is destructive to the tissues of the body. Further, the effect is cumulative over the period of a person's entire lifetime. For example, approximately 40 to 50 standard units of radiation (**rads**) to the corneas of the eye can produce cataracts in later life. It does not matter whether the dose is received from a single exposure of 40 rads or forty exposures of a single rad over a time period of several years. It is well known that a sufficiently high level of radiation is lethal. It has been calculated that a total body dose of approximately 600 rads is lethal; however, much higher doses can be given to small areas of the body without resulting in death. Thus both the amount of radiation to any specific part of the body and the total dose to the entire body are important determiners of risk. The point is that exposure of subjects to x-irradiation involves risks to those subjects. Therefore, studies involving this method must be carefully designed to involve negligible risk and must only be done when the information to be gained is worth the risk involved, however small that risk may be. For this reason, radiological studies of normal subjects are few in number, and most involve the use of patients who have been irradiated for some medical purpose unrelated to research. One obvious question is whether the medical problem that gave rise to the need for irradiation will in any way compromise the results of the research study.

The value of x-ray investigations in determining anatomical configuration and patterns of motion in living persons is obvious. There are, however, shortcomings associated with the nature of the information obtainable. In a standard x-ray, all of the structures of the head that lie in the path of the x-ray beam are superimposed upon one another. Also, the densities of adjacent tissues may not be sufficiently different to be observable on the x-ray film. For this reason, it is relatively easy to visualize the outlines of bones and air columns, but it is not possible to distinguish muscles, since the density of the muscle is too similar to that of the surrounding soft tissue.

In order to take motion picture x-rays, the radiation must be increased. **Cineradiography** (x-ray motion pictures) may require two to five times the amount of radiation needed for standard x-ray, depending on the exposure time required to capture the motion. This has been partially overcome by the use of videofluoroscopy. **Fluoroscopy** is a radiological method requiring less radiation than standard x-ray, since the electron beams are used to illuminate a cathode ray tube screen rather than to impress an image on film. Originally, the disadvantage of standard fluoroscopy was that it was not possible to obtain a permanent image of good quality, since permanent images could only be obtained by photographing the image on the cathode ray tube. With the advent of television, however, this problem was largely solved, since the electron beam could be used to impress the image on videotape. This tape could then be replayed. It is still true, however, that while videofluoroscopy results in less radiation than cineradiography, cineradiography produces clearer images and these images may be traced to obtain measurements.

Recent advances in technology have also helped to solve the problem of the superimposition of images in standard x-ray procedures. This has been made possible by the advent of tomography (also called laminagraphy). **Linear tomography** (Figure 2-38) involves motion of the x-ray source in one direction while the film is moved in the opposite direction, so that the paths travelled by the beams from the moving x-ray source cross within the target body plane. All structures that lie outside of the plane in which the x-ray beam paths cross are blurred, and only those structures lying within that plane are left clear. The resulting image gives more information than the standard x-ray if the structures to be studied lie within the particular plane of the body that is in focus. However, any structure that lies parallel to the direction of travel of the beam and film can result in serious artifacts in the film, giving the appearance of structures that are not present.

Circular tomography (Figure 2-39) involves movement of both the x-ray source and the film in a circular direction. Since few structures would lie parallel to this direction of travel, the quality of the image obtained is significantly enhanced.

Triradial tomography (Figure 2-40) involves moving the x-ray source through a spiral motion. This, once again, results in a somewhat better defined image. Tomograms give information regarding a plane through the body that is only 1 mm thick. Therefore, for the study of any particular structure, a number of laminagrams may be necessary. Since each laminagram exposes the same area of the body, the radiation level to the subject can become significantly increased. Even in the case of very small structures or structures requiring only a single laminagram, several laminagrams may be necessary in order to locate the exact plane of interest.

An additional problem common to all types of laminagraphy is that tissue contrasts within the plane in focus are reduced by the blurring effect from planes not in focus, because the x-ray beams pass through the whole structure and not just through the plane of interest. Thus even though planes out of focus are not imaged clearly, their presence does affect the quality of the image of the plane in focus.

Within the last few years, a revolutionary new method of x-ray has been introduced. This is called **computed tomography** (**CT**) (Figure 2-41). In this method, a large number of finely focused x-rays are taken around the circumference of the body in a given plane. A computer then summates the information obtained from the individual x-ray beams and reconstructs an image of that plane, which is then portrayed as a tomographic slice of extraordinary clarity. This method is so sensitive to tissue density differences that individual muscles and nerves can be visualized. In addition, since radiation is delivered discretely to the plane of interest, the total amount of radiation

---

2-38. *Linear sagittal tomogram of adult human head: b, Brain; s, Soft palate; v, Vertebra; m, Mandible. Tomograms shown in Figures 2-38 through 2-41 were all taken through the same plane of the same head. (Reproduced, with permission, from Dickson DR, Maue-Dickson W: Velopharyngeal structure and function: A model for biomechanical analysis. In Lass NJ (Ed):* Speech and Language: Advances in Basic Research and Practice, *Vol. 3. P. 167, 1980. Copyright by Academic Press, New York.)*

2-39. *Circular sagittal tomogram of adult human head. b, Brain; s, Soft palate; v, Vertebra; m, Mandible. (Reproduced, with permission, from Dickson DR, Maue-Dickson W: Velopharyngeal structure and function: A model for biomechanical analysis. In Lass NJ (Ed):* Speech and Language: Advances in Basic Research and Practice, *Vol. 3. P. 167, 1980. Copyright by Academic Press, New York.)*

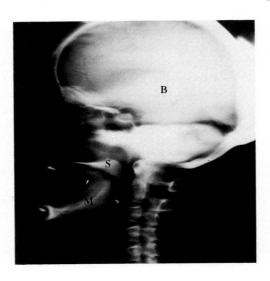

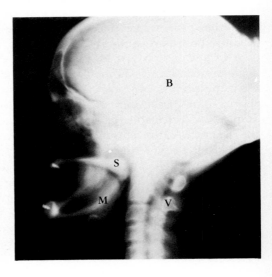

received by the subject in the imaging of contiguous slices does not increase as it does in standard tomographic x-ray procedures. The disadvantage of CT scanning, as with all other still forms of x-ray, is that motion cannot be studied.

In the study of physiology, it is obvious that cineradiography or videofluoroscopy are the only x-ray methods currently available that show structures during function. It should be remembered, however, that while the movement of structures can be observed with these methods, they still do not provide any direct evidence with regard to specific muscles involved in a given activity. For example, using x-ray motion pictures, we can observe the nature of motion of the mandible. The observation of the motion combined with the study of anatomy may provide us with reasonable hypotheses with regard to which muscles are responsible for the activity, but it cannot tell us which muscles are active and which muscles are inactive during any particular activity.

Electromyography

Electromyography (EMG) records the electrical potentials developed by muscles when they contract. This can be done either by placing an electrode on the skin over a superficial muscle or by placing an electrode directly into the muscle. In either case, EMG simply reveals when a muscle is contracting and when it is not. It does not necessarily indicate whether the muscle is acting as a prime mover, synergist, stabilizer, or even antagonist to the action under study.

It is possible to determine relative degrees of contraction of a single muscle by the magnitude of its electrical signal. However, the methods in standard use cannot demonstrate the relative intensity of contraction of two or more muscles or the absolute level of activity of any one muscle. The reasons for this are quite simple. If an electrode is placed over the surface of a muscle while the muscle is in a state of contraction, the greatest amount of electrical activity will be recorded at

2-40. *Triradial sagittal tomogram of adult human head: b, Brain; p, Soft palate; v, Vertebra; m, Mandible. (Reproduced, with permission, from Dickson DR, Maue-Dickson W: Velopharyngeal structure and function: A model for biomechanical analysis. In Lass NJ (Ed): Speech and Language: Advances in Basic Research and Practice,* Vol. 3. P. 167, 1980. Copyright by Academic Press, New York.)

2-41. *Computed sagittal tomogram of adult human head: b, Brain; p, Soft palate; v, Vertebra. (Reproduced, with permission, from Dickson DR, Maue-Dickson W: Velopharyngeal structure and function: A model for biomechanical analysis. In Lass NJ (Ed):* Speech and Language: Advances in Basic Research and Practice, *Vol. 3. P. 167, 1980. Copyright by Academic Press, New York.)*

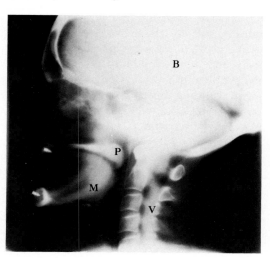

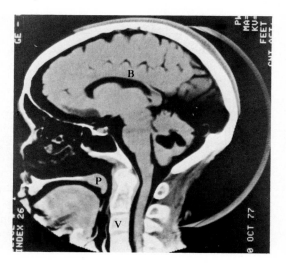

the myoneural junction, also called, for this reason, the **motor point.** The level of activity will diminish with increasing distance from the motor point. Thus, unless electrodes in two or more muscles have identical proximity to the motor point, valid conclusions regarding their relative levels of activity cannot be made. Such determination is further complicated by the fact that different muscles have different levels of activity to start with and differ in the number and arrangement of their fibers.

The principal advantage of surface electromyography is that the skin does not have to be punctured in order to obtain electrical recordings. The disadvantage is that if other muscles intervene between the target muscle and the electrode, it may be impossible to determine which muscle is undergoing contraction. The advantage of intramuscular electromyography is that the electrode is positioned within the target muscle, instead of being placed on the surface of the body. Therefore, there should be little doubt as to which muscle is being recorded, except in the case where two or more muscles interweave their fibers. The difficulty with the placement of intramuscular electrodes is how to be certain that the electrode, which is usually in the form of the tip of a needle, is located within the specific target muscle. In very large or superficial muscles this does not usually present a problem. However, in deep muscles, and most particularly when those deep muscles are small or thin, this can pose a problem. This situation is complicated still further when a small thin target muscle lies in close proximity to other muscles.

Unfortunately, some investigations of this type have employed circular reasoning with regard to electrode placement when there is some question as to whether a muscle is active in a particular activity. The needle electrode presumably is inserted into the target muscle, the activity is performed, and if a recording is obtained, it is presumed that the electrode is in fact in the target muscle. In any evaluation of electromyographic research, considerable attention must be given to electrode placement and to its validation. Obviously, this validation becomes extremely difficult if the anatomy of the area under study is not well known.

The earliest intramuscular electrodes were made from needles and were called **needle electrodes.** The entire needle, except for its tip, was coated with insulation. This type of electrode is still in common use but has two disadvantages: First, it is somewhat painful for the subject; and second, if the experiment necessitates bodily motion, this may set the needle into motion within the muscle. The motion itself may generate an electrical signal, which may make it impossible to ascertain when the signal is emanating from the muscle. If the motion required is of any significant degree, it may increase the discomfort to the subject considerably, and may also dislodge the needle. The matter of discomfort is of considerable importance. Subjects in sufficient discomfort may become tense and, in doing so, may not contract the musculature under study as they would normally for the function being observed. Thus, it may become impossible to achieve valid results.

It was for these reasons that hooked-wire electrodes were developed. **Hooked-wire electrodes** are made of thin, flexible wires insulated except for their tip. They are inserted into the shaft of a hypodermic needle, and the end of the wire is bent over the needle tip. The needle is inserted into the target muscle and is then withdrawn. The hook of the wire snags within the muscle and is left there. The extremely small diameter of these wires precludes most discomfort, and their flexibility overcomes some of the problem of motion. Conversely, precise placement within a muscle is more difficult with the hooked-wire than with the needle electrode.

Another important consideration in electromyographic research is the posture of the subject during the recording. As indicated previously, gravity may have an effect on whether, or to what degree, a muscle functions in a given activity. For example, examination of the muscles of respiration while the subject is lying supine (on the dorsal surface of his rib cage) may affect the muscular mechanics of respiration.

Other Methods

In addition to dissection, x-ray, and electromyography, a number of other methods have been used by investigators to study the functions involved in the speech and hearing processes. Some of these have involved direct or indirect methods of viewing structures in motion. Extremely high-speed motion pictures that can be viewed in slow motion have been taken of the vocal folds, since their movements are too fast to be observed in real time. Fiberoptic devices permit direct view of structures such as the nasopharynx and larynx through a thin, flexible fiberoptic bundle. In some cases, motion of deep structures has been viewed either during surgery or after surgical removal of superficial structures. For example, direct view of the nasopharynx has been possible in cases where parts of the face have been removed because of cancerous growths.

Oral and pharyngeal structures and the results of movement have been examined by a variety of methods that yield casts of those structures. Another method, palatography, involves "dusting" the palate with powder, followed by articulation of a sound in order to view what part of the palate was touched by the tongue during the articulation.

Several methods have been employed to study movements of the chest wall and abdomen during respiration. These have typically involved the use of a device that straps around the body and responds to changes in circumference. Other techniques involve the use of electromagnetic coils, where the magnetic field detected by one coil is a function of its distance from another. Movements of this type have also been measured by volume-displacement. This is done by enclosing part of the body in an airtight container and measuring the flow in and out of the container as a person breathes.

Devices sensitive to pressure or to strain placed on them have also been used to study movements associated with speech and with hearing (such as movement of the eardrum).

The use of **ultrasound** in the study of speech was introduced by Kelsey, Hixon, and Minifie in 1969 [12]. This involves the generation of an acoustic signal, which is reflected back to a detector by an interface where there is an abrupt change in density. If the unit is applied to the side of the neck, for example, reflection will occur at the tissue-air interface at the lateral wall of the throat. Thus movements of that wall can be charted. In some instances this method has replaced x-ray methods but is of limited use if bony structures lie between the ultrasound source and the target structure.

Several methods of examining neuromuscular relationships have been used. Neural activity and conduction velocity can be measured by placing electrodes along the path of the nerve to be studied. One method of studying sensory function uses topical (surface) anesthetic and nerve block (local anesthetic) techniques. Topical anesthetics can be used to deaden touch sensation. Nerve blocks have been used to study the result of blocking motoneuron transmission to a specific muscle. With great care, this method can be used to block transmission of the small gamma efferents without blocking the larger sensory or alpha motor neurons. These methods obviously require demonstration of the validity of the assumption about what has been blocked and what has not.

The foregoing discussion is not meant to be all inclusive. The types of techniques listed have been used for special purposes in the study of specific parts of the speech and hearing mechanism. They will be described where appropriate in succeeding chapters.

Two other general types of methodology should be mentioned. Both are used to measure the output of the biomechanical systems, which will be covered in subsequent chapters. One of these concerns the measurement of air flow and pressure within the vocal tract, and the other has to do with measures of the acoustic result of vocal tract activity. While these two areas are, in general, beyond the scope of this volume, they, and data stemming from their use, will be referred to in certain instances. This will be necessary since we cannot properly understand the structure and function of the vocal mechanism without some understanding of the output of that mechanism.

REFERENCES

1. Abbs JH: The influence of the gamma motor system on jaw movements during speech: A theoretical framework and some preliminary observations. *J Speech Hear Res* 16:175, 1973.
2. Baken RJ: Neuromuscular spindles in the intrinsic muscles of a human larynx. *Folia Phoniatr* (Basel) 23:204, 1971.
3. Baken RJ, Noback CR: Neuromuscular spindles in intrinsic muscles of a human larynx. *J Speech Hear Res* 14:513, 1971.
4. Baum J: Beitrage zur Kenntniss der Muskelspindeln. *Anat Hefte* 13:251, 1900.
5. Bowden REM, et al: The afferent innervation of facial and laryngeal muscles. *Anat Rec* 136:168, 1960.
6. Ganong WF: *Review of Medical Physiology.* Los Altos, Calif., Lange Medical Publications, 1979.
7. Goerttler K: Die Anordnung Histologie und Histogenese der guergestreiften Muskulatur in menschlich Stimmband. *Z Anat Entw Gesch* 115:352, 1950.
8. Gracheva MS: Sensory innervation of locomotor apparatus of the larynx. *Fed Proc Trans* [Suppl] 22:1120, 1963.
9. Gregor A: Uber die Verteilung der Muskelspindeln in der Muskulatur des menschlichen Fötus. *Arch Anat Entw Gesch* 112:196, 1904.
10. Grim M: Muscle spindles in the posterior cricoarytenoid muscle of the human larynx. *Folia Morphol* (Praha) 15:124, 1967.
11. Keene WF: Muscle spindles in human laryngeal muscles. *J Anat* 95:25, 1961.
12. Kelsey CAT, Hixon TJ, Minifie FD: Ultrasonic measurement of lateral pharyngeal wall displacement. *IEEE Trans Biomed Eng* April, 1969, p. 143.
13. Konig WF, von Leden H: The peripheral nervous system of the human larynx. Part I. The mucous membrane. *Arch Otolaryngol* 73:1, 1961.
14. Konig WF, von Leden H: The peripheral nervous system of the human larynx. Part II. The thyroarytenoid (vocalis) muscle. *Arch Otolaryngol* 74:153, 1961.
15. Paulsen K: Uber Vorkommen und Zahl von Muskelspindeln in innern Kehlkopfmuskeln des Menschen. *Z Zell Forsch* 48:349, 1958.
16. Rossi G, Cortesina G: Morphological study of the laryngeal muscles in man. *Acta Otolaryngol* 59:575, 1964.
17. Smith J: Fusimotor neuron block and voluntary arm movements in man. University of Wisconsin, PhD dissertation, 1969.
18. Wyke B: Laryngeal myotatic reflexes and phonation. *Folia Phoniatr* (Basel) 26:249, 1974.

Respiration

The process of bringing oxygen into the bloodstream and removing carbon dioxide from it is called **respiration.** This process takes place across the membranous linings of the smallest subdivisions of the lung. These membranes separate lung tissue from the capillaries of the vascular system. The air brought into the lungs is high in oxygen content and low in carbon dioxide content, while the blood that has circulated through the body and is returned to the capillaries of the lungs is high in carbon dioxide content and low in oxygen content. By a process of diffusion, these gases are exchanged across the thin walls of the lungs and capillaries. The oxygenated blood is then returned to the body system and the oxygen-depleted air is expelled from the lungs.

This process requires the movement of air into and out of the lungs during inhalation and exhalation. Air movement through the vocal system during exhalation makes voice production possible. Also important to speech production is the ability to vary both air flow and air pressure during exhalation. This chapter will examine the forces that control air flow and pressure.

During inhalation air enters the mouth and/or nose (Figure 3-1). Within the mouth, but more particularly within the nose, the temperature and humidity of the air are moderated and foreign materials are filtered from the air. From the nose and mouth, the air passes into the **pharynx,** which links the nasal and oral cavities to the larynx and esophagus. The **esophagus** is a muscular tube that extends from the inferior part of the pharynx to the stomach. Just below the base of the tongue, the pharynx opens into the larynx anteriorly. The larynx lies between the pharynx superiorly and the trachea inferiorly.

The **larynx** is a musculocartilaginous structure the primary function of which is to open and close during various biologic and phonatory functions. It closes during swallowing to prevent food and liquid from entering the trachea and lungs. During

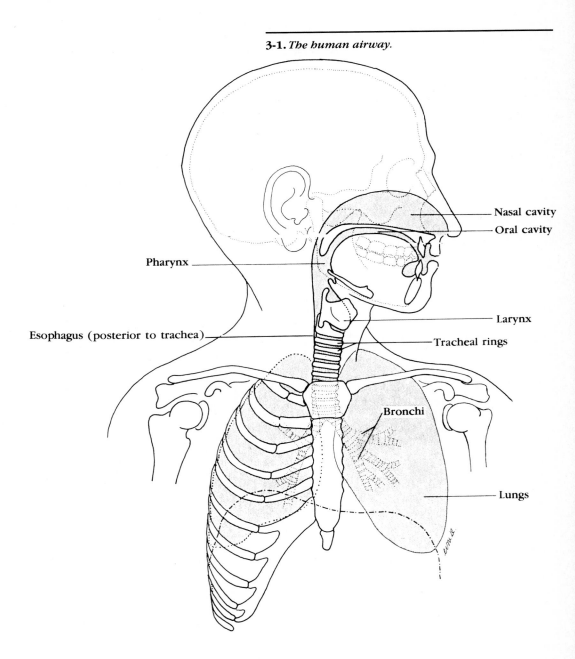

3-1. *The human airway.*

Nasal cavity

Oral cavity

Pharynx

Larynx

Esophagus (posterior to trachea)

Tracheal rings

Bronchi

Lungs

respiration the larynx remains open to permit air flow to and from the lungs. The larynx is situated at the top of the **trachea,** a membranous tube surrounded and held open by rings of cartilage. Inhaled air passes from the larynx into the trachea. At the level of the top of the rib cage, the trachea divides into two somewhat smaller tubes called **bronchi.** Each bronchus supplies air to one of the two lungs.

The **lungs** lie within membranous sacs located in the thorax (Figure 3-2) and are surrounded by the bony rib cage. The left lung is slightly smaller than the right, thus making room for the heart. The **rib cage** is composed of twelve pairs of ribs con-

nected to the **sternum** (breastbone) anteriorly. The floor of the **thorax** (chest) is formed by a large, rounded circumpennate muscle called the **diaphragm,** which separates the thorax from the abdominal cavity below. The diaphragm attaches to the sternum, the lower ribs, and the vertebrae. In addition to the lungs and heart, the thoracic cavity also contains several major blood vessels and nerves and the esophagus.

Within each lung, the bronchi subdivide into smaller bronchi and again into smaller tubes called **bronchioles** (Figure 3-3). These continue to subdivide into smaller and smaller bronchioles, then into still smaller tubes called **alveolar ducts,**

3-2. Structural relationships in the thorax. A, Mid-sagittal section; B, Transverse section through the plane of the arrow in A.

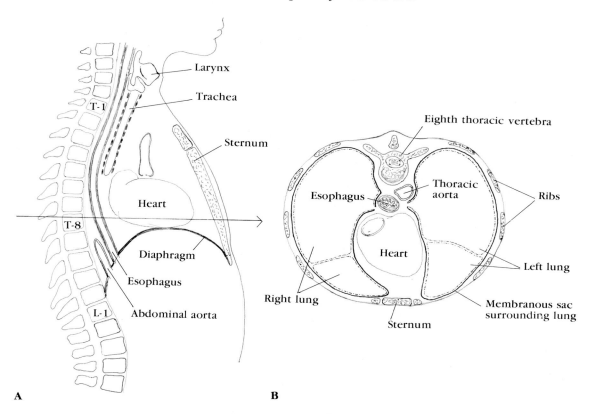

A   B

3-3. *Components of the respiratory tract.*

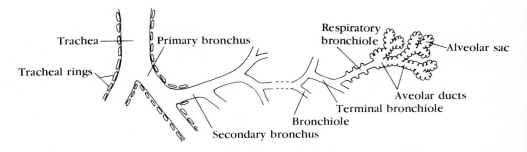

Trachea

Primary bronchus

Tracheal rings

Respiratory bronchiole

Alveolar sac

Aveolar ducts

Terminal bronchiole

Bronchiole

Secondary bronchus

3-4. *Skeletal framework for respiration, posterior view.*

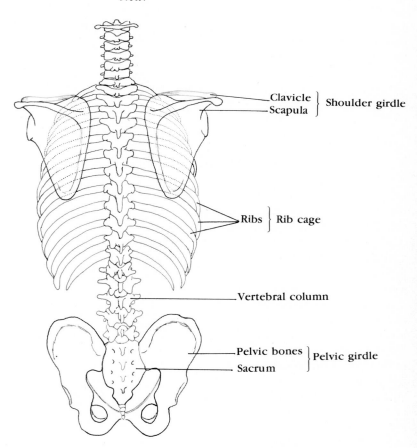

Clavicle ⎤
Scapula ⎦ Shoulder girdle

Ribs ⎤ Rib cage

Vertebral column

Pelvic bones ⎤
Sacrum   ⎦ Pelvic girdle

which open into **alveolar sacs,** terminating in hollow bubble-like structures called **alveoli.** It is here that the gaseous exchange of respiration takes place. The human lungs contain 300 million alveoli with a total surface area of about 70 m².

SKELETAL FRAMEWORK

The skeletal framework for respiration includes the vertebral column, rib cage, shoulder girdle, and pelvic girdle (Figure 3-4).

Vertebral Column

The vertebral column (Figure 3-5) consists of a number of individual bones that surround and protect the spinal cord. These are named for their location within the body. The first seven vertebrae, which lie between the base of the cranium and the top of the thorax are called **cervical** (neck) vertebrae. The next twelve vertebrae are called **thoracic** vertebrae and lie at the back of the thorax. In the space between the inferior terminus of the thorax and the top of the pelvis (the part of the body called the loin) are the five **lumbar** vertebrae. The next five vertebrae are fused together to form a plate of bone called the **sacrum,** which forms the posterior part of the **pelvis.** The origin of the term sacrum is not known, but is supposed to have come from the word "sacred," since this was thought to be the point of entry of the soul. Below the sacrum are three or four bits of bone that are rudimentary vertebrae. Together they are called the **coccyx,** so named because an anatomist thought they were in the shape of the beak of the cuckoo bird. In lower animals these bits of bone form the beginning of the tail. In man they are vestigial.

The cervical, thoracic, and lumbar vertebrae are called the **true vertebrae.** The vertebrae that form the sacrum and coccyx below this level are modified in structure. The true vertebrae have several major anatomical features in common. A few comments about the purposes served by the vertebrae will help to make sense out of those common features. First, the vertebrae serve to surround and protect the spinal cord. Second, the vertebrae form a movable bony pillar for support of the trunk, the shoulder girdle, and the head. Third, the vertebrae serve as points of muscular attachment.

A number of structural features might be anticipated to meet these needs: first, a bony ring to surround and protect the spinal cord; second, an enlarged bony portion to bear weight; third, joints to permit intervetebral motion; fourth, processes (extensions) for the attachments of muscles; and fifth, intervertebral cartilages to absorb shock.

3-5. *Vertebral column, lateral view of left side.*

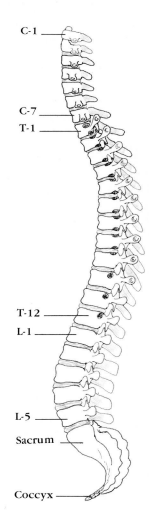

C-1

C-7
T-1

T-12
L-1

L-5

Sacrum

Coccyx

Without some shock absorbing mechanism, all of the pressure developed when one's foot strikes the floor in walking would be transmitted directly to the skull. Also, bony fractures would be much more likely to occur.

Now let us examine a typical vertebra, as seen in Figure 3-6. The anterior part of the vertebra is composed of a large bony mass called the **centrum (body)**. Posterior to the vertebral body is a bony ring called the **neural arch,** which surrounds the **neural foramen** (hole), through which the spinal cord passes. This bony arch has two parts on each side: The more anterior part is rounded and is called the **pedicle** (foot), and the more posterior portion is flattened and is therefore called the **lamina** (plate). At the juncture of the lamina and pedicle on each side there is a lateral process (projection or peninsula) called the **transverse process.** At the point where the two laminae join posteriorly, there is another process that projects posteroinferiorly called the **spinous process.** These processes provide surfaces for the attachment for muscles.

Superior articular processes project upward from the pedicle and have smooth **articular facets.** In general, an articular (pertaining to a joint) process is a projection from a bone with an articular surface that forms part of a joint with another bone. These articular facets meet with the inferior articular facets of the next vertebra above to form synovial joints. An **inferior articular facet** is located on each side of the deep surface of the lamina. It is at these paired joints that most of the intervertebral motion takes place.

The superior and inferior surfaces of the body of the vertebra are slightly concave. These surfaces are separated from the opposing surfaces of the adjacent vertebrae by fibrocartilaginous **intervertebral disks.** Adjacent vertebral bodies and their intervening disks form a symphysis that permits a slight amount of movement.

In lateral view, it can be seen that the vertical surface of the vertebral body is also slightly concave. This gives added strength to the vertebra because the primary forces acting upon it are from above and below. Given the functional requirements placed on the vertebrae, it would be difficult if not impossible to design a series of bones better adapted to their purposes.

Individual vertebrae and groups of vertebrae have specialized forms to meet specialized needs by virtue of their position. In general, the vertebrae become more delicate as one ascends toward the head and more massive as one descends to-

3-6. *Typical vertebra. A, Superolateral view; B, Superior view.*

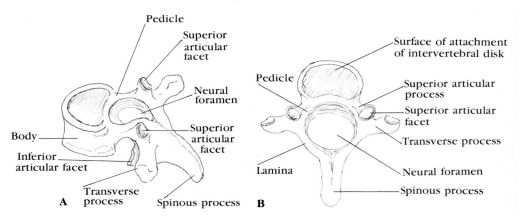

ward the pelvis. This is reasonable in terms of the increased load applied to the more inferior vertebrae. As another generalization, the intervertebral articular facets are more horizontal in the superior vertebrae and become more vertically inclined in the inferior vertebrae.

Cervical vertebrae (Figure 3-7) have two characteristics that make them easy to identify. One is a foramen in each transverse process for the passage of blood vessels. The other is a bifid (divided) spinous process. The first and second cervical vertebrae are unique in structure (Figure 3-8). The first cervical vertebrae (also called the **atlas**) is devoid of a body and spinous process and instead possesses small anterior and posterior projections called tubercles. Two large articular facets are located on the superior surface of the atlas. These articulate with the base of the skull. There is an additional articular facet located on the deep surface of the anterior tubercle. The second cervical vertebra (also called the **axis**) has a body that projects superiorly into the large central foramen of the first cervical vertebra to articulate with the facet located on the deep surface of the anterior tubercle. This projected body is called the **odontoid process** (also called the **dens**) and is named for its toothlike appearance.

Thoracic vertebrae (Figure 3-9) also have several unique characteristics. Among these are articular facets that form joints with the ribs. Typically, a thoracic vertebra possesses **demifacets** (half facets) located superiorly and inferiorly on each side of its body near the junction of the body and pedicle. Each superior demifacet joins with the inferior demifacet of the vertebra above to form a whole facet, which receives the head (posterior end) of a rib. Each transverse process contains a facet for articulation with a rib slightly distal to the rib head. Each rib descends slightly from its point of contact with the vertebral bodies to its point of contact with the transverse process. This means, for example, that the fifth rib articulates with the bodies of the fourth and fifth vertebrae at their contiguous demifacets, and with the transverse process of the fifth vertebra. The joints

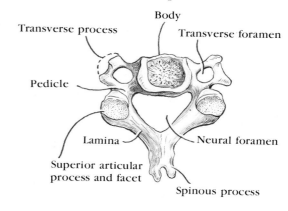

3-7. *Typical cervical vertebra, superior view.*

Body
Transverse process
Transverse foramen
Pedicle
Lamina
Neural foramen
Superior articular process and facet
Spinous process

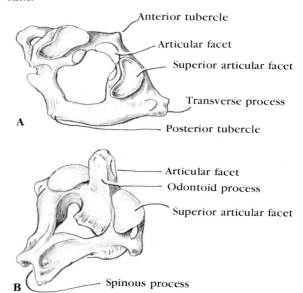

3-8. *First and second cervical vertebrae. A, Atlas; B, Axis.*

Anterior tubercle
Articular facet
Superior articular facet
Transverse process
A
Posterior tubercle

Articular facet
Odontoid process
Superior articular facet

B
Spinous process

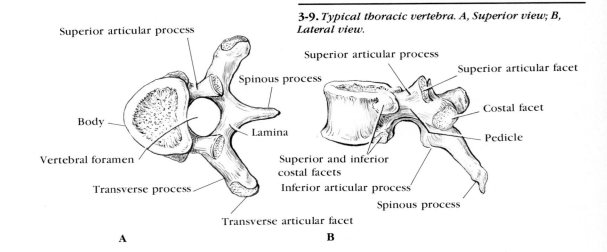

Superior articular process

Spinous process

Body

Lamina

Vertebral foramen

Transverse process

Transverse articular facet

A

3-9. *Typical thoracic vertebra. A, Superior view; B, Lateral view.*

Superior articular process

Superior articular facet

Costal facet

Pedicle

Superior and inferior costal facets

Inferior articular process

Spinous process

B

3-10. *Transverse computed tomogram of costovertebral articulations.*

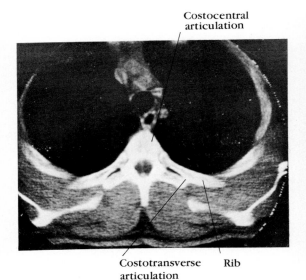

Costocentral articulation

Costotransverse articulation   Rib

3-11. *Transverse computed tomogram of costovertebral articulations.*

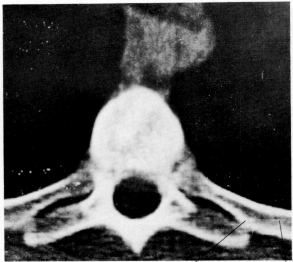

Costotransverse articulation   Rib

formed by the vertebral bodies and the head of a rib are called **costocentral articulations,** and those formed by the transverse process of a vertebra and the shaft of a rib are called **costotransverse articulations** (Figures 3-10, 3-11).

The superior and inferior thoracic vertebrae have an atypical arrangement of their articular facets. Since ribs do not normally articulate with cervical vertebrae, the first thoracic vertebra has a whole facet on the side of its body to receive the head of the first rib, and an additional demifacet on the inferior margin of the body which, with its counterpart on the second thoracic vertebra, receives the head of the second rib. A diagrammatic representation of rib-vertebral relationships is shown in Figure 3-12.

The ninth thoracic vertebra has superior demifacets for the ninth rib but typically lacks inferior demifacets. The tenth, eleventh, and twelfth thoracic vertebrae have whole facets on each side for the heads of the corresponding ribs. The eleventh and twelfth thoracic vertebrae typically lack articular facets on their transverse processes. Thus, the eleventh and twelfth ribs lack costotransverse joints.

The sacral vertebrae (Figure 3-13) are fused into a single wedge-shaped piece, which forms the back of the pelvis. They are characterized by very

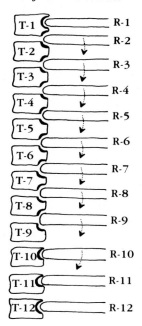

3-12. *Diagrammatic representation of rib-vertebral relationships. Arrows indicate costotransverse articulations between ribs and subadjacent vertebrae.*

3-13. *Sacrum. A, Anterior view; B, Posterior view.*

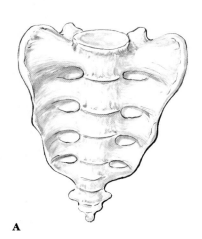

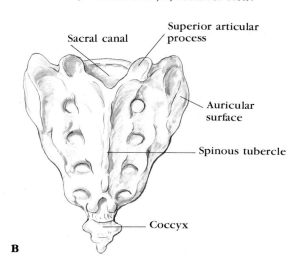

A   B

large fused transverse processes, small fused spinous processes, and fused bodies that diminish in size from superior to inferior. At the lateral boundaries of the fused transverse processes there are large articular facets that form symphyses with the pelvis.

For the purposes of this text, it is not relevant to pursue any further the intervertebral joints or their motions. The costocentral and costotransverse joints will be discussed with the sternal joints in greater detail after considering the anatomy of the sternum and ribs.

Sternum

The sternum (Figure 3-14) is a roughly triangular, blade-shaped structure consisting of three parts. Its most superior part is the **manubrium** (handle), which forms a cartilaginous joint with the larger mid-portion of the sternum, called the **corpus** (body). Inferiorly, the corpus is fused with the small cartilaginous portion called the **xiphoid process** (also called the **ensiform process**). The sternum lies in a plane slightly oblique to the vertical, with the manubrium being slightly more posterior than the xiphoid process. There are two pairs of articular facets on the manubrium. The first is on the superolateral margins for articulation with the clavicle, and the second is on each lateral portion for articulation with the cartilage of the first rib. A third pair of articular facets is found laterally at the junction of the manubrium and corpus for articulation with the cartilage of the second rib. There are five other pairs of articular facets on the lateral margins of the corpus for articulation with the cartilages of ribs three through ten. The cartilages from ribs eight, nine, and ten join the cartilage from rib seven, which attaches to the sternum. The cartilages of ribs eleven and twelve are very short and do not articulate with the sternum.

Ribs

Ribs (Figure 3-15) are elongated, flattened shafts of bone. Typically, the posterior end of a rib is wedge-shaped and has dual articular facets that articulate with two adjacent vertebral bodies and

their intervertebral disk. A short distance from the end of the rib (called the **head**) is an enlargement, the **tubercle,** which lies on the superficial surface of the rib. The tubercle has an articular surface that forms a joint with the transverse process of the corresponding vertebra. The area between the head and tubercle is called the **neck** of the rib.

3-14. *Sternum, anterior view.*

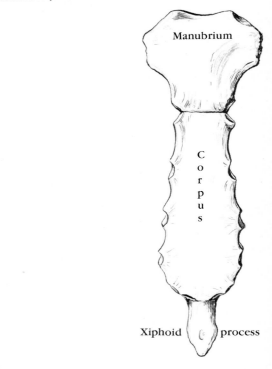

3-15. *Typical rib, posterior view.*

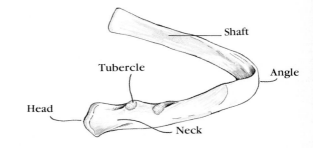

That part of the rib that extends from the tubercle to the anterior end of the rib is called the **shaft.** Since the ribs are flattened, they have two surfaces, inner and outer, and two edges, superior and inferior.

Typically, a rib extends posterolaterally from its costocentral articulation until it reaches the coronal plane of the posterior tips of the vertebral spinous processes. Here the rib turns anterolaterally, and then anteromedially (Figure 3-16). The first curvature, that at the rib's most posterior point, is called the **angle** of the rib.

Between its posterior and anterior ends, the rib also is directed somewhat inferiorly so that its anterior end is lower than its posterior end (Figure 3-17). In addition, most of the ribs undergo a twist from posterior to anterior. Posteriorly, the external surface of the rib is directed somewhat superiorly, while anteriorly it faces outward (Figure 3-17). The lengths of the ribs increase from the first, which is the shortest, through the seventh, and then decrease in length through the twelfth (Figure 3-18).

The first rib is atypical in that it is broad and flat, with its surfaces facing superiorly and inferiorly

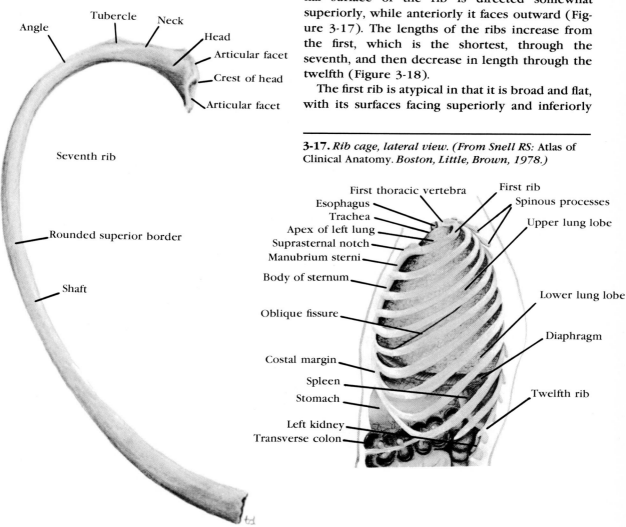

3-16. Seventh rib, superior view. (From Snell RS: Atlas of Clinical Anatomy. Boston, Little, Brown, 1978.)

Angle

Tubercle

Neck

Head

Articular facet

Crest of head

Articular facet

Seventh rib

Rounded superior border

Shaft

3-17. Rib cage, lateral view. (From Snell RS: Atlas of Clinical Anatomy. Boston, Little, Brown, 1978.)

First thoracic vertebra

First rib

Esophagus

Spinous processes

Trachea

Apex of left lung

Upper lung lobe

Suprasternal notch

Manubrium sterni

Body of sternum

Oblique fissure

Lower lung lobe

Diaphragm

Costal margin

Spleen

Stomach

Twelfth rib

Left kidney

Transverse colon

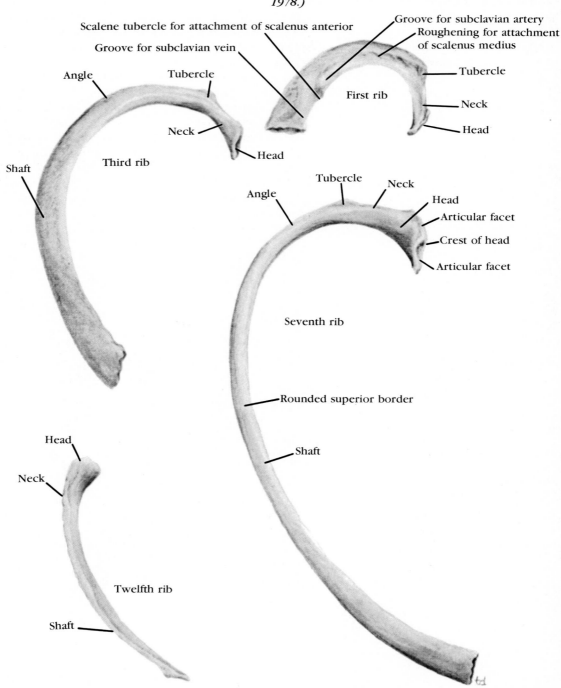

3-18. *Representative ribs, superior view. (From Snell RS:* Atlas of Clinical Anatomy. *Boston, Little, Brown, 1978.)*

Scalene tubercle for attachment of scalenus anterior

Groove for subclavian vein

Groove for subclavian artery

Roughening for attachment of scalenus medius

Angle

Tubercle

Tubercle

First rib

Neck

Neck

Head

Head

Shaft

Third rib

Tubercle

Neck

Head

Angle

Articular facet

Crest of head

Articular facet

Seventh rib

Rounded superior border

Head

Neck

Shaft

Shaft

Twelfth rib

Shaft

and its edges facing inward and outward. The second rib is also atypical in that it lacks the twist of the lower ribs. Each rib articulates anteriorly with its costal cartilage. For ribs one through ten, the **costal cartilages** extend medially to attach to the sternum. The costal cartilages of ribs eight, nine, and ten each articulate with the cartilage of the supraadjacent rib. Due to the inferior inclination of the ribs as they extend anteriorly, the anterior ends of ribs five or six are at the level of the in-ferior end of the body of the sternum. Thus, the costal cartilages of the lower ribs are directed superomedially to articulate with the sternum. The costal cartilage of ribs eleven and twelve are very short and end freely in the lateral wall of the thorax.

Joints of the Sternum

The joint between the manubrium and corpus of the sternum (Figure 3-19) is typically cartilag-

3-19. *Joints of the sternum. (From Snell RS:* Atlas of Clinical Anatomy. *Boston, Little, Brown, 1978.)*

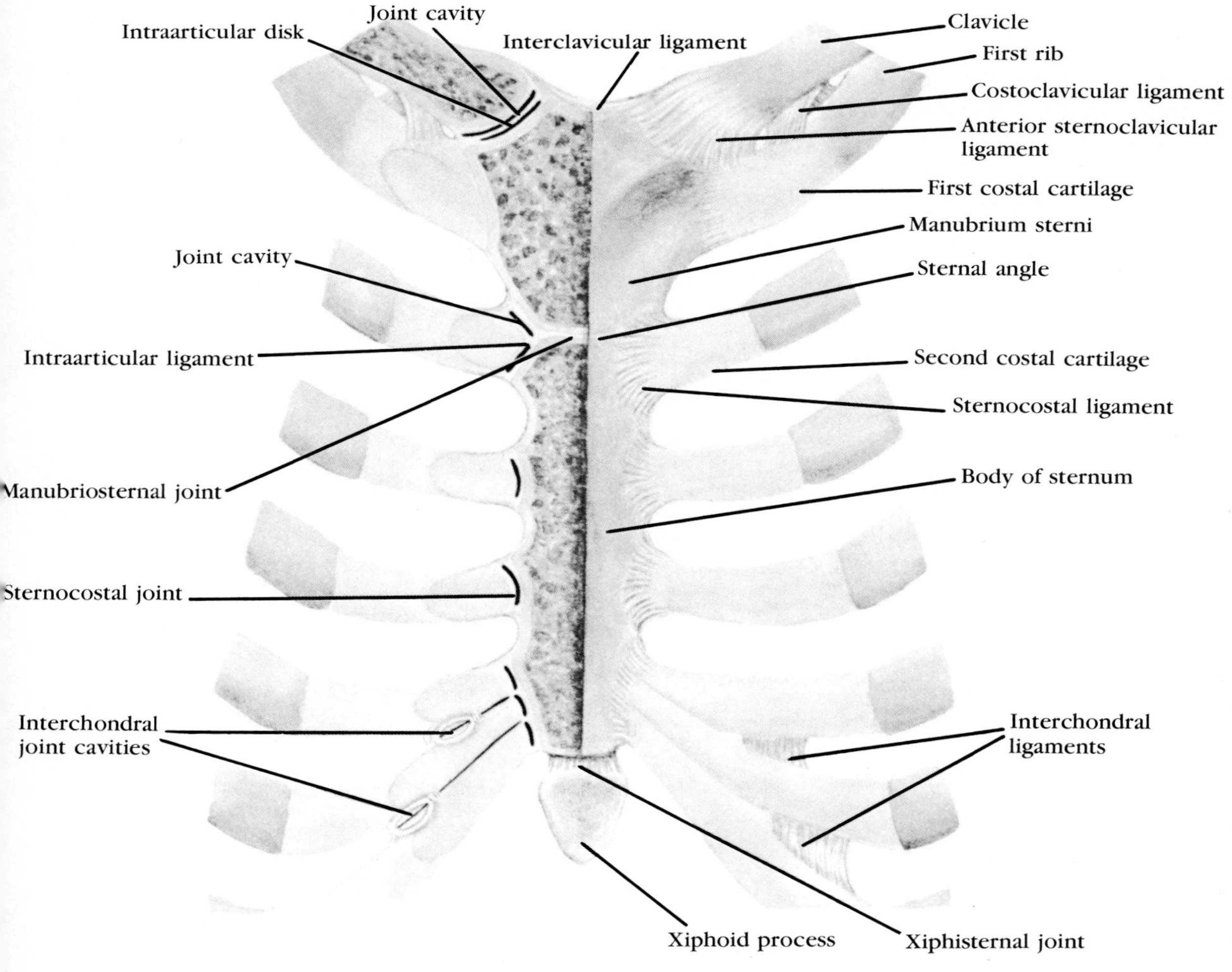

Intraarticular disk
Joint cavity
Interclavicular ligament
Clavicle
First rib
Costoclavicular ligament
Anterior sternoclavicular ligament
First costal cartilage
Manubrium sterni
Sternal angle
Joint cavity
Intraarticular ligament
Second costal cartilage
Sternocostal ligament
Manubriosternal joint
Body of sternum
Sternocostal joint
Interchondral joint cavities
Interchondral ligaments
Xiphoid process
Xiphisternal joint

inous and occasionally ossifies in later life. In some cases a synovial cavity occurs in this joint and may permit slight hinge-like movement in the sagittal plane. The joint between the corpus and xiphoid process is a symphysis early in life but typically ossifies by the age of 15 years.

Costosternal Joints

The cartilage of the first rib is fused with the sternum. The other costosternal articulations form plane synovial joints, which permit some motion. Each of the joints is surrounded by an articular capsule that is strongest superiorly and inferiorly (Figures 3-20). **Radiate ligaments** extend from the anterior and posterior surfaces of the cartilages to broad attachments on the adjacent anterior and posterior surfaces of the sternum. The second costosternal joint contains an **intraarticular sternocostal ligament,** which extends from the medial end of the costal cartilage to the fibrocartilage that lies between the manubrium and corpus. This

ligament divides the synovial joint into two parts. **Costoxiphoid ligaments** extend from the regions of the seventh costal cartilage to the sternum in a form similar to the radiate ligaments. In addition to these joints, there are plane synovial joints between contiguous borders of the lower costal cartilages. Each is enclosed in an articular capsule and is strengthened by **interchondral ligaments** laterally and medially.

Costovertebral Joints

The costocentral articulations form plane synovial joints with articular capsules, radiate ligaments, and intraarticular ligaments (Figure 3-21). The **articular capsules,** which consist of short strong fibers, are strongest superiorly and inferiorly. The **radiate ligament** extends from the anterior surface of the rib head to the vertebral bodies and intervertebral disk associated with the joint. On the first, tenth, eleventh, and twelfth ribs, the radiate ligaments extend to the vertebrae with

3-20. *Costosternal joints.*

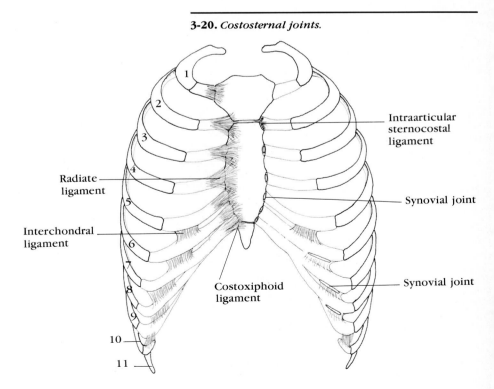

which the ribs articulate and to the immediately superior vertebra. The **intraarticular ligaments** are analogous to the intraarticular sternocostal ligaments.

The costotransverse articulations are also plane synovial joints with articular capsules and several associated ligaments. The **articular capsule** is thin. The **superior costotransverse ligament** is broad and extends from the superior border of the rib neck to the inferior surface of the supraadjacent transverse process. A weak band of fibers forms the **posterior costotransverse ligament,** which extends from the rib neck to the inferior articular process of the supraadjacent vertebra. The **ligament of the tubercle,** which is short, strong, and thick, extends from the apex of the transverse process laterally to the tubercle distal to the joint. These ligaments prevent proximal-distal sliding but allow superior-inferior sliding.

Joint Motion

Little if any motion is permitted between the manubrium and corpus of the sternum. Costosternal motion is slight owing to very tight anterior and posterior radiate ligaments which severely limit motion in any direction. The costovertebral joints permit motion but more at the costotransverse than at the costocentral joint. The nature of motion permitted at the costotransverse joints is rotational in the upper six ribs, since the articular facets on the transverse processes of the vertebrae in this region are concave from superior to inferior (Figure 3-22). They form a very tight saddle joint whose axis of rotation is through the neck of the rib. For ribs seven through ten, the articular facets are flat and lie in an oblique plane from postero-superior to anteroinferior. Thus these joints permit sliding of the neck of the rib superiorly and posteriorly or inferiorly and anteriorly. Ribs eleven and twelve lack costotransverse joints and analysis of their motion potential based only on the structure of the costocentral articulation is difficult.

The motion of the ribs resulting from motion at their necks varies somewhat from rib to rib owing to differences in their length and shape. The first

---

3-21. *Costovertebral joints and ligaments. A, Costocentral articulations, lateral view; B, Costotransverse articulations, superior view.*

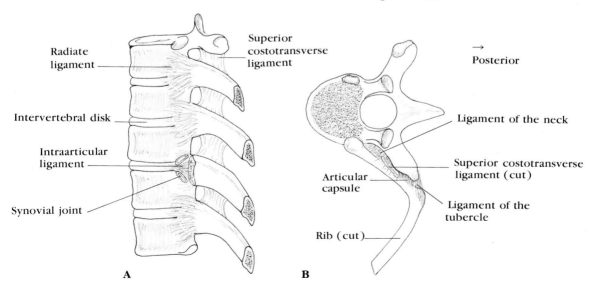

Radiate ligament

Superior costotransverse ligament

→ Posterior

Intervertebral disk

Ligament of the neck

Intraarticular ligament

Articular capsule

Superior costotransverse ligament (cut)

Synovial joint

Ligament of the tubercle

Rib (cut)

A   **B**

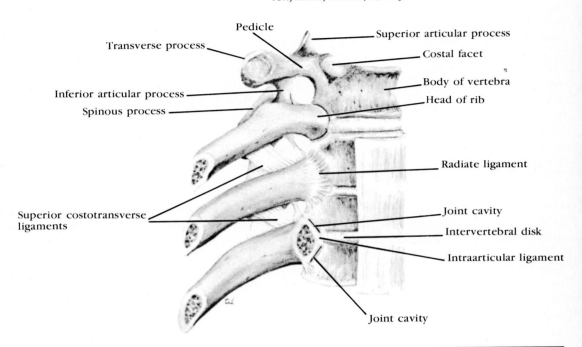

3-22. *Costovertebral joints and ligaments, lateral view. (From Snell RS:* Atlas of Clinical Anatomy. *Boston, Little, Brown, 1978.)*

Pedicle

Transverse process

Inferior articular process

Spinous process

Superior articular process

Costal facet

Body of vertebra

Head of rib

Radiate ligament

Superior costotransverse ligaments

Joint cavity

Intervertebral disk

Intraarticular ligament

Joint cavity

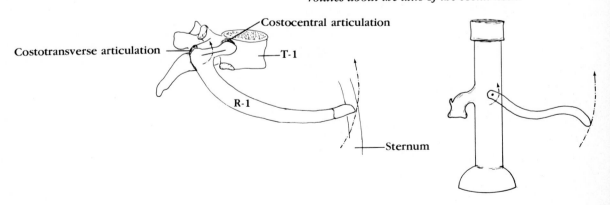

3-23. *"Pump-handle" motion of an upper rib as it rotates about the axis of the costal neck.*

Costocentral articulation

Costotransverse articulation

T-1

R-1

Sternum

rib is flat, and its sternal end is lower than its vertebral end. Therefore, slight rotation of the rib's neck raises or lowers the shaft, anterior cartilage, and consequently the sternum. Since the rib is the arm of a lever with its fulcrum at its posterior end, the greatest motion of the rib is at the sternum. Moving down the rib cage from the first rib to the seventh, the ribs increase in length and the most lateral part of each rib is placed increasingly lower relative to its vertebral and sternal ends. Thus the anterior ends of the ribs and the sternum move obliquely from inferoposterior to superoanterior (Figure 3-23). This is referred to as a **pump-handle** type of motion. The lateral parts of the ribs move obliquely from inferomedial to superolateral (Figure 3-24). This movement is described as being similar to the movement of a **bucket handle.** Thus the volume of the thorax can be changed by rib movement, which can increase and decrease both the anteroposterior and lateral dimension of the thorax.

Shoulder Girdle

The shoulder girdle is composed of the scapulae and clavicles (Figure 3-25). Each clavicle articulates laterally with the corresponding scapula and

medially with the manubrium of the sternum. Each scapula articulates with the clavicle and with the **humerus,** which is the long bone of the upper arm.

The **clavicle** (Figure 3-26) is shaped like an elongated shallow "S" lying in the horizontal plane with its anterior convexity lying medially and its posterior convexity lying laterally. It articulates medially with the manubrium of the sternum in a plane synovial joint containing a cartilagenous articular disk (Figure 3-27). Its ligaments permit a limited amount of motion in all directions. The lateral end of the clavicle articulates with the scapula at the **claviculoscapular joint,** which will be described below.

The **scapula** (Figure 3-28) is a large, flattened, triangular bone that lies superficial to the ribs posteriorly and extends superolaterally and anteriorly to articulate with the clavicle and humerus at the shoulder. The large triangular portion of the scapula is slightly convex on its superficial (posterior) surface and slightly concave on its deep (anterior) surface. The longest side of its triangular form is its **medial border.** Viewed from the back, the medial borders of the two scapulae face each other and lie to either side of the posterior midline. The point of the triangular form is directed

3-24. *"Bucket-handle" motion of a lower rib as it rotates about an axis passing through the dorsal and ventral ends of the costal arch.*

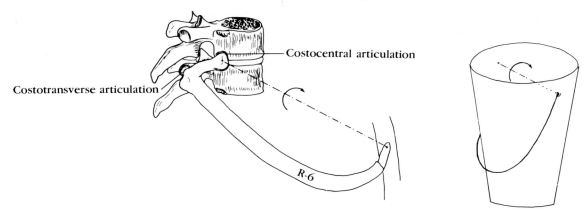

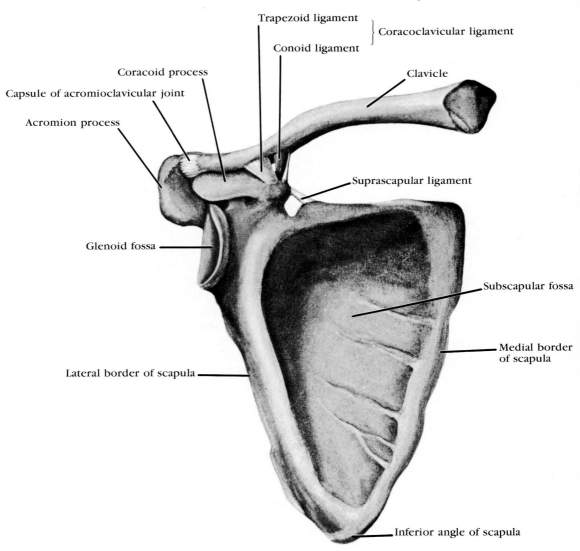

3-25. *Shoulder girdle, anterior view. (From Snell RS: Atlas of Clinical Anatomy. Boston, Little, Brown, 1978.)*

Trapezoid ligament

Conoid ligament

Coracoclavicular ligament

Coracoid process

Clavicle

Capsule of acromioclavicular joint

Acromion process

Suprascapular ligament

Glenoid fossa

Subscapular fossa

Medial border of scapula

Lateral border of scapula

Inferior angle of scapula

3-26. *Left clavicle, anterior view.*

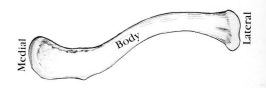

Medial

Body

Lateral

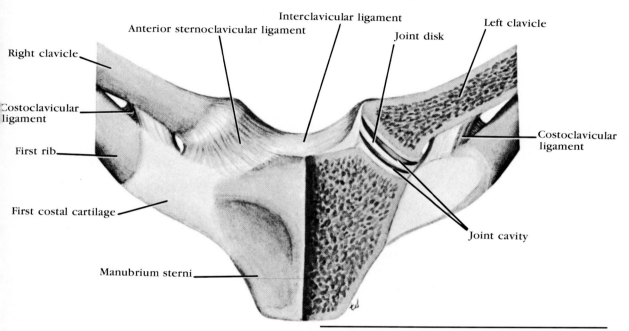

3-27. *Sternoclavicular joint. On the right, the clavicle and sternum have been cut and the joint opened. (From Snell RS:* Atlas of Clinical Anatomy. *Boston, Little, Brown, 1978.)*

Right clavicle

Costoclavicular ligament

First rib

First costal cartilage

Manubrium sterni

Anterior sternoclavicular ligament

Interclavicular ligament

Joint disk

Left clavicle

Costoclavicular ligament

Joint cavity

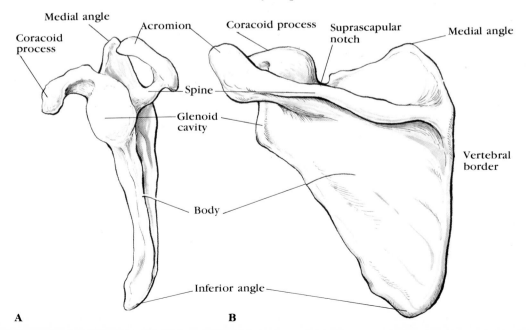

3-28. *Scapula. A, Lateral view and B, posterior view of the left scapula.*

Coracoid process

Medial angle

Acromion

Coracoid process

Suprascapular notch

Medial angle

Spine

Glenoid cavity

Vertebral border

Body

Inferior angle

A

B

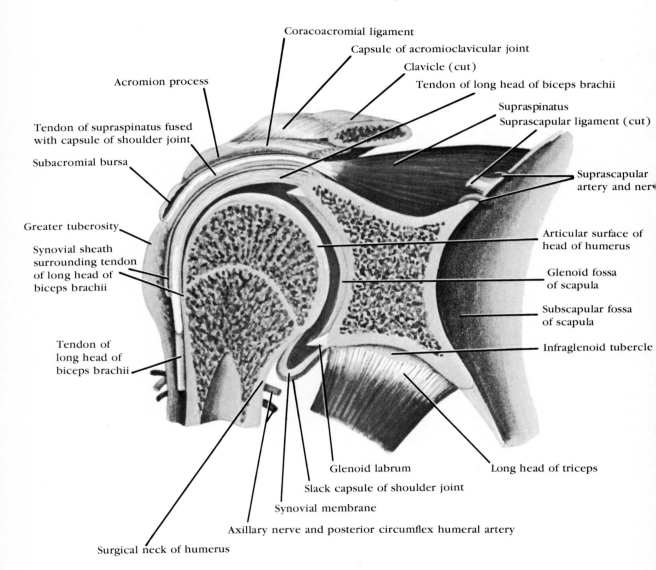

3-29. *Shoulder joint. A, Coronal section of the humero-scapular joint; B, Coronal section of the acromio-clavicular joint.* (*From Snell RS:* Atlas of Clinical Anatomy. *Boston, Little, Brown, 1978.*)

Coracoacromial ligament

Capsule of acromioclavicular joint

Clavicle (cut)

Tendon of long head of biceps brachii

Supraspinatus

Suprascapular ligament (cut)

Acromion process

Tendon of supraspinatus fused with capsule of shoulder joint

Subacromial bursa

Suprascapular artery and nerve

Greater tuberosity

Articular surface of head of humerus

Synovial sheath surrounding tendon of long head of biceps brachii

Glenoid fossa of scapula

Subscapular fossa of scapula

Tendon of long head of biceps brachii

Infraglenoid tubercle

Glenoid labrum

Long head of triceps

Slack capsule of shoulder joint

Synovial membrane

Axillary nerve and posterior circumflex humeral artery

Surgical neck of humerus

A

downward and is called the **inferior angle.** The **lateral border** of the scapula extends from the inferior angle upward and laterally to the lower limit of the **glenoid cavity,** the articular cavity that receives the head of the humerus. The **superior border** and the medial border meet at the **superior angle.**

The posterior triangular surface of the scapula is traversed by the **scapular spine,** which ends superolaterally in an enlarged process called the **acromion,** which forms the roof of the shoulder joint. Another large process, the **coracoid process,** extends anteriorly from the juncture of the superior border and glenoid portion to form a hook that is open laterally and is positioned inferior to the anterior concavity of the clavicle.

The lateral end of the clavicle forms a sliding synovial joint with the medial part of the acromion of the scapula (Figure 3-29). The humerus forms a ball and socket synovial joint with the glenoid cavity of the scapula. While the detailed anatomy of these joints is not important to an understanding of respiration, it should be noted that movement of the shoulder involves the lateral end of the clavicle and that the sternoclavicular joint is the only point of articulation between the shoulder girdle and the rest of the skeleton.

Pelvic Girdle

The pelvic girdle (Figure 3-30) is composed of the paired hip bones (also called the **os innominata**) and the sacrum. The sacrum has already been described as part of the vertebral column. Each **hip bone** articulates with the corresponding femur, the long bone of the upper leg, and anteriorly the two hip bones articulate with each other at the **pubic symphysis.** The hip bone is composed of three smaller bones: the ilium, the ischium, and the pubis. These three bones are fused in the adult and form the lateral and anterior parts of the pelvis. The three parts of the hip bone come together at the **acetabulum,** the socket that receives the head of the **femur.**

The **ilium** is the large expanded upper part of the hip bone. The superior rim of the ilium is called the **iliac crest,** which ends anteriorly at the **anterior superior iliac spine** and posteriorly at the **posterior superior iliac spine.** Posteriorly, the ilium articulates with the sacrum. Anteriorly, the ilium is characterized by a large notch that separates the anterior superior spine from the pubic symphysis. Along this concavity is a projection called the **anterior inferior iliac spine,** below which is an eminence that marks the fusion of the ilium and pubis.

The **ischium** forms the posterior inferior part of the hip bone and articulates with the pubic bone both at the acetabulum and posteriorly in the ring of bone surrounding a large opening in the hip bone called the **obturator foramen.**

The **pubis** forms the anterior inferior portion of the hip bone and meets anteriorly with the pubis of the opposite side at the pubic symphysis. Extending laterally from the anterior superior margin is the **pubic crest.**

3-29 (*continued*)

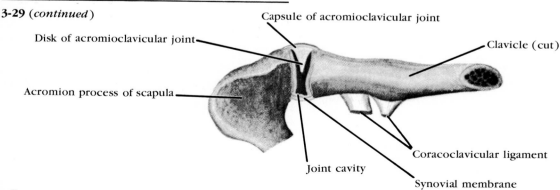

Capsule of acromioclavicular joint

Disk of acromioclavicular joint

Clavicle (cut)

Acromion process of scapula

Coracoclavicular ligament

Joint cavity

Synovial membrane

B

3-30. *Pelvic girdle. A, Anterior view; B, lateral view of the left os innominatum.*

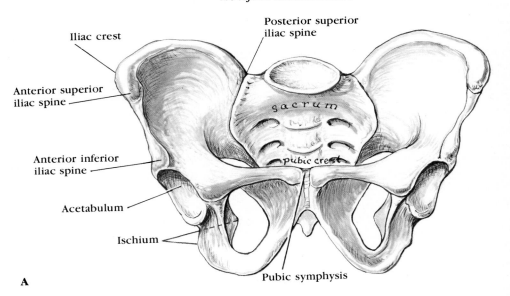

Iliac crest

Posterior superior
iliac spine

Anterior superior
iliac spine

sacrum

Anterior inferior
iliac spine

pubic crest

Acetabulum

Ischium

Pubic symphysis

A

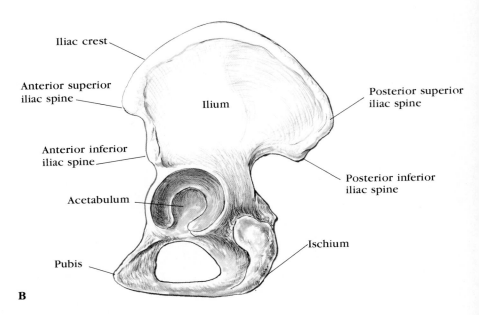

Iliac crest

Anterior superior
iliac spine

Ilium

Posterior superior
iliac spine

Anterior inferior
iliac spine

Posterior inferior
iliac spine

Acetabulum

Ischium

Pubis

B

RELATIONSHIPS OF THE LUNG, THORAX, AND ABDOMEN

Motion of the rib cage and diaphragm cause the volume of the thorax to increase and decrease during respiration (Figure 3-31). The external surfaces of the lungs are linked to the deep surfaces of the thoracic walls and the superior surface of the diaphragm. This linkage is a function of a fluid interface between two membranes called pleura. One of these, the **visceral pleura,** invests the lung on each side of the thorax. The other, the **parietal pleura,** lines the inside of the left and right halves of the thoracic cavity. Between the visceral and parietal pleura is a fluid-filled potential space called the **pleural cavity.** Thus, motions of the thoracic wall and diaphragm cause increases and decreases in lung volume. As the volume of the lungs increases, air pressure within the lungs begins to drop, causing air to flow into the lungs via the upper airway to balance external and al-

veolar air pressure. This is the process of inhalation. These events reverse during exhalation.

The relationships among lung volume, air flow, and alveolar (lung) pressure are illustrated in Figure 3-32. As lung volume increases during inhalation, alveolar pressure drops by about 1 cm H_2O, and flow of air into the lungs increases to about 0.5 liter per second. Toward the end of inhalation, alveolar pressure returns to atmospheric pressure, and flow stops. This process is reversed during exhalation.

During normal quiet breathing, the respiratory system is at rest at the end of exhalation. The rest position of the respiratory system is a function of the independent rest positions of the system components (i.e., the thoracic wall including the rib cage, the lungs, diaphragm, abdominal wall, and abdominal contents) and the linkages binding them together. The most critical linkage is that between the visceral and parietal pleura. If that link-

3-31. *Motion of the rib cage and diaphragm during respiration. A, Anterior view; B, Lateral view. Solid lines and light shading = inspiration; broken lines and dark shading = expiration.*

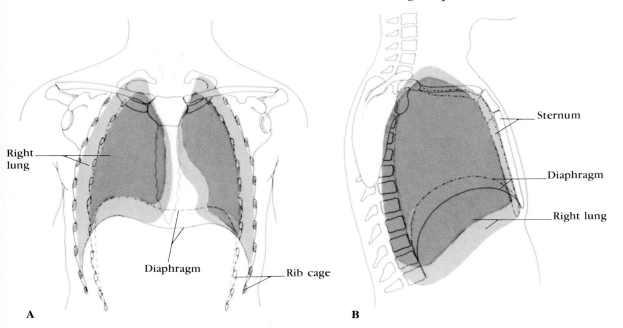

Right lung

Diaphragm

Rib cage

Sternum

Diaphragm

Right lung

A

B

age is broken by opening the pleural cavity to atmospheric pressure, the lungs collapse, the rib cage expands, and the dome of the diaphragm descends (Figure 3-33). The rest position of the respiratory system is a balance point between the tendency of the lungs and the tissues surrounding them to recoil away from one another due to their individual elastic properties. This balance is maintained by the pleural linkage.

It is commonly held that this linkage is a function of the surface tension of the fluid contained within the pleural space [10,14]. This is analogous to the surface tension between wet sheets of glass placed in contact with one another; they resist separation but still slide freely upon one another. However, there is evidence that surface tension is insufficient to account for pleural linkage, but that

---

3-32. *Relationships among lung volume, air flow, and alveolar pressure during one inspiration-expiration cycle. (Reproduced, with permission, from Comroe JH Jr:* Physiology of Respiration, *2nd ed. Copyright © 1974 by Year Book Medical Publishers, Inc, Chicago.)*

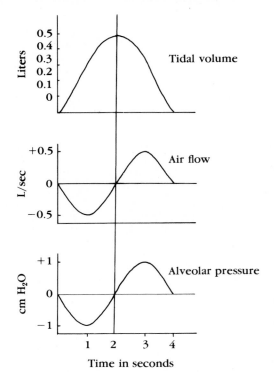

instead the linkage is a function of fluid transport out of the pleural space combined with elasticity of the pleura itself [2]. The latter explanation is more likely since the pleural linings are permeable to the intrapleural fluid.

Linkage also exists between the diaphragm and the rib cage, since the diaphragm attaches to the inferior margin of the rib cage. As the rib cage expands, the circumference of the diaphragm increases. Also, since the muscle fibers of the diaphragm course superiorly toward the dome of the diaphragm from their costal attachments, contraction of the diaphragm could elevate the lower margin of the rib cage. Clearly, the actions of the rib cage and diaphragm are not independent.

The diaphragm is also linked to the abdominal wall via the interposed abdominal viscera (Figure 3-34). The abdominal cavity is bounded by two moveable walls: the diaphragm above, and the muscular abdominal walls anteriorly and laterally. Because the abdominal contents are essentially noncompressable, lowering of the diaphragm increases abdominal pressure, which drives the abdominal wall outward. In addition, the degree of motion of the abdominal wall is affected by motion of the rib cage, which forms the superior attachment of the abdominal wall.

In order to describe the results of these linkages and elastic forces and the pressures which result from them, it is helpful to express various subdivisions of the total air capacity of the lungs according to standard definitions (Figure 3-35) [21]. The quantity of air remaining in the lungs after as much air as possible has been expelled by exhalation is called the **residual volume.** This has been estimated at about 25% of the **total lung capacity** [2]. The maximum volume of air that can be exchanged during respiration is the difference between the total lung capacity and the residual volume and is called the **vital capacity. Tidal volume** is the quantity of air exchanged during any particular breath and thus will vary according to oxygen requirements and activity. **Inspiratory reserve volume** and **expiratory reserve volume** refer to that part of the vital capacity still available at the end of any given inhalation or exhalation, respectively. **Inspiratory capacity** is

3-33. *Natural position of the lungs (light shading) and position after opening the pleural spaces to atmospheric pressure (dark shading).*

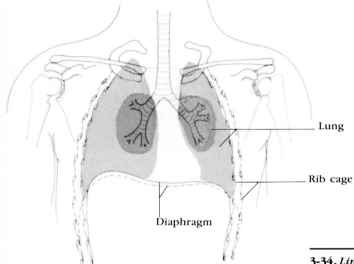

Lung

Rib cage

Diaphragm

3-34. *Linkage of the abdominal wall and diaphragm via the interposed abdominal viscera, lateral view.*

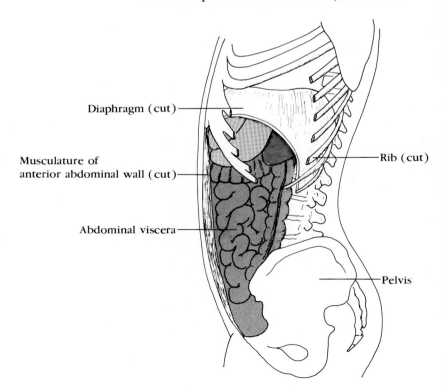

Diaphragm (cut)

Musculature of
anterior abdominal wall (cut)

Abdominal viscera

Rib (cut)

Pelvis

the amount of air that can be inhaled from rest position of the respiratory system. The amount of air in the lungs at rest position is called the **functional residual capacity.**

Pressures that result from nonmuscular forces acting on the respiratory system are called **relaxation pressures** and can be measured at various lung volumes by measuring breath pressure within a closed airway at various levels of respiration with all muscles relaxed. A typical relaxation pressure diagram is shown in Figure 3-36. It can be seen that zero pressure (which occurs at the end-expiratory rest position) occurs at approximately 35% of vital capacity, so that inspiratory capacity is approximately 65%. At higher levels of vital capacity, positive pressure exists within the closed

respiratory system since recoil forces are developed when the respiratory system is expanded from its rest position. Alternatively, at lower levels of vital capacity, negative pressure exists within the closed respiratory system because of the recoil forces of the system that has now been compressed from its rest position.

Figure 3-37 demonstrates the effect of disrupting the pleural linkage and allowing the components of the respiratory system to assume their independent rest positions. Zero pressure for the rib cage rises to approximately 55% of the vital capacity and zero pressure for the lungs drops to near 0% of total lung capacity [2]. Consequently, during inhalation from rest position to about 55% of vital capacity, the lungs are moving away from

3-35. *Subdivisions of the total air capacity of the lungs.*

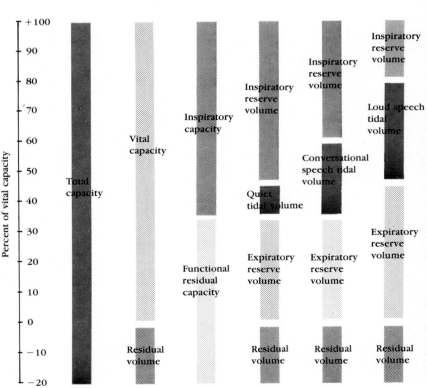

Respiratory functions

3-36. *Static volume-pressure curves of the total respiratory system during relaxation in the upright posture, with a spirometer tracing showing the pulmonary subdivisions. The slanting broken lines indicate the volume change during relaxation against an obstruction due to gas compression at total lung capacity and expansion at resting volume. The curve was extended to include the full vital capacity range by means of externally applied pressures. (Reprinted, with permission, from Agostoni E, Mead J: Statics of the respiratory system. In Fenn WO, Rahn H (Eds):* Handbook of Physiology, *Section 3,* Respiration, *Vol 1. Copyright 1964 by the American Physiological Society, Bethesda, Maryland.)*

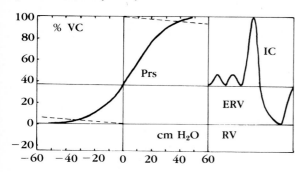

3-37. *The effect of disrupted pleural linkage on the rib cage and lungs.*

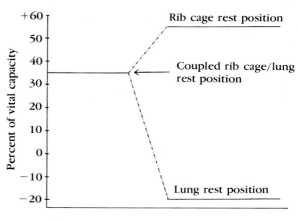

3-38. *Respiratory motions of the rib cage and lungs relative to their rest positions.*

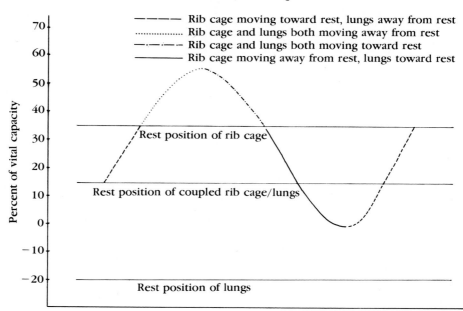

their rest position, but the rib cage is moving toward its rest position. As vital capacity exceeds 55%, both the rib cage and lungs move away from their rest position. During exhalation above 55% vital capacity, both the lungs and rib cage move back toward their rest position, but below that level, the rib cage moves away from its rest position (Figure 3-38).

The forces at work are reflected in the **pleural pressure** (the pressure within the interpleural space). With the respiratory system at rest, pleural pressure is about −5 cm of H_2O. During quiet inhalation the pleural pressure drops to about −11cm of H_2O and during heavy exercise it may drop to as low as −30 cm of H_2O. During exercise, pleural pressure may become positive during the peak of expiration [20].

As illustrated in Figure 3-39, quiet respiration has been calculated to occur between 35 and 45% vital capacity [14], that is, between the respiratory system rest position and the rib cage rest position. Hixon [14] goes on to point out that normal conversational speech typically occurs within the range of 35 to 60% vital capacity. Thus inhalation for conversational speech extends slightly beyond the rib cage rest volume. Very loud speech, he reported, involves inhalation of up to 80% vital capacity. He also points out that "in the upright posture, breathing phrases are usually terminated slightly above or at the resting respiratory level (around 40–35% VC) during conversational utterances of normal loudness, with occasional phrases encroaching modestly upon the expiratory reserve volume." He also reported that ". . . loud utterances are frequently terminated at lung volumes above the resting expiratory level, sometimes appreciably above."

Thus both quiet breathing and conversational speech are typically accomplished within small proportions of the vital capacity. In examining the static (nonmuscular) forces involved, Agostoni and Mead [2] found that recoil forces alone will not account for the events of exhalation in either case. Figure 3-40 demonstrates that exhalation occurs much more slowly than it would if recoil forces were unchecked by muscular activity. This

is even more true of speech, during which exhalation is prolonged for several seconds (see Figure 3-39). Thus not only are inhalatory muscular forces required to move the respiratory system away from its rest position during inhalation, those muscular forces must continue into exhalation to provide a braking action.

Exhalatory muscular forces are needed in two instances: when exhalation continues below the resting respiratory system level (about 35% vital capacity), and when more alveolar pressure is required than is provided by relaxation pressure at any respiratory level (e.g., for speech). Alveolar (and, therefore, sublaryngeal) pressure translates into loudness of the voice. Therefore, if constant

3-39. *Lung volume changes characteristic of conversational and loud speech in the upright posture. Duration of utterance is shown by the bracketed time segments above each of the tracings. (From Minifie FD, Hixon TJ, Williams F (Eds):* Normal Aspects of Speech, Hearing and Language, © *1973, p. 115. Reprinted by permission of Prentice-Hall, Inc., Englewood Cliffs, New Jersey.)*

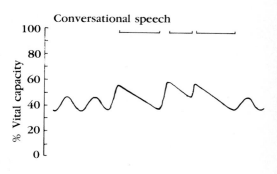

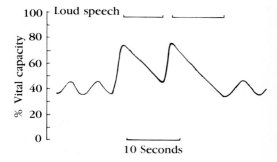

loudness is to be maintained, constant pressure must be maintained. Assuming that constant pressure is required for a particular utterance, the circumstances during speech under which inspiratory and expiratory muscle forces would be needed may be determined by combining the data of Hixon [14] and Agostoni and Mead [2], as presented in Figure 3-41. Under these circumstances, we can see that inspiratory muscle forces would be required for inhalation and for the initial part of exhalation for speech. However, during the latter part of the utterance described, the need for some exhalatory muscle force is indicated. This latter condition occurs when the curves for required alveolar pressure for speech descend and cross the relaxation curve, indicating that more alveolar pressure is required than would be produced by relaxation pressure.

In particular, increasing exhalatory muscle force would be required during loud utterances that continue until the respiratory system reaches its rest position. This may be why we typically end loud utterances at levels well above the respiratory rest position.

3-41. Top, *Lung volume-alveolar pressure relations during relaxation and during an isolated vowel utterance of normal loudness produced throughout most of the vital capacity. Hatched area shows muscular pressure required for the utterance. Relaxation curve from Figure 3-36.* Bottom, *Lung volume-muscular pressure relations replotted from data of the upper graph. Negative values represent net inspiratory forces and positive values represent net expiratory forces. (From Minifie FD, Hixon TJ, Williams F (Eds.):* Normal Aspects of Speech, Hearing and Language. © *1973, p. 102. Reprinted by permission of Prentice-Hall, Inc., Englewood Cliffs, New Jersey.)*

3-40. *Volume and flow during spontaneous breathing (solid lines) and as they would be if only static forces were operating (broken lines). (Redrawn, with permission, from Mead J, Agostoni E: Dynamics of breathing. In Fenn WO, Rahn H (Eds):* Handbook of Physiology, *Section 3,* Respiration, *Vol 1. Copyright 1964 by the American Physiological Society, Bethesda, Maryland.)*

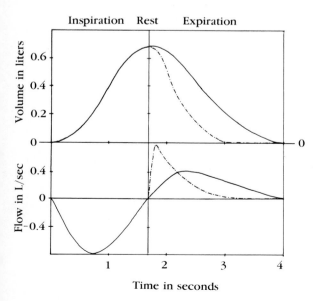

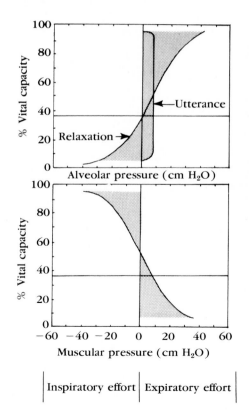

Motion of the Rib Cage versus Diaphragm-Abdomen

Motion of the rib cage produced by respiratory muscles and static forces results in inhalation and exhalation. Inhalation and exhalation can also be accomplished by motion of the diaphragm and its antagonistic muscles of the abdominal wall. Before describing the individual muscles that may be involved in respiration, it will be helpful to examine what is known about the motions of the rib cage and diaphragm-abdomen. These motions have been studied radiologically as well as by means of magnetometers (electromagnetic coils placed on the back and on the thoracic and abdominal walls) and by plethysmographic methods [13]. There is general agreement [1] that at least in quiet respiration the diaphragm typically produces the major portion of the tidal volume. However, as pointed out by Hixon [14], ". . . it is possible to move air both in and out of the lungs through a wide variety of relative displacements of the thoracic cage and diaphragm-abdomen." The relative degree to which these two components are utilized during speech varies greatly among individuals.

Important changes in the relative use of the rib cage and diaphragm-abdomen occur developmentally. Infants, perhaps in part due to developmental neurological factors and/or the lack of rib curvature, are primarily diaphragmatic breathers.

Body position has a dramatic effect upon the events of respiration owing to the effect of gravity. Moving from the upright to the supine position principally affects the diaphragm. In the upright posture, the pull of gravity on the abdominal contents is inferior. This would tend to displace the diaphragm inferiorly and accounts for much of the static force that balances the recoil forces of the lungs. In the supine posture, gravity pulls dorsally which tends to displace the diaphragm cephalically (Figure 3-42). This changes the resting level of the respiratory system from 35% of the vital capacity to about 20% of the vital capacity [14].

3-42. *Effect of gravity on the diaphragm and abdominal wall. (Modified and reproduced, with permission, from Agostoni E, and Mead J: Statics of the Respiratory System. In Fenn WO, and Rahn H (Eds):* Handbook of Physiology, Section 3, Respiration, Vol 1. *Copyright 1964 by the American Physiology Society, Bethesda, Maryland.)*

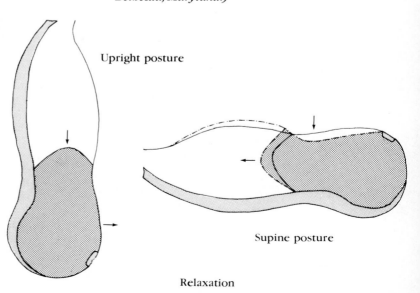

Upright posture

Supine posture

Relaxation

Furthermore, whereas in the upright posture the static inspiratory force of gravity on the diaphragm helps to control alveolar pressure (such as during exhalation for quiet speech), this force must now be provided by active contraction of the diaphragm.

Hixon and associates [15] found that during rest breathing the relative motion of the rib cage and abdomen followed the relaxation curve and that the contribution of the rib cage far exceeded that of the abdomen. The work of Goldman and Mead [11] suggests that the diaphragm, acting alone, will drive the rib cage and abdomen along the relaxation curve. Thus the findings of Hixon and associates is consistent with the notion that diaphragmatic activity predominates in rest breathing. The authors further reported that in the supine position, the rib cage-abdomen relationship reverses, with the contribution of the abdomen far exceeding that of the rib cage.

These same authors also studied the rib cage-abdomen relationships during speech, reading, and singing at various loudnesses. They found that for all utterances in the upright posture, ". . . forces were operating to make the rib cage larger

and the abdomen smaller than they were during relaxation at the prevailing lung volume" [15].

Bloomer [3], in a radiological study of motion of the rib cage during respiration, found that over the range of vital capacity all of the ribs move simultaneously and in the same direction. This contradicted unsupported statements in the literature suggesting that the first and/or twelfth rib may serve as stable anchors during respiration. He also found that the greatest degree of elevation of the posterior part of the ribs occurred in the upper rib cage (ribs two or three) and decreased from that level downward. However, the lateralmost points on the ribs moved to a similar extent from the first rib to the twelfth. Thus the fact that the longer ribs exhibit a greater arc of motion than shorter ribs (given the same degree of motion at the neck of the rib) is compensated for by greater motion of the necks of the shorter ribs. In addition, Bloomer found neither a change in the angle of the sternum with the body axis nor any change in the manubrial-corpal angle over the range of vital capacity (Figure 3-43). The motion of the sternum was anterosuperior during inhalation and posteroinferior during exhalation.

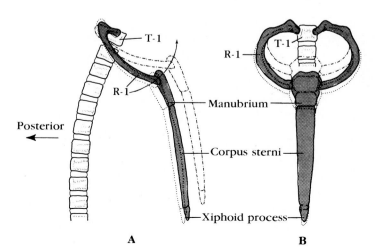

3-43. *Position of the first rib and sternum during respiration. Shaded areas indicate normal rest position.*

Respiratory System Regulation

During quiet breathing, the upper airway remains open and respiratory rate and depth are controlled in response to blood gas levels (oxygen and carbon dioxide). As will be seen in subsequent chapters, the size of the nasal airway changes in response to environmental conditions. In addition, there are small rhythmic changes in the dimensions of the pharyngeal and laryngeal airway during respiration. However, during conversational speech dramatic changes occur in the upper airway with great rapidity. During phonation the larynx alternately opens and closes many times per second. During articulation, structures of the oral and pharyngeal cavities repeatedly open, close, and impede the airway. As the upper airway closes, the load on the respiratory system increases, and as it opens, the load is decreased. Thus we need to examine the way in which the respiratory system responds to or interacts with these changes.

Hixon and associates [15] stated that "We know that during running speech, changes in alveolar pressure can be relatively large, yet we did not see substantial motion on the [rib cage-abdomen relative motion] diagram corresponding to these pressure changes (that is, the tracings were relatively smooth and did not show major 'jogs' for the pressure changes)." They interpreted their data to mean that ". . . the general distortion of the chest wall from its relaxed configuration constitutes a form of posturing of the system, off of which the speaker then minimally distorts the chest wall to provide the rapid compressional volume changes (pressure fluctuations) needed to drive the larynx and upper airway."

MUSCLES OF RESPIRATION

Current research on the muscular physiology of respiration has not yet fully defined either the specific function of muscles known to be involved in respiration or which of the muscles with functional potential for respiration actually serve that function. For this reason it is necessary to study all of the muscles believed to have this functional po-

tential. We will first examine the anatomy and potential function of each muscle, then the probable muscle functions based on what is known currently from electromyographic research.

It might seem reasonable to categorize the muscles as those with potential for inhalation and those with potential for exhalation. Even here, however, there is disagreement in the literature. Thus the anatomy of the muscles will be covered by region, an approach that will also clarify the interrelationships among adjacent structures.

Muscles of the Neck

Two muscles of the neck, the sternocleidomastoid and scalene, have one of their attachments on the rib cage and thus may provide for rib motion.

STERNOCLEIDOMASTOID. The sternocleidomastoid (Figure 3-44) is a broad, thick muscle that lies superficially in the lateral part of the neck. It originates by two heads, one from the anterior surface of the manubrium of the sternum, and the other from the sternal end of the clavicle. It extends superiorly and posteriorly to insert on the side of the skull behind the ear. The specific insertions are the mastoid process and the superior nuchal line (Figure 3-45). The **mastoid process** is an inferior projection from the temporal bone. The **superior nuchal line** extends across the posterior aspect of the occipital bone. The medial edges of the inferior tendons can be felt in a "V" shape above the manubrium of the sternum.

The functional potential of this muscle can be analyzed by assessing the nature of the lever systems upon which it operates. If its action on the skull is viewed from a lateral perspective (Figure 3-46A), it can be seen that the muscle attaches posterior to the fulcrum of head motion, which occurs at the articulation of the first cervical vertebra with the skull. This articulation is at the same coronal plane as the transverse process of C-1, which can be palpated just below the ear between the mandible and the sternocleidomastoid muscle. The result is a class 1 lever, with the muscle pulling down on the back of the head, resulting in elevation of the chin.

3-44. *Sternocleidomastoid muscle, anterolateral view.*

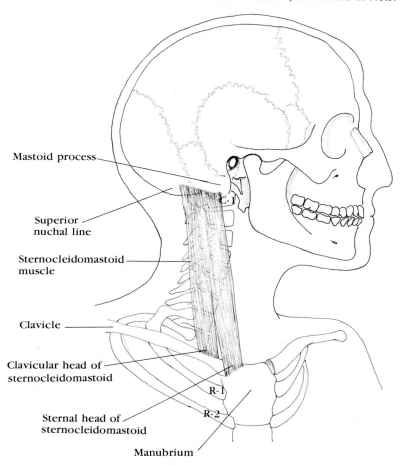

Mastoid process

Superior
nuchal line

Sternocleidomastoid
muscle

Clavicle

Clavicular head of
sternocleidomastoid

Sternal head of
sternocleidomastoid

Manubrium

C-1

R-1

R-2

Viewed from the front (Figure 3-46B), we again have a class 1 lever, with the two sides of the muscle pulling downward on each end of the lever arm. The fulcrum is in midline at the odontoid process of the second cervical vertebra. Thus contraction of alternate sides of the muscle will tilt the head from side to side. The fact that the inferior attachment of the muscle is anterior to the superior attachment means that contraction of one side of the muscle will move the mastoid process of that side downward and forward, thus tilting the face upward and to the opposite side.

If the skull were stabilized by other muscles, the sternocleidomastoid would exert its force on the sternum and clavicle and, therefore, the rib cage. In doing so it would operate as a class 2 lever. Its efficiency would be low, since its direction of pull differs from the direction of motion of the anterior rib cage by at least 45 degrees. The power of the muscle would be transmitted to the ribs indirectly via the sternum and clavicle.

3-45. *Mastoid process (MP) and superior nuchal line (arrows and dotted line). A, Lateral view; B, Inferior view.*

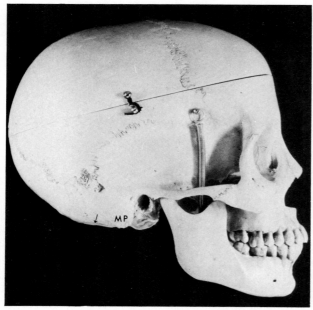

A

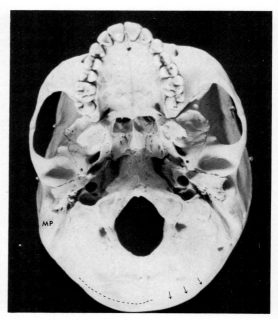

B

3-46. *Functional potential of the sternocleidomastoid muscle. A, Lateral view; B, Anterior view.*

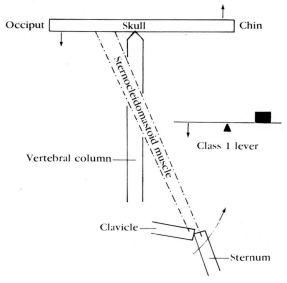

A

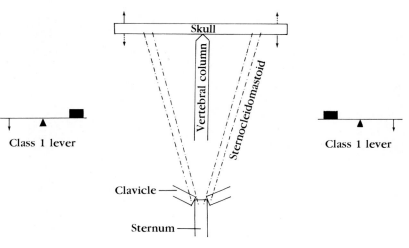

B

SCALENES. This group of muscles, which lies deep in the lateral part of the neck (Figure 3-47), includes the **anterior, medius, posterior,** and **minimus scalenes.** In general, their course is from the transverse processes of the cervical vertebrae to the lateral parts of the first and second ribs. The origins of this group of muscles are distributed over the transverse processes of all seven cervical vertebrae: the anterior scalene from C-3 to C-6; the middle scalene from C-2 to C-7; the posterior scalene from C-5 to C-7; and the scalene minimus from C-6 to C-7. The anterior and middle scalenes attach to the upper surface of the lateral part of the first rib. The posterior scalene attaches to a similar area on rib two. The scalene minimus varies in size and may even be replaced by connective tissue strands. It extends from the transverse processes of the lower one or two cervical vertebrae and sends fibers to rib one and to the pleura overlying the upper dome of the lung. With the two sides acting together, the scalenes may either stabilize the head or elevate the upper ribs. One side acting alone may flex the cervical vertebral column to the same side. As shown in Figure 3-48, the direction of pull of the scalenes on the first two ribs is almost vertical. Thus these muscles may provide for elevation of the first two ribs during inhalation, particularly if the head is maintained in the upright position. This action could be interfered with, however, during lateral flexion of the cervical spine.

In vertebral column motion, and in their potential for rib motion, the scalenes would act as part of a class 3 lever (Figure 3-49).

3-47. *Scalene muscles. A, Lateral view of the left scalenes with anterior to the left; B, Anterior view. AS, anterior scalenes; MS, middle scaleness; PS, posterior scalenes; ELM, extrinsic laryngeal muscles.*

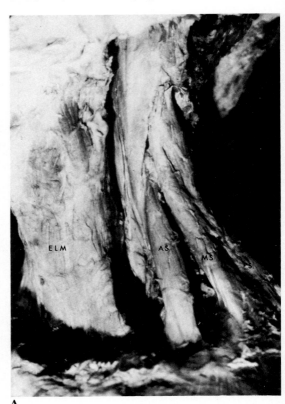

A

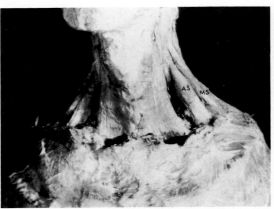

B

3-48. *Vector of pull of the scalenes on the ribs.*

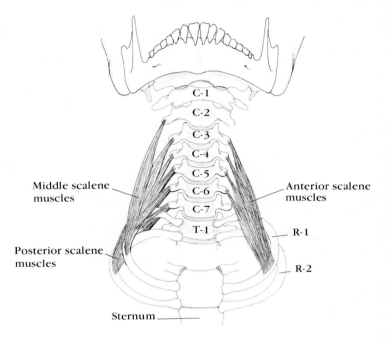

3-49. *Functional potential of the scalene muscles, anterior view.*

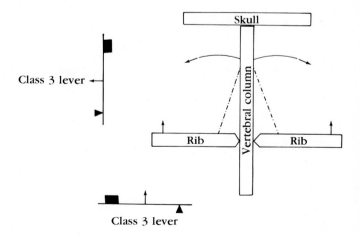

Muscles of the Anterior Thorax

The anterior thoracic wall contains several muscles, which will be examined from superficial to deep. As in other parts of the body, the skin covers a layer of superficial fascia of variable thickness. This layer collects fat and therefore is thick in obese persons and thin in slender persons. Typically, the abdominal fascia collects more fat than the thoracic fascia. The most superficial layer of muscle lies deep to the superficial fascia. In the female, the mammary gland also lies superficial to the musculature of the thoracic wall.

PECTORALIS MAJOR. The pectoralis major (Figure 3-50), the most superficial muscle of the anterior thoracic wall, is a broad, thick, powerful muscle composed of laminae that arise from the medial half of the clavicle and from the superficial surface of the sternum and the adjacent costal cartilages. The fibers converge to insert onto the humerus just below its head. Thus the fibers from the clavicle are oblique and travel inferolaterally to the humerus, while the sternal fibers are essentially horizontal, and the most inferior fibers have a superolateral course. This muscle can easily be palpated at the anterior border of the **axillary triangle** (the underarm area).

The muscle's most obvious functional potential is adduction and slight rotation of the arm as part of a class 3 lever (Figure 3-51). Since it attaches to the thorax, it has been assigned a potential role in respiration. However, its primary direction is lateralward, while the sternum moves anterosuperiorly. Thus only the most inferior fibers could provide thoracic lifting, and then only if the arm were fixed. It is interesting to note that in one form of artificial respiration the arms are elevated above the head to provide for inhalation. This puts stretch on the pectoralis major, which assumes a more vertical direction and elevates the rib cage. Thus the use of this muscle for respiration would apparently necessitate alternately raising and lowering the arms.

3-50. *A and B, Pectoralis major muscle, anterior view. PM-C, clavicular head; PM-S, sternal head; Arrow, humeral attachment; P, platysma muscle; SCM, sternocleidomastoid muscle; DL, deltoid muscle; S, sternum; RA, rectus abdominis muscle.*

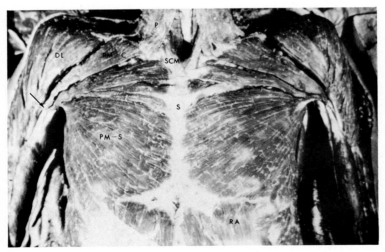

A

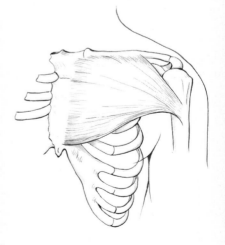

B

PECTORALIS MINOR. The pectoralis minor muscle (Figure 3-52) lies just deep to the pectoralis major. It originates as a broad lamina that attaches to the anterior surfaces of ribs three through five just lateral to their costochondral junctions and to the intervening intercostal fascia. The muscle courses superiorly and slightly laterally to insert onto the coracoid process of the scapula.

One functional potential of this muscle is depression of the shoulder by pulling downward on the scapula as part of a class 3 lever (Figure 3-53). It could also elevate the ribs if the scapula were prevented from descending by other muscles. In respiration, this muscle would exert an almost vertical pull on ribs three through five. Its vector is less appropriate to rib motion than to shoulder motion since its pull is more lateral than the direction of rib motion.

SUBCLAVIUS. The subclavius (see Figure 3-52) is a small cylindrical muscle that lies deep to the pec-

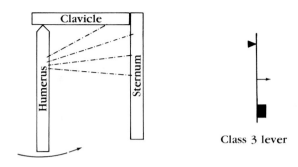

3-51. *Functional potential of the pectoralis major muscle.*

Class 3 lever

3-52. *A and B, Pectoralis minor (PM) and subclavius (SC) muscles, anterior view. Pectoralis major has been removed on the subject's right side. SCM, sternocleidomastoid muscle; Arrow, coracoid process of the scapula; S, sternum; 3,4,5, ribs; CH, interchondral portion of the internal intercostal muscles.*

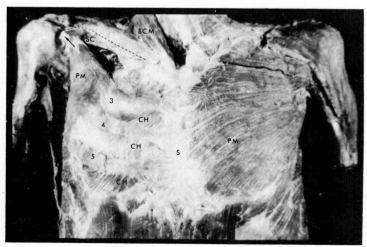

A

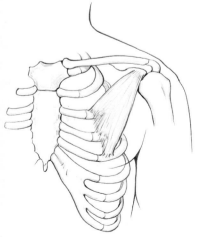

B

toralis minor and extends beneath the length of the clavicle. It arises from the junction of the first rib and its costal cartilage and inserts onto the inferior border of the lateral part of the clavicle.

Since the subclavius lies along the long axis of the clavicle, its vector of pull is poor for any activity. As can be seen in Figure 3-54, this muscle's attachment to the first rib is very near the sternoclavicular joint, virtually precluding any leverage for lifting the rib. If, on the other hand, the

costal attachment is seen as its functional origin, the insertion (the lateral end of the clavicle) can swing in around the sternoclavicular–first rib junction. In either case, this muscle has no potential for respiratory function.

SERRATUS ANTERIOR. The serratus anterior (Figure 3-55) lies, in its most anterior part, deep to the pectoralis major. A very broad, thick muscle, it arises by small slips of muscle (the term serratus means saw-toothed) from the external surfaces of the upper eight or nine ribs anterior to the most lateral curvature of the ribs. These muscle slips join into a broad sheet of muscle that wraps around the external surface of the rib cage as it proceeds posteriorly and then medially. It continues deep to the scapula and lies between the scapula and the rib cage. Its insertion is over the entire length of the medial border of the scapula from the superior angle to the inferior angle. About half of the muscle fibers insert onto the inferior angle. The fibers from ribs one through four are nearly horizontal and attach to the superior angle and medial border. Fibers from ribs five through nine travel more obliquely with a superior inclination as they approach and attach to the inferior angle of the scapula.

3-53. *Functional potential of the pectoralis minor muscle, anterior view.*

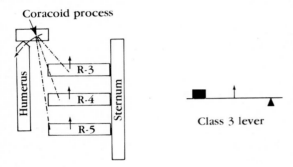

3-54. *Subclavius muscle (A) and its functional potential (B).*

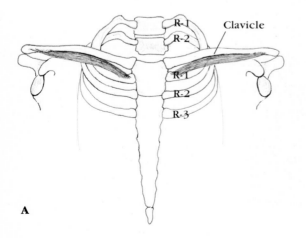

A

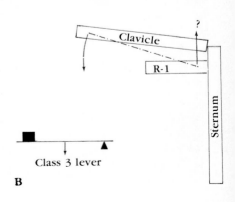

B

3-55. *Serratus anterior muscle. A, Anterolateral view of right side. PM, pectoralis major muscle; S, sternum; EAO, external abdominal oblique muscle; Arrows, anterior attachment of the serratus anterior. B. Dorsolateral surface of the serratus anterior muscle (SA) and the scapula (SC) detached from the rib cage. C, Left lateral view.*

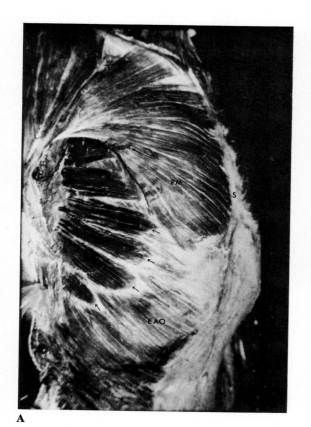

A

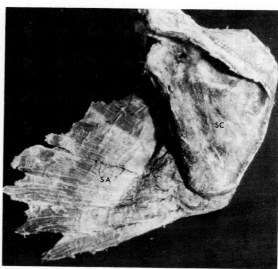

B

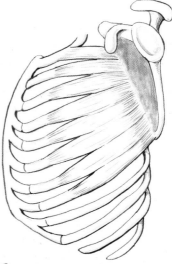

C

3-56. *Functional potential of the serratus anterior muscle. A, Superior view; B, Lateral view.*

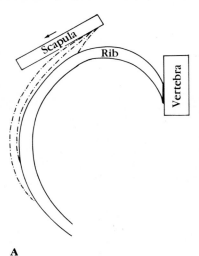

A

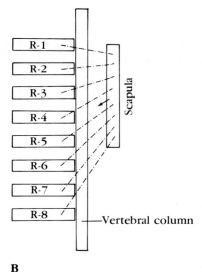

B

This muscle could move the scapula laterally, thereby adducting the shoulder and projecting it anteriorly as part of a class 2 lever action (Figure 3-56). The preponderant inferior fibers could move the inferior angle of the scapula laterally and tip the acromion to elevate the humerus above the horizontal. A respiratory function is possible for the lower part of the muscle since these fibers descend from the scapula to the lower ribs and could therefore elevate them in a class 2 lever action. Their angle, however, is more lateral than superior, and so this action would require relatively great force in addition to stabilization of the shoulder. The superior fibers are horizontal and would have little or no leverage for rib motion.

EXTERNAL INTERCOSTALS. The external intercostal muscles (Figure 3-57) are composed of short fibers that extend from the inferior margin of one rib to insert onto the superior margin of the subadjacent rib. The orientation of the fibers is oblique, since their superior attachment is nearer the vertebral end of the rib than is their inferior attachment. They are found between all of the ribs and extend from the vertebral column posteriorly to the costochondral junction anteriorly.

The muscle fascicles extend from rib to rib and form part of a class 3 lever with either rib (Figure 3-58). However, the fascicles will operate

3-57. *Intercostal muscles. A, Anterolateral view of the left side. Ribs two through nine are numbered. The brackets indicate the anterior ends of the bony parts of ribs five and six. The position of the external intercostals (EI) is indicated by the dotted line between ribs three and four. The external intercostals have been removed between ribs five and eight to show the internal intercostals. The arrow indicates the line of separation between the interchondral (CH) and interosseous (OS) portions of the internal intercostals. S, sternum; CC, costal cartilage. B, Artist's rendering. C, Left lateral view of the rib cage showing the external and internal intercostal muscles. The external intercostals (EI) have been removed in one intercostal space (arrow) to show the internal intercostals. R = ribs. D, The external intercostals (arrows). Several of the ribs are indicated (R); SA = serratus anterior; PL = pelvis.*

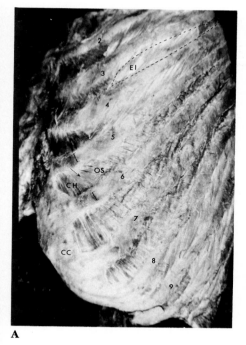

A

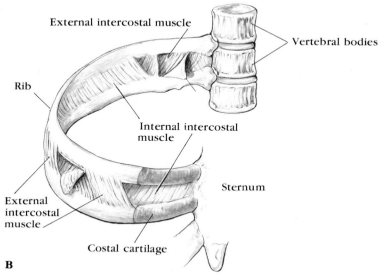

External intercostal muscle

Vertebral bodies

Rib

Internal intercostal muscle

External intercostal muscle

Sternum

Costal cartilage

B

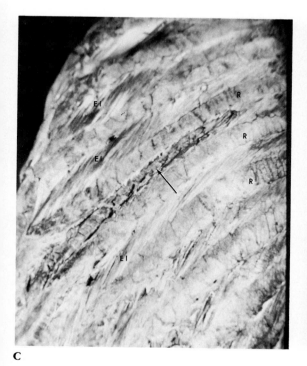

C

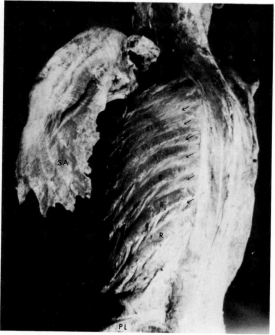

D

3-58. *Functional potential of the external intercostal muscles.*

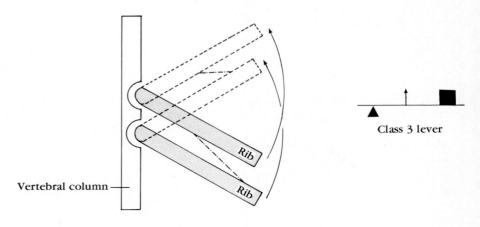

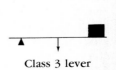

Class 3 lever

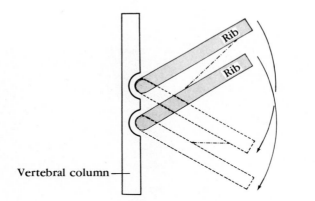

Class 3 lever

much more efficiently on the attachment furthest from the posterior fulcrum, that is, on the lower rib. For this reason they have a much greater capacity for raising the lower rib than for depressing the upper rib. In fact, as illustrated in Figure 3-58, the muscle fascicles can only shorten if both ribs rise, since their attachments move through an arc. If the ribs are lowered, the fascicles are stretched. Thus, the functional potential of these muscles is to raise the ribs.

INTERNAL INTERCOSTALS. The internal intercostals (see Figure 3-57) lie deep to the external intercostals and are quite similar to them with only two exceptions. First, they extend from the rib angles posteriorly to the sternum anteriorly and thus occupy, in part, the interchondral spaces. Second, their obliquity is opposite to that of the external intercostals. The superior attachment of the internal intercostals is more distant from the vertebral column than is the inferior attachment.

They, too, form class 3 levers with the ribs to which they attach (Figure 3-59). However, with regard to the interosseous parts of the muscle, the distance relationship of the attachment to the posterior fulcrum is reversed. The upper attachment is more distant from the fulcrum than is the lower; therefore, the function must also reverse. The functional potential of the interosseous portions of the internal intercostal muscles is to lower the ribs.

Hamberger [12] first described these relationships relating to potential function of the intercostals in 1748. He suggested that the functional potential of the interchondral portion of the internal intercostals is the same as that of the external intercostals, that is, to raise the ribs. This is logical because the downward slope of the ribs from posterior to anterior ends at the costochondral junction. The costal cartilages rise to the sternum and, therefore, the fulcrum would be at the sternum

rather than the vertebral articulation. In summary, Hamberger has pointed out that, based on the biomechanics of the system, the external intercostals and the interchondral portions of the internal intercostals would be inspiratory muscles, while the interosseous portions of the internal intercostals would be expiratory muscles.

TRANSVERSE THORACIC. The transverse thoracic muscle, located on the deep surface of the anterior thoracic wall (Figure 3-60), is a thin muscle that varies from person to person in the amount of muscle tissue it contains. It arises from the deep surface of the sternum and inserts onto the costal cartilages and intercostal fascia above its point of origin.

3-60. *Transverse thoracic muscle, posterior view of the anterior thoracic wall.*

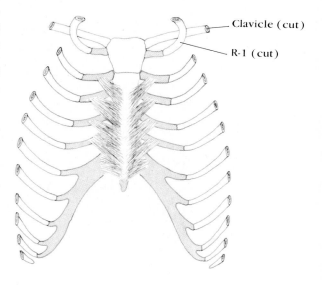

Clavicle (cut)

R-1 (cut)

3-61. *Functional potential of the transverse thoracic muscle.*

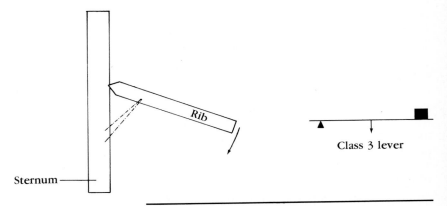

Sternum

Rib

Class 3 lever

3-62. *A and B, Posterior view of the superficial muscles of the back. TR, trapezius muscle; LD, latissimus dorsi muscle; LDF, lumbodorsal fascia; Arrow, acromion.*

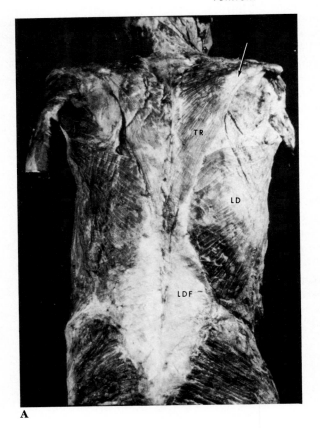

TR

LD

LDF

A

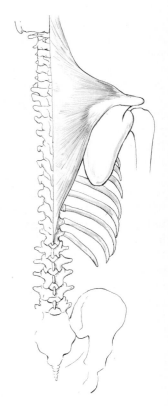

B

Shortening of the fibers of the transverse thoracic muscle would lower the costal cartilages to which they attach, functioning as a class 3 lever (Figure 3-61). Given the lack of a freely moveable costosternal joint, however, and the close approximation of the costal attachment of the muscle and the fulcrum (costosternal articulation), it would seem that this muscle has little functional potential.

Muscles of the Posterior Thorax

Five layers of muscles of the back could have (or are said to have) potential function in respiration. These five layers are composed of eight separate muscles or muscle groups, as follows.

TRAPEZIUS. The trapezius (Figure 3-62) is a thick, broad, trapezoid-shaped muscle that lies superficially in the upper back. It has multiple origins, including the cranial base, cervical vertebrae, and the thoracic vertebrae. Its most superior origin is from the external occipital protuberance and the adjacent portion of the superior nuchal line on the posterior aspect of the occipital bone. Below that, it arises indirectly from the spinous processes of the cervical vertebrae by means of the nuchal ligament, which covers those processes. Still lower, it arises from the spinous processes of the thoracic vertebrae. From this extensive line of origin, the fibers converge to attach to the scapular spine, acromion, and lateral third of the clavicle. Thus, its upper fibers extend obliquely downward and laterally while its inferior fibers extend obliquely upward and laterally. While it has no direct attachment to the rib cage, it could act as a stabilizer of the scapula in the event that the pectoralis minor were to act from the coracoid process of the scapula to elevate the ribs.

LATISSIMUS DORSI. The latissimus dorsi (Figure 3-63), is a broad, thick, powerful muscle of the lower back. It arises from the spinous processes of the lower six thoracic vertebrae, the spinous processes of all of the lumbar and sacral vertebrae, and from the fascial sheets into which the muscles of the lower back insert. These fascial sheets are collectively called the **lumbodorsal fascia.** At its origin from the thoracic vertebra, this muscle lies deep to trapezius. The fibers from this extensive line of origin converge to insert onto the humerus posterior to the attachment of the pectoralis major. The latissimus dorsi lies against the inferoposterior part of the rib cage, and some of its deep fibers arise from the external surfaces of the lower three or four ribs. Other fibers arise from the adjacent part of the iliac crest. It is important to note that below the point of attachment to the lower ribs and iliac crest this muscle is tendinous and its muscle fascicles extend from this level to the humerus.

The most obvious function of this muscle would be to adduct and rotate the arm and to draw the shoulder inferiorly and posteriorly as a part of a class 3 lever (Figure 3-64). A potential respiratory function has been ascribed to it by some authors because of the attachment of some of its deep fibers to the lower ribs, also forming a class 3 lever. Let us evaluate this. The rib attachment occurs at the junction of the muscle fascicles with the inferior tendon of the muscle. This means that there are no muscle fibers extending from the ribs downward, thus ruling out an exhalatory function. But it also means that those few fibers attaching to the ribs and rising to the humerus would have to stretch the lower tendon in order to elevate the ribs. Since tendons do not stretch, this muscle has no respiratory potential.

SERRATUS POSTERIOR SUPERIOR. The serratus posterior superior (Figure 3-65), which lies deep to the trapezius, is a short, thin slip of muscle. It arises by a long tendon from the nuchal ligament and the spinous processes of the seventh cervical and upper two or three thoracic vertebrae. It inserts onto the upper borders of ribs two through five just beyond their angles.

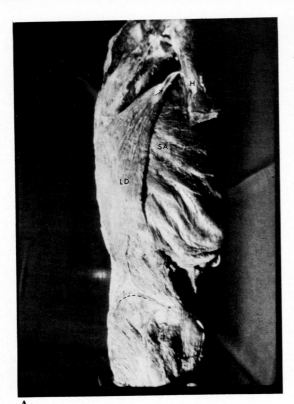

3-63. *Latissimus dorsi muscle (LD). A, Lateral view. SA, serratus anterior muscle; dotted line, iliac crest; Arrow, superior tendon of the latissimus dorsi attaching to the humerus (H). B, Dorsolateral view of the inferior attachment. LDF, lumbodorsal fascia; R, ribs; SA, serratus anterior muscle; Arrows, attachment to the rib cage; Dotted line, iliac crest. C, Artist's rendering.*

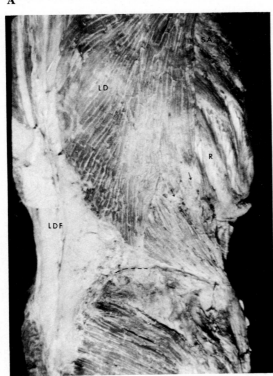

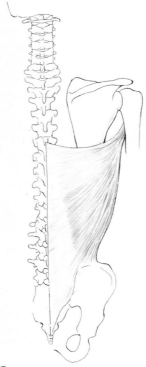

3-64. *Functional potential of the latissimus dorsi muscle.*

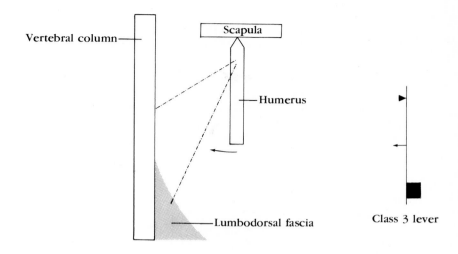

Vertebral column

Scapula

Humerus

Lumbodorsal fascia

Class 3 lever

3-65. *A and B, Upper back with the trapezius muscle and the left side of the latissimus dorsi muscle removed to reveal the serratus posterior superior muscle. Arrow, musculotendinous junction; SC, scapula; SS, sacrospinal muscles; LD, right latissimus dorsi muscle.*

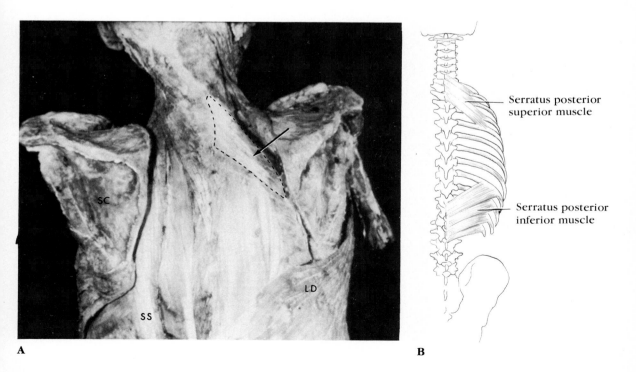

SC

SS

LD

Serratus posterior superior muscle

Serratus posterior inferior muscle

A

B

This muscle forms a class 3 lever with both the cervical spine and the ribs to which it attaches. Thus it has potential for both lateral flexion of the lower cervical and upper thoracic spine and elevation of the ribs two through five (Figure 3-66). Its power to flex the vertebral column appears to be slight, since little flexion occurs between the lower cervical and upper thoracic vertebrae and since the muscle itself is quite short and thin. It could act as a stabilizer of the vertebral column or as a rib elevator.

SERRATUS POSTERIOR INFERIOR. The serratus posterior inferior (Figure 3-67) is nearly a mirror image of the serratus posterior superior and is located in the lumbodorsal area. However, it is more muscular than the superior muscle, and its fascicles are longer. It arises by long tendons from the spinous processes of the lower two or three thoracic and upper two or three lumbar vertebrae. It extends

superolaterally to attach to the inferior borders of the lowest four ribs just beyond their angles.

This muscle forms a class 3 lever with the lower thoracic–upper lumbar spine and with the lower ribs (Figure 3-68). Thus it would have potential in lateral flexion of this part of the vertebral column or in lowering the ribs to which it attaches. However, little flexion occurs within the span of vertebrae covered by this muscle. It does have some potential for stabilization or lowering the ribs to which it attaches.

SACROSPINALS. The sacrospinals are a large, thick, powerful group of muscles that extends lateral to the vertebral column from the cervical to the lumbar area. Muscles of the lateral part of this group attach, in part, to the rib cage and are known collectively as the iliocostal muscles (Figure 3-69). The iliocostal muscles are divided into cervical, thoracic, and lumbar components.

3-66. *Functional potential of the serratus posterior superior muscle.*

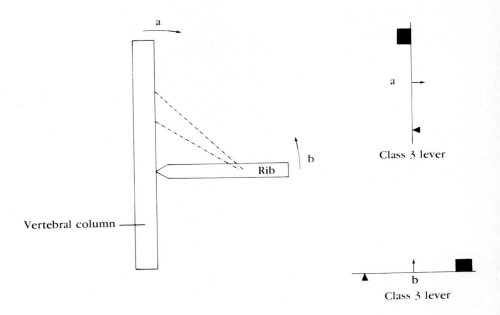

3-67. *Lower back with the latissimus dorsi muscle removed on the left side to reveal the serratus posterior inferior muscle (SPI). The tendinous origin of the upper bundle of the muscle has been elevated slightly (arrows). SA, serratus anterior muscle; LD, latissimus dorsi muscle.*

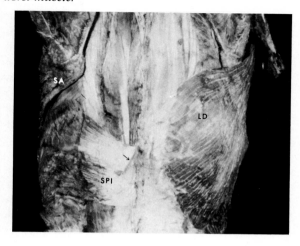

3-68. *Functional potential of the serratus posterior inferior muscle.*

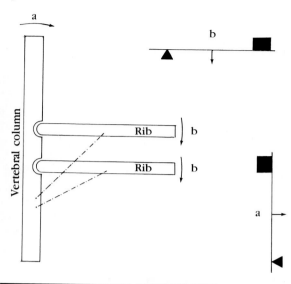

3-69. *A and B, Dissection of the back with the trapezius, latissimus dorsi, and posterior serratus muscles removed. Arrows indicate the sacrospinal muscles laterally and the erector spinae muscles medially.*

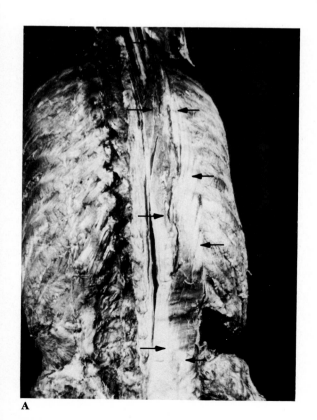

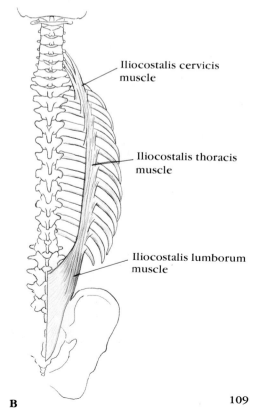

Iliocostalis cervicis muscle

Iliocostalis thoracis muscle

Iliocostalis lumborum muscle

A

B

109

The cervical component, called the **iliocostalis cervicis,** arises from the superficial surfaces of the angles of the third through sixth ribs and inserts on the transverse processes of the fourth through sixth cervical vertebrae. The thoracic component, called the **iliocostalis thoracis,** arises from the superior borders of the lower six ribs at their angles and inserts onto the lower borders of the upper six ribs beyond their angles. The lumbar component, called the **iliocostalis lumborum,** arises from the lumbodorsal fascia (and thereby indirectly from the lumbar vertebrae) and from the posterior part of the iliac crest. It inserts into the inferior borders of the lower six ribs at their angles.

As a group, the iliocostal muscles form a complex class 3 lever with the vertebral column (Figure 3-70) and have potential for lateral flexion of the vertebral column. The cervical portion would act on the cervical spine, and the lumbar portion on the lumbar spine. The thoracic portion could be synergistic, thus preventing separation of the

upper and lower ribs during lateral flexion of the vertebral column. The cervical portion of the muscle group also forms a class 3 lever with the upper ribs, and has potential for elevating them; however, the angle of pull would be superomedial, whereas rib motion is superior or superolateral. The lumbar portion forms a class 3 lever with the lower ribs and could depress them. The vector of the lumbar component (with potential for exhalation) is more efficient than is the vector of the cervical component (with potential for inhalation).

COSTAL LEVATORS. The costal levators (Figure 3-71) consist of twelve pairs of short muscles deep to the sacrospinals. They arise from the transverse processes of the seventh cervical and upper eleven thoracic vertebrae. Typically they extend downward and slightly laterally to insert on the subadjacent rib between its tubercle and angle. Some of the lower costal levators pass over one rib to insert on the next lower rib.

3-70. *Functional potential of the iliocostal muscles.*

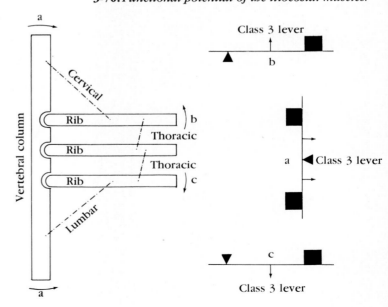

3-71. *A and B, Costal levator muscles (CL) of the left half of the posterior thorax. Asterisks indicate the transverse processes of the vertebrae. Ribs are numbered.*

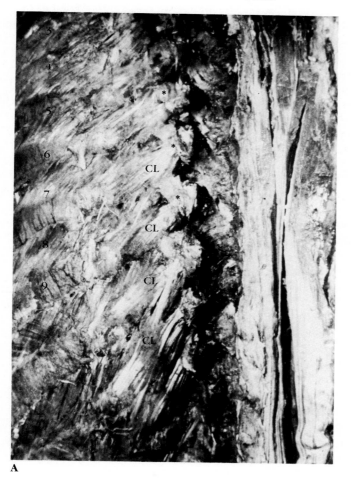

A

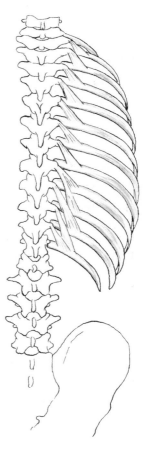

B

The costal levators form a class 3 lever with both the vertebrae and the ribs (Figure 3-72). Thus they could elevate the ribs; assist in extension of the thoracic part of the vertebral column (if both sides act together); or assist in lateral flexion of the thoracic spine (with one side acting alone). Since these muscle fibers are short, rib motion at the point of their attachment to the ribs is slight. However, because the costal levators attach near the fulcrum of rib motion, slight elevation of the rib at this point of attachment results in a much greater range of motion of the lateral and anterior parts of the rib. In all of these functions, however, the costal levators act against a severe mechanical disadvantage.

QUADRATUS LUMBORUM. The quadratus lumborum, a large, powerful quadrilateral muscle, lies deep in the lumbodorsal area between the twelfth rib and the iliac crest (Figure 3-73). It arises from the posterior half of the iliac crest and inserts onto the transverse processes of the upper four lumbar vertebrae and the posterior half of the twelfth rib. Its fibers course in a vertical direction.

This muscle forms a class 3 lever with both the lumbar vertebrae and with the twelfth rib (Figure 3-74). One side acting alone could produce lateral flexion of the lumbar spine. Downward pull on the twelfth rib could assist in exhalation. It has also been suggested that this muscle stabilizes the twelfth rib against the pull of the diaphragm, which also attaches to it. The quadratus lumborum would function as a synergist to the diaphragm only during "diaphragmatic breathing" in the absence of a thoracic component. Its combined attachment to the lumbar vertebrae and the twelfth rib suggests a postural function rather than a respiratory one, though it could function for both.

SUBCOSTALS. The subcostals are thin slips of muscle that lie on the deep surface of the posterior thoracic wall (Figure 3-75). They are quite variable in form and extent and are sometimes absent in the upper thorax. They arise from the deep surfaces of several ribs near the vertebral column and insert onto the deep surfaces of the second or

third rib above their origin near the rib angles. Thus, the subcostals rise obliquely in a superolateral direction, parallel to the internal intercostals.

The subcostals could provide the same function as the interosseous part of the internal intercostals that they parallel, thus acting to lower the ribs to which they attach (Figure 3-76).

3-72. *Functional potential of the costal levator muscles.*

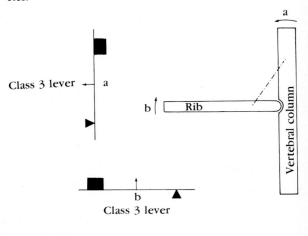

3-73. *Quadratus lumborum muscle shown on the left side, posterior view.*

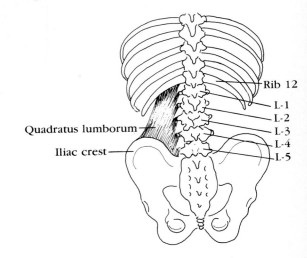

3-74. *Functional potential of the quadratus lumborum muscle.*

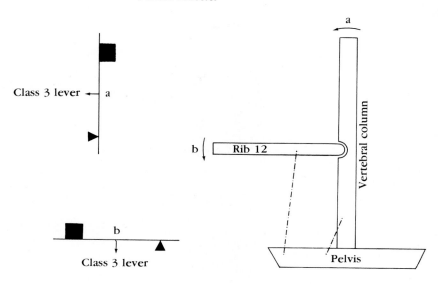

Class 3 lever ← a

b

Class 3 lever

3-75. *Subcostal muscle, right side, anterior view.*

3-76. *Functional potential of the subcostal muscle.*

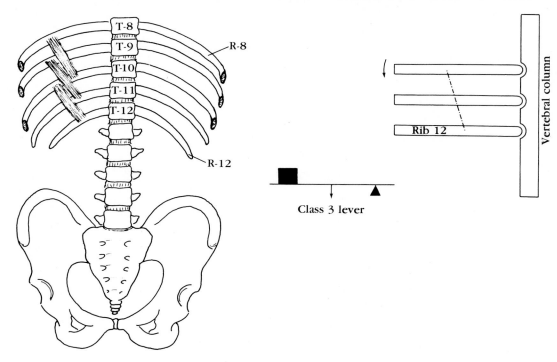

T-8

T-9

T-10

T-11

T-12

R-8

R-12

Class 3 lever

3-77. *Diaphragm, inferior view. VC, vena caval foramen; ES, esophageal hiatus; AA, abdominal aorta; RC, rib cage; S, sternum; CT, central tendon of the diaphragm; Arrows, radiating fibers of the diaphragm. B, Anterior view. C, Sagittal section.*

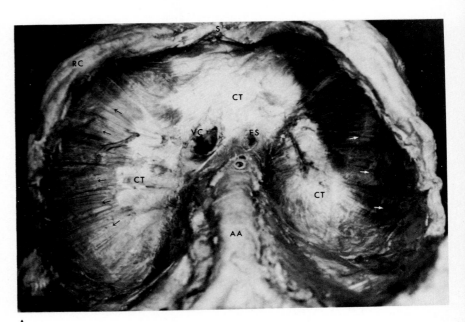

A

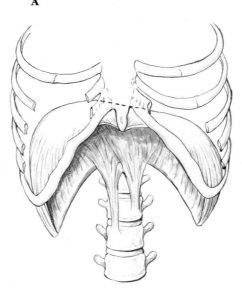

B

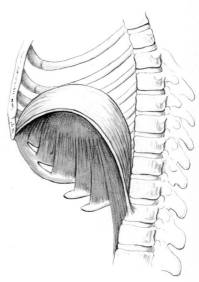

C

Muscles of the Abdomen

The abdominal muscles are located within the anterior and lateral parts of the abdominal wall. While not properly an abdominal muscle, the diaphragm will be included in this group since a part of its function is closely linked with that of the muscles of the abdominal wall.

DIAPHRAGM. The diaphragm (Figure 3-77), a large circumpennate muscle, divides the thoracic from the abdominal cavity. It attaches to the lower perimeter of the rib cage and rises to an elevated central tendon. Thus it is dome-shaped, with the lungs and heart above and the liver and other abdominal viscera below. The central dome is slightly higher on the right than on the left. The diaphragm is penetrated by the **esophagus,** which goes to the stomach; by the **aorta,** the large artery that supplies the lower part of the body; and by the venous counterpart of the aorta, the **inferior vena cava.** The diaphragm originates from the deep surface of the xiphoid process of the sternum, the anterior ends of ribs seven to eleven and their cartilages, the twelfth rib, and the bodies of the upper four lumbar vertebrae. The muscle fibers rise vertically along the deep surface of the lower thoracic wall and turn centrally to insert into the large tri-leafed central tendon.

The most apparent functional capacity of the diaphragm is to lower its elevated central tendon, which would increase the vertical dimension of the thorax and thus provide for inhalation (Figure 3-78). In doing so, it would displace the abdominal viscera. This results in the bulging of the abdominal wall that is apparent in diaphragmatic inhalation. Two other observations may be made, however. First, it is possible to draw the abdominal wall inward voluntarily during inhalation. Second, with very deep inhalation the abdominal wall is drawn inward as the chest rises. One of three things may account for this. First, the diaphragm may not be contracting during these maneuvers. Second, the vertical stretching of the abdominal wall that occurs during deep inhalation may provide the increase in abdominal cavity size necessary. Third, the muscular action of the diaphragm in these instances may elevate the lower perimeter of the rib cage and thus may assist in respiration. The diaphragm's most apparent function, that is, lowering of its central tendon, would serve two purposes. The first, as described above, would be to increase the thoracic space and therefore function for inhalation. The second would be to increase abdominal pressure if the abdominal wall were made tense by other muscles. An increase in abdominal pressure occurs during forced urina-

---

3-78. *Functional potential of the diaphragm. A, Anteroposterior view. B, Lateral view. d', diaphragm relaxed; d², diaphragm contracted; rc', rib cage at rest; rc², rib cage elevated.*

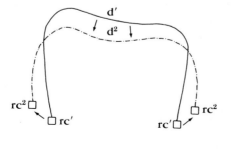

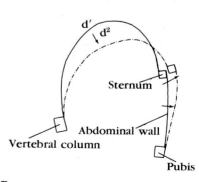

A   B

tion, defecation, vomiting, and parturition. However, its potential to increase abdominal pressure would not imply that the diaphragm is not principally involved in respiration since the two activities do not happen simultaneously. During those activities that require increased abdominal pressure, respiration ceases.

RECTUS ABDOMINIS. The rectus abdominis is a large thick muscle that extends vertically in the anterior abdominal wall just lateral to midline (Figure 3-79). It arises from the pubic crest and inserts onto the superficial surfaces of costal cartilages five through seven. Over its vertical course it is partially divided into four short segments by tendinous insertions. As in a multipennate muscle, this increases the power of the muscle. However, since the segments are in series, its range of motion is not restricted. The rectus abdominis is surrounded by a dense connective tissue sheath except in its lower third, where the sheath is incomplete on the deep surface of the muscle. The rectus sheaths from each side come together in the vertical midline of the abdominal wall. This single layer of connective tissue separating the left and right rectus muscles is called the **linea alba** (Figure 3-80). Laterally, the rectus sheath gives rise to the three broad, flat tendons of the lateral abdomi-

3-79. *A, Anterolateral thoracoabdominal wall, right side. EAO, external abdominal oblique muscle; IC, iliac crest; IL, inguinal ligament; LA, linea semilunaris; REC, rectus abdominus muscle. B, Rectus abdominis muscle, anterior view.*

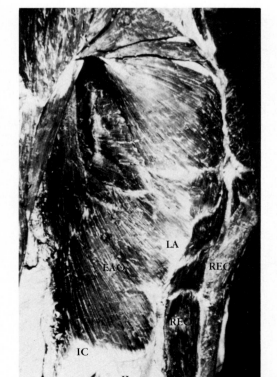

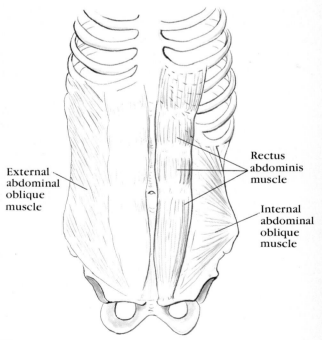

External abdominal oblique muscle

Rectus abdominis muscle

Internal abdominal oblique muscle

A

B

3-80. *Transverse section of the anterior abdominal wall.*

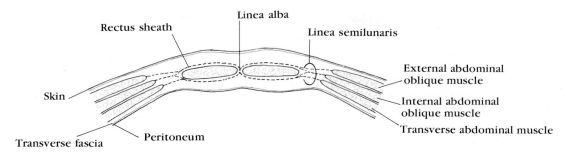

Linea alba

Rectus sheath

Linea semilunaris

External abdominal oblique muscle

Skin

Internal abdominal oblique muscle

Transverse abdominal muscle

Transverse fascia

Peritoneum

3-81. *Functional potential of the rectus abdominis muscle.*

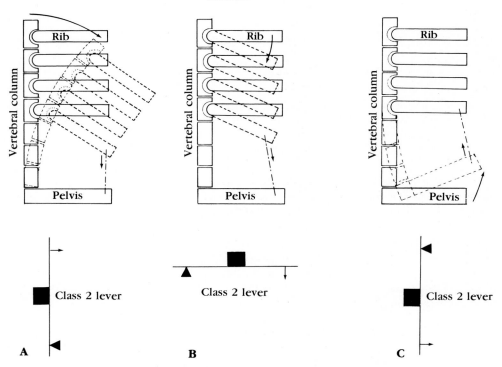

A

B

C

nal muscles: external abdominal oblique, internal abdominal oblique, and transverse abdominal. The area of tendon separating the rectus muscle from the lateral abdominal muscles is called the **linea semilunaris.** The inferior edge of this tendinous sheet is thickened, extends from the anterior superior iliac spine to the lateral part of the pubic crest, and is called the **inguinal ligament.** The linea alba, rectus sheath, linea semilunaris, and inguinal ligament together are called the **abdominal aponeurosis.**

The rectus abdominis forms a class 2 lever with the lower ribs (Figure 3-81). It is a powerful vertical muscle and so has great mechanical advantage for lowering the ribs. In addition, it is in a position to act as an antagonist to the diaphragm. Also, if the extensors of the vertebral column are relaxed, the rectus abdominis may act as a class 2 lever with the lumbar spine. In this case it could provide for anterior flexion, an action apparent during "sit-ups."

EXTERNAL ABDOMINAL OBLIQUE. The external oblique muscle is the thickest of the three muscles of the lateral abdominal wall and is also the most superficial (Figures 3-79, 3-82). It arises from the linea alba, the lateral half of the inguinal ligament, and the anterior half of the iliac crest. Its fibers are directed superolaterally and insert onto the inferior borders and superficial surfaces of the lower eight ribs.

The potential functions of this muscle are similar to those of the rectus abdominis. In addition, contraction of one side of the external oblique would result in circumflexion. That is, the thorax of the same side would be drawn downward and medially in a twisting motion (Figure 3-83). Owing to its large surface area, the external oblique has greater potential to affect abdominal pressure and thus greater potential as an antagonist to the diaphragm than the rectus muscle.

3-82. *External abdominal oblique muscle.*

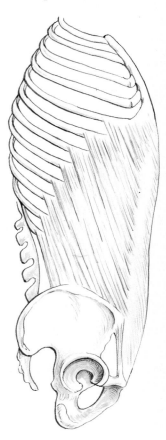

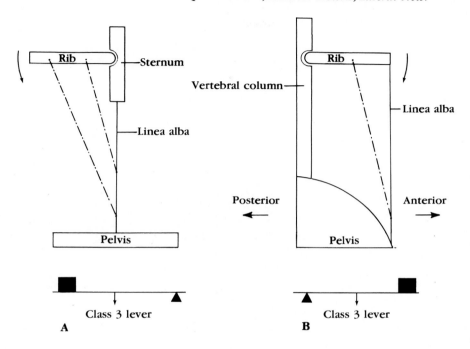

3-83. *Functional potential of the external abdominal oblique muscle. A, Anterior view. B, Lateral view.*

INTERNAL ABDOMINAL OBLIQUE. The internal oblique (Figure 3-84) lies deep to the external oblique and courses at nearly a right angle to it. It arises from the lateral half of the inguinal ligament, the anterior two-thirds of the iliac crest, and the lower part of the lumbodorsal fascia. Its fibers are directed principally superomedially and insert into the linea alba and onto the lower borders of the lowest three or four costal cartilages.

The functional potential of this muscle is similar to that of the external oblique (Figure 3-85). The exception is that if one side were to contract, it would draw the thorax of the opposite side downward and medially.

3-84. *A, Anterolateral thoracoabdominal wall, right side, external abdominal muscle removed. IAO, internal abdominal oblique muscle; AA, abdominal aponeurosis; IC, iliac crest; IL, inguinal ligament. B, Internal abdominal oblique muscle.*

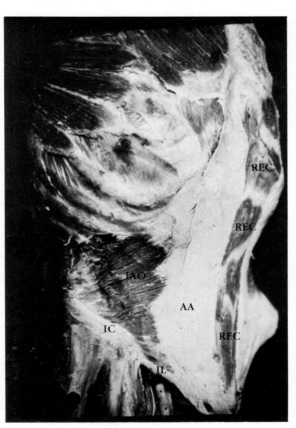

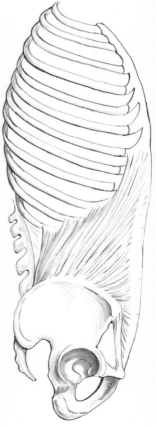

A   B

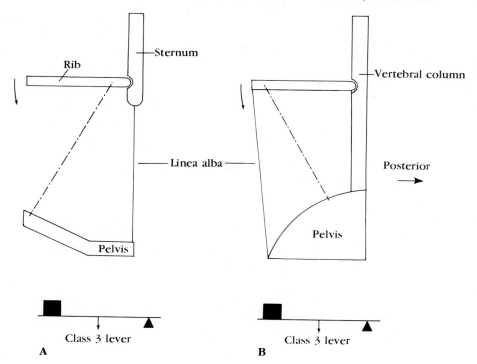

3-85. *Functional potential of the internal abdominal oblique muscle. A, Anterior view. B, lateral view.*

3-86. *Transverse abdominal muscle.*

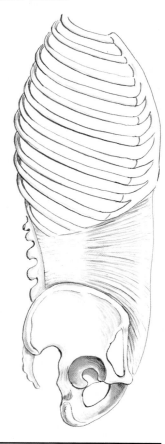

3-87. *Functional potential of the transverse abdominal muscle.*

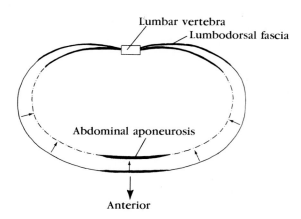

TRANSVERSE ABDOMINAL. The transverse abdominal (Figure 3-86) is the deepest and thinnest of the three lateral abdominal muscles. It arises from the lumbodorsal fascia, the anterior three-fourths of the iliac crest, and lateral third of the inguinal ligament. Its fibers fan out superiorly and inferiorly, but are principally horizontal. They insert into the linea alba and the deep surfaces of the lower six costal cartilages, where they interdigitate with fibers of the diaphragm.

The transverse abdominal muscle can be thought of as encircling the abdomen from the lumbar area of one side to the lumbar area of the other with an intermediate tendon (the abdominal aponeurosis) at midline (Figure 3-87). Its only apparent functional potential, unlike other abdominal muscles, is to act as antagonist to the diaphragm, either in respiration or in increasing abdominal pressure. It does not appear to be capable of postural adjustments.

Innervation

The muscles of the neck and trunk are innervated by spinal nerves that exit from the spinal cord and typically supply muscles at or near the level of exit. A long muscle commonly receives innervation from a number of spinal nerves. Table 3-1 shows the pattern of motor innervation for the muscles covered in this chapter. In general, successively lower muscles of the trunk are innervated by spinal nerves from successively lower segments of the spinal cord. An exception is the innervation of the diaphragm, which will be discussed later. Note that the subcostals, costal levators, and intercostals are innervated by a nerve from each thoracic segment. Each spinal nerve is named for the vertebra above its exit. An exception is the cervical area, where the first cervical nerve (C-1) exits above the atlas. Thus there are eight cervical nerves. In the adult, the spinal cord is shorter than the vertebral column. Thus, the corresponding levels of the cord and column do not match, particularly in the lower part of the cord.

In the cervical and lumbar areas, the spinal nerves join and branch to form **plexuses.** A

Table 3-1. Innervation Patterns of Muscles of Respiration

Muscle	Spinal Nerves																					
	C-1	C-2	C-3	C-4	C-5	C-6	C-7	C-8	T-1	T-2	T-3	T-4	T-5	T-6	T-7	T-8	T-9	T-10	T-11	T-12	L-1	L-2
Sternocleidomastoid	X	X																				
Trapezius	X	X	X																			
Scalenes		X	X	X	X	X	X	X														
Iliocostalis cervicis				X	X	X	X	X	X	X	X	X										
Diaphragm			X	X	X																	
Subclavius					X	X												X	X	X		
Serratus anterior					X	X	X															
Pectoralis major					X	X	X	X	X													
Pectoralis minor						X	X	X														
Lastissimus dorsi						X	X	X														
Serratus posterior superior										X	X											
Transverse thoracic										X	X	X	X	X								
Costal levators								X	X	X	X	X	X	X	X							
Iliocostalis thoracis									X	X	X	X	X	X	X	X	X	X	X			
Subcostals									X	X	X	X	X	X	X	X	X	X	X			
Intercostals									X	X	X	X	X	X	X	X	X	X	X			
Rectus abdominis															X	X	X	X	X	X		
Transverse abdominal															X	X	X	X	X	X	X	
Iliocostalis lumborum															X	X	X	X	X	X	X	
External abdominal oblique																X	X	X	X	X	X	X
Internal Abdominal oblique																X	X	X	X	X	X	
Serratus Posterior inferior																	X	X	X	X		
Quadratus lumborum																				X	X	X

123

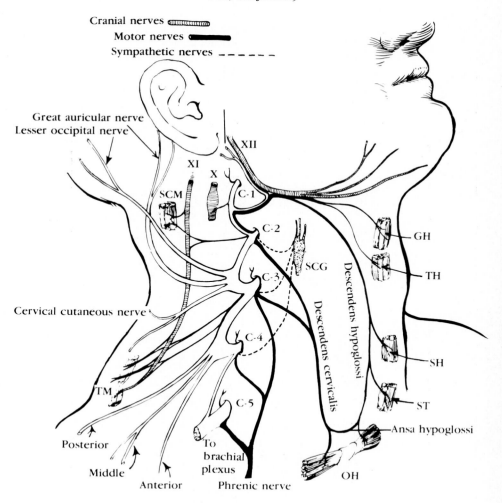

3-88. *Left, Cervical plexus. SCM, sternocleidomastoid muscle; TM, trapezius muscle; SCG, superior cervical ganglion; GH, geniohyoid muscle; TH, thyrohyoid muscle; SH, sternohyoid muscle; ST, sternothyroid muscle; OH, omohyoid muscle. Right, Brachial plexus. MAC, medial antebrachial cutaneous nerve; MBC, medial brachial cutaneous nerve; IN, intercostal nerves; LP, lateral pectoral nerve; MP, medial pectoral nerve. The upper part of the brachial plexus is labelled to show the organization of the plexus into roots (R), trunks (T), divisions (D), cords (C), and nerves (N). (Modified, with permission, after Chusid JG:* Correlative Neuroanatomy and Functional Neurology, *17th ed. Copyright 1979 by Lange Medical Publications, Los Altos, California.)*

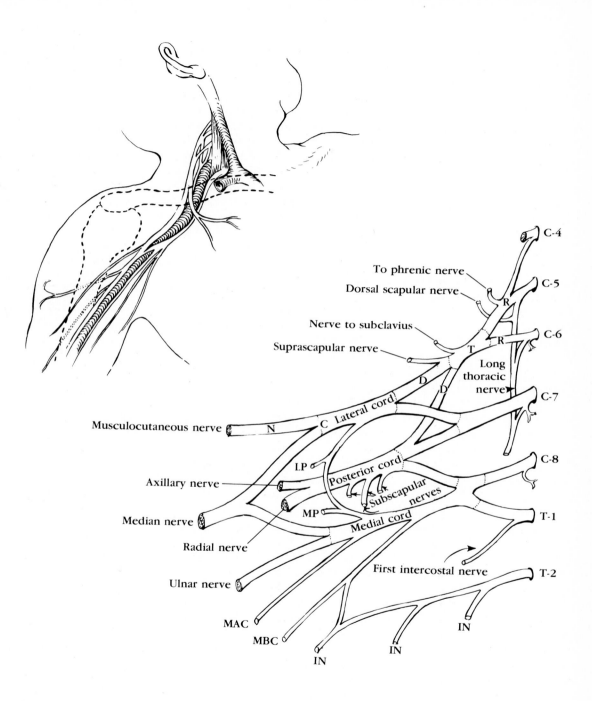

number of nerves, some of which are named for the course they take, are a combination of two or more spinal nerves. In the cervical area there are two nerve plexuses: the cervical plexus and the brachial plexus. These are summarized in diagrammatic form in Figure 3-88. The **brachial plexus** supplies the muscles of the arm, while the **cervical plexus** supplies many of the muscles of the neck. One of the nerves formed from the cervical plexus is a combination of branches from C-1 to C-5. These branches rise together as the **spinal accessory nerve.** The spinal accessory nerve ascends the neck, passes through the **foramen magnum** (the hole in the skull through which the spinal cord passes) and joins the eleventh cranial nerve (**accessory nerve**). This combined nerve then descends and divides again. The cranial portion joins the tenth cranial nerve, while the spinal portion descends to innervate the sternocleidomastoid muscle and the trapezius muscle.

Another nerve from the cervical plexus is formed from branches of C-3, C-4, and C-5; called the **phrenic (diaphragmatic) nerve,** it descends to a large portion of the diaphragm. The remainder of the diaphragm is innervated by **intercostal nerves,** which arise from the ventral rami of spinal nerves. This is an important protective mechanism. Injury to the spinal cord in the lower cervical or thoracic region may disrupt the muscles of costal respiration, but only a high cervical lesion will denervate the diaphragm.

The specific innervations to each of the muscles of respiration are listed in Table 3-2.

Functional Potential for Respiration

It is apparent from the preceding information that a large number of muscles have potential for respiratory movements. From a biomechanical standpoint, some of these muscles have potential for inhalation and others for exhalation. Within each of these two groups some muscles have greater potential or a higher probability of respiratory function than others. However, we must remember that determination of degree of functional potential does not, in itself, tell us which muscles actually perform specific functions. Nonetheless, such determinations will be of assis-

tance in guiding our way through the physiological evidence that will be presented later in this chapter.

INHALATION. Studies of the patterns of respiratory motion cited earlier in this chapter have demonstrated that inhalation can be accomplished by elevation-expansion of the rib cage and/or lowering of the diaphragm. There has been general agreement that the diaphragmatic action typically predominates. Because the muscular fibers of the

Table 3-2. Specific Innervation of Muscles of Respiration

Muscle	Innervation
Sternocleidomastoid	C2–C4 (spinal accessory)
Scalenes	C2–C8
Pectoralis major	C5–C8 (anterior thoracic nerve)
Pectoralis minor	C5–C8 (anterior thoracic nerve)
Subclavius	C5–C6
Serratus anterior	T2–T3, C5–7 (long thoracic nerve)
Intercostals	T1–T11
Transverse thoracic	T2–T6
Trapezius	C1–C5 (spinal accessory)
Latissimus dorsi	C6–C8 (thoracodorsal nerve, C7–C8)
Serratus posterior superior	T2–T3
Serratus posterior inferior	T9–T12
Sacrospinals	C4–L2
Costal levators	C8–T11
Quadratus lumborum	T12–L2
Subcostals	T1–T11
Diaphragm	C3–C5 (phrenic nerve), T10–T12
Rectus abdominis	T7–T12
External abdominal oblique	T8–L1
Internal abdominal oblique	T8–L1
Transverse abdominal	T7–T12

diaphragm are vertical, diaphragmatic contraction could result in elevation of the inferior margin of the rib cage as well as descent of the central tendon. In addition, the nonrespiratory function of the diaphragm (increasing abdominal pressure) normally takes place during suspended respiration. Thus, of all of the individual muscles studied, the diaphragm has the greatest independent potential for inhalation.

Muscles with potential for rib cage elevation and expansion include the scalenes, sternocleidomastoid, pectoralis minor, external intercostals, interchondral part of the internal intercostals, serratus anterior, serratus posterior superior, iliocostalis cervicis, and costal levators. A number of these have obvious potential for postural adjustment that would have to be eliminated by stabilization in order for them to function in respiration. These include

Scalenes—Lateral flexion of the cervical spine
Sternocleidomastoid—Rotation and tilting of the head
Pectoralis minor—Depression of the shoulder
Serratus anterior—Anterior movement and rotation of the shoulder
Iliocostalis cervicis—Lateral flexion and possibly extension of the spine

Two of these muscles, the serratus anterior and, to a lesser extent, the sternocleidomastoid, pull at an angle quite oblique to the direction of rib motion. Of the other muscles, the serratus posterior superior would function at a considerable mechanical disadvantage because of its oblique angle and its function as a class 3 lever. Thus, it would need to exert considerable power to function primarily in rib cage elevation; it is, however, a very thin, short muscle. The costal levators function at a very considerable mechanical disadvantage with their attachment at the fulcrum of movement. It is possible that all of the back muscles work together in postural movements.

It has been suggested that the intercostals may also serve a postural function with the intercostals of one side providing lateral flexion of the spine by decreasing the distances between the ribs on that side. Simultaneous contraction of the external and internal intercostals would be necessary and may result in fixation rather than compression of the ribs.

From the foregoing discussion, the external and interchondral internal intercostals appear to have the greatest probability of providing for rib cage elevation-expansion for several reasons: This may be their singular function, they are uniquely able to act on the entire rib cage, and they have the mechanical capability to provide the required function.

The question then arises as to whether muscles that can lift the rib cage from structures external to it provide the primary force that is translated to the entire rib cage by the intercostals. Of all of the muscles available, two stand out as having a high degree of potential for rib cage elevation because of their vector of pull and their anterior or lateral (rather than posterior) attachment to the ribs. These are the scalenes and the pectoralis minor.

EXHALATION. This process requires muscles that are antagonistic to the diaphragm and/or depress the rib cage. The abdominal muscles, as a group, have the potential for providing both of these functions. Other muscles that may have potential for rib cage lowering are the interosseous internal intercostals, transverse thoracic, subcostals, serratus posterior inferior, iliocostalis lumborum, and quadratus lumborum. The latter three muscles may be more important in postural adjustments than in respiration. Analysis of the potential of serratus posterior inferior and iliocostalis lumborum parallels the analysis of the serratus posterior superior and iliocostalis cervicis. The transverse thoracic and subcostal muscles seem to have limited capacity for independently producing motion of the rib cage because of their limited extent, but are mechanically similar to the internal intercostals.

Of all of the muscles listed above, two stand out as having a high probability of having a principal function in respiration. The interosseous internal intercostals assume importance for the reasons discussed with regard to the external intercostals.

The transverse abdominal muscle is the only one of the abdominal groups that does not have an obvious potential for postural movements but rather seems capable only of increasing abdominal pressure. However, if lowering of the rib cage requires muscles that attach external to the rib cage, the abdominal oblique muscles and the rectus abdominis are obviously capable of providing the necessary force while also aiding in abdominal compression.

The above discussion has omitted consideration of the pectoralis major, subclavius, and latissimus dorsi. None of these muscles appear to have potential for respiratory activity.

Electromyographic Evidence

For a number of the muscles considered in this chapter there is insufficient electromyographic data to draw any conclusions. These are the subclavius, subcostals, serratus posterior superior and inferior, the iliocostals, costal levators, and quadratus lumborum. Most studies of the lateral abdominal muscles have viewed them as a unit, and no separate data are available for the external oblique, internal oblique, and transverse abdominal muscles.

The latissimus dorsi was found to be inactive at rest and at moderate levels of respiration [4]. The serratus anterior is inactive even at high levels of ventilation [4,7]. Four of the muscles studied are electrically active during respiration, but only at the end of maximum inhalation. These are the sternocleidomastoid muscles [5,22], pectoralis major and minor, and trapezius muscles [4]. It is not reasonable to term a muscle respiratory solely on the basis of its activity at the extremes of vital capacity. Many muscles that serve a bracing function, including those of the back and legs, may be active at the extremes of respiratory effort. If we are to understand respiration, it behooves us to look for those muscles for which there is evidence of direct involvement in the respiratory process. For instance, while the sternocleidomastoids can be seen to contract during extreme respiratory distress, they do not, acting alone, prevent cyanosis [9].

There is some evidence that the scalenes are ac-
tive during inhalation. Some investigators [5,17, 18,22] report scalene activity even during quiet inhalation. Others [25,26] fail to support this. Campbell [5] found activity to occur when tidal volume exceeded 2 liters (quiet tidal volume is 0.5 liter) with ventilation in excess of 40 liters per minute (quiet ventilation is 7 to 8 liters per minute). It is interesting to note that the degree of rib motion is not affected in some patients who have had the scalenes surgically removed [16]. Thus, while the scalenes may be functional during costal respiration, they are not essential to it.

The intercostal muscles have been studied extensively [6,8,19]. There is ample data to support Hamberger's hypothesis [12], that is, that the external and interchondral internal intercostals are inspiratory, while the interosseous internal intercostals are expiratory. There is further evidence that only the intercostals in the upper intercostal spaces function in quiet respiration. Intercostals in successively lower intercostal spaces are recruited as the depth of respiration is increased. The external intercostals are active for inhalation and gradually reduce their contraction during the initial stages of exhalation for speech as predicted by the muscle pressure studies cited previously. The internal (interosseous) intercostals contract only when relaxation pressure is insufficient to account for necessary alveolar pressure. In addition, it has been observed that activity of the external intercostals is linearly related to the total inhalatory muscle force [6]. Evidence from the work of Sears and Davis [23] suggests that responses to changes in load on the respiratory system during speech are controlled at least in part reflexively by the activity of muscle spindles in the intercostals and the associated gamma efferent system.

The transverse thoracic muscle has been found to be active during forced exhalation [24] and probably functions with the interosseous internal intercostals. In this activity the transverse thoracic complements the latter muscles in the interchondral spaces.

There is ample evidence from many sources that the diaphragm is a principal muscle of inhalation [6]. The degree to which its contraction may elevate the rib cage in addition to lowering the cen-

Table 3-3. Summary of Evidence for Muscle Function for Inhalation

Muscle	Functional Potential		Electromyographic Evidence			
	Possible	Probable	Rest	Normal Speech	Effort	Maximum Effort
Diaphragm	+	+	+	+	+	+
External intercostals	+	+	+	+	+	+
Internal intercostals (interchondral)	+	+	+	+	+	+
Scalenes	+	+	±	+	+	+
Sternocleidomastoid	+	−	−	−	−	+
Pectoralis major	−	−	−	−	−	+
Pectoralis minor	+	+	−	−	−	+
Serratus posterior superior	+	−				
Iliocostalis cervicis	+	−				
Costal levators	+	+				
Trapezius	+	−	−	−	−	+
Subclavius	−	−				
Serratus anterior	+	−	−	−	−	−
Latissimus dorsi	−	−	−	−		

Table 3-4. Summary of Evidence for Muscle Function in Exhalation

Muscle	Functional Potential		Electromyographic Evidence			
	Possible	Probable	Rest	Normal Speech	Effort	Maximum Effort
Internal intercostals (interosseous)	+	+	−	+	+	+
Transverse thoracic	+	+			+	+
Rectus abdominis	+	+	−	−	+	+
External abdominal oblique	+	+	−	−	+	+
Internal abdominal oblique	+	+				
Transverse abdominal	+	+				
Serratus posterior inferior	+	−				
Quadratus lumborum	+	−				
Subcostals	+	+				
Iliocostalis lumborum	+	−				
Latissimus dorsi	−	−	−	−		

tral tendon is a matter of speculation. As discussed previously, however, its contraction moves the respiratory system along the relaxation line, suggesting that it does act on the rib cage to some degree.

The rectus abdominis has been found to contract at the end of a long utterance and during loud speech [8]. It comes into play after the internal intercostals and is followed in activity by the external abdominal oblique.

The summary presented in Tables 3-3 and 3-4 show that a great deal is still unknown about specific muscle function in respiration. The importance of the diaphragm and the intercostals is clear. Other muscles, such as the scalenes in inhalation and the transverse abdominal in exhalation, probably come into play in conversational speech, but the evidence is incomplete.

REFERENCES

1. Agostoni E: Action of respiratory muscles. In Fenn WO, Rahn H (Eds): *Handbook of Physiology, Section 3: Respiration, Vol. I.* Washington, DC, American Physiological Society, 1964.
2. Agostoni E, Mead J: Status of the respiratory system. In Fenn WO, Rahn H (Eds): *Handbook of Physiology, Section 3: Respiration, Vol. I.* Washington, DC, American Physiological Society, 1964.
3. Bloomer HH: A roentgenographic study of the mechanics of respiration. *Speech Monographs* 3:118, 1936.
4. Campbell EJM: The muscular control of breathing in man. University of London, PhD dissertation, 1954.
5. Campbell EJM: The role of the scalene and sternomastoid muscles in breathing in normal subjects. An electromyographic study. *J Anat* 89:378, 1955.
6. Campbell EJM, Agostoni E, Davis JN: *The Respiratory Muscles, Mechanics and Neural Control.* Philadelphia, WB Saunders, 1970.
7. Catton WT, Gray JE: Electromyographic study of the action of the serratus anterior muscle in respiration. *J Anat* 85:412, 1951.
8. Draper MH, Ladefoged P, Whitteridge D: Respiratory muscles in speech. *J Speech Hear Res* 2:16, 1959.
9. Duchenne GBA: *Physiologie des mouvements démontrée à l'aide de l'expérimentation électrique et de l'observation clinique, et applicable à l'étude des paralysies et des déformations.* Paris, Baillière, 1887.
10. Ganong WF: *Review of Medical Physiology.* Los Altos, Calif., Lange Medical Publications, 1979.
11. Goldman M, Mead J: The passive volume-pressure characteristics of the rib cage. *Physiologist* 13:208, 1970.
12. Hamberger GE: Dissertatio de respirationis mechanismo et usu genuino. Jena, Germany, 1748.
13. Hixon TJ: Some new techniques for measuring the biomechanical events of speech production. One laboratory's experience. *ASHA Reports* 7:68, 1972.
14. Hixon TJ: Respiratory function in speech. In Minifie FD, Hixon TJ, Williams F (Eds): *Normal Aspects of Speech, Hearing, and Language.* Englewood Cliffs, Prentice-Hall, 1973.
15. Hixon TJ, Goldman MD, Mead J: Kinematics of the chest wall during speech production: Volume displacements of the rib cage, abdomen, and lung. *J Speech Hear Res* 16:78, 1973.
16. Joly H, Vincent Ph-A: Rôle respiratoire des muscles scalènes et inter-costaux étudié en fonction de la collapsotherapie pulmonaire. *Arch Med-Chir Appar Resp* 12:392, 1937.
17. Jones DS, Beargie RJ, Pauly JE: An electromyographic study of some muscles of costal respiration in man. *Anat Rec* 117:17, 1953.
18. Jones DS, Pauly JE: Further electromyographic studies on muscles of costal respiration in man. *Anat Rec* 128:733, 1957.
19. McClung JA: An electromyographic investigation of the internal intercostal muscles during respiration. University of Pittsburgh, PhD dissertation, 1970.
20. Mead J, Agostoni E: Dynamics of breathing. In Fenn WO, and Rahn H (Eds): *Handbook of Physiology, Section 3: Respiration, Vol. I.* Washington, DC, American Physiological Society, 1964.
21. Pappenheimer JR, Comroe JH Jr, Cournand A, Ferguson JKW, Filley GF, Fowler WS, Gray JS, Helmholz HF Jr, Otis AB, Rahn H, Riley RL: Standardization of definitions and symbols in respiratory physiology. *Fed Proc* 9:602, 1950.
22. Raper AJ, Thompson WT, Shapiro W, Patterson JL Jr: Scalene and sternomastoid muscle function. *J Appl Physiol* 21:497, 1966.
23. Sears TA, Davis JN: The control of respiratory muscles during voluntary breathing. *Ann NY Acad Sci* 155:183, 1968.
24. Taylor A: The contribution of the intercostal muscles to the effort of respiration in man. *J Physiol (Lond)* 151:390, 1960.
25. Thompson WT Jr, Patterson JL, Shapiro W: Observations on the scalene respiratory muscles. *Arch. Intern. Med.* 113:856, 1964.
26. Varene P, Richard P, Jacquemin C: Electromyography of the diaphragm during transverse accelerations in man. *CR Acad Sci* [D] (*Paris*) 256:4975, 1963.

The **larynx** is the organ of phonation. Located in the anterior part of the neck at the top of the trachea, it serves three functions: airway protection, pressure-valving, and phonation. Within the larynx there are two pairs of folds, one muscular and one glandular, which extend into the airway from the side walls of the larynx. These folds can be approximated to prevent or restrict airflow, or separated to permit airflow.

The larynx is suspended by membranes, ligaments, and muscles from a free-floating bone, the hyoid bone, which is horseshoe-shaped and positioned in the neck just below the tongue. The hyoid bone is in turn suspended from the skull by muscles and ligaments (Figure 4-1).

The larynx is surrounded on three sides, posteriorly and laterally, by the lower part of the pharynx (Figure 4-2). The pharyngeal spaces lateral to the larynx are called the **pyriform sinuses.** The entire area of the pharynx surrounding the larynx, including the pyriform sinuses, is called the **laryngopharynx.** The anterior wall of the larynx extends superiorly behind the root of the tongue. This superior extension of the anterior wall of the larynx is formed from a leaf-shaped cartilage called the **epiglottis.** The posterior wall of the larynx does not extend as far superiorly as does the anterior wall. Thus the larynx opens posteriorly into the pharynx.

The pharynx empties into the esophagus at the same level that the larynx empties into the trachea (Figure 4-3). Thus the larynx lies within the anterior pharynx, and the trachea lies anterior to the esophagus. The esophagus passes inferiorly through the thoracic cavity and diaphragm to the stomach.

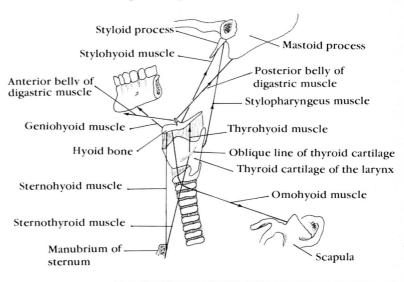

4-1. *Suspension of the hyoid bone and larynx. (Adapted from an original painting by Frank H. Netter, M.D. from CLINICAL SYMPOSIA, copyright by CIBA Pharmaceutical Company, Division of CIBA-GEIGY Corporation.)*

Styloid process

Stylohyoid muscle

Mastoid process

Anterior belly of digastric muscle

Posterior belly of digastric muscle

Stylopharyngeus muscle

Geniohyoid muscle

Thyrohyoid muscle

Hyoid bone

Oblique line of thyroid cartilage

Thyroid cartilage of the larynx

Sternohyoid muscle

Omohyoid muscle

Sternothyroid muscle

Manubrium of sternum

Scapula

4-2. *Posterior view of the pharynx with its posterior wall opened.*

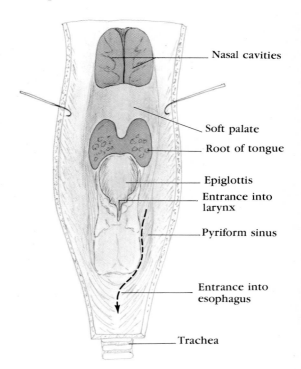

Nasal cavities

Soft palate

Root of tongue

Epiglottis

Entrance into larynx

Pyriform sinus

Entrance into esophagus

Trachea

TOPOGRAPHY OF THE LARYNX

In sagittal section, the folds within the larynx are revealed (Figure 4-4). The superior folds are called the **ventricular folds** and are glandular. The inferior folds are called the **vocal folds** and are muscular. Each vocal fold contains a longitudinal muscle called the **vocalis muscle.** The superior opening of the larynx is called the **laryngeal aditus.** The **aryepiglottic folds** form the lateral rim of the laryngeal aditus. The **vestibule** of the larynx is its superior part bounded above by the aditus and below by the ventricular folds. That portion of the larynx between the level of the ventricular folds and the level of the vocal folds is called the **ventricle.** That part of the larynx below the vocal folds is called the **inferior division.** The space between the paired vocal folds is the **glottis.**

4-4. *Midsagittal section through the larynx.*

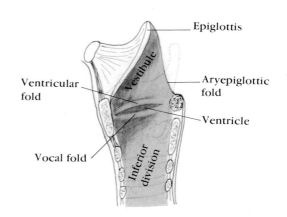

4-3. *Sagittal section through the head and neck showing the airway (solid line) and food channel (dashed line).*

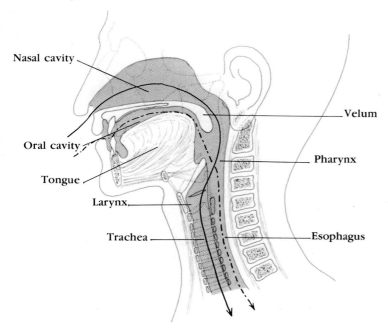

The ventricle of the larynx (Figure 4-5) was first described in detail by Morgagni in 1741 and so is frequently called the **ventricle of Morgagni.** Laterally, the ventricle opens into a small sac, the **laryngeal saccule** (also called the **laryngeal appendix**), on each side. The lining of the saccule contains numerous mucosal glands, which supply mucus to the area of the vocal folds.

The entire airway of the larynx is lined with mucous membrane, which is continuous with that of the pharynx above and the trachea below. The mucous membrane lining most of the airway is covered by columnar epithelium, with the exception of the superior part of the ventricular fold, the medial part of the vocal fold, and the superior half of the epiglottis, which are covered by stratified squamous epithelium. As we will see, those parts of the vocal and ventricular folds covered by squamous epithelium are the parts that come into contact during laryngeal function.

FUNCTIONS OF THE LARYNX

Figure 4-6 shows the vocal folds in the open and closed positions. When the vocal folds are open, the glottis is wedge-shaped, with the vocal folds approximated anteriorly and widely separated posteriorly. The posterior ends of the vocal folds are attached to the arytenoid cartilages, which can move the posterior ends of the vocal folds toward each other (adduction) or away from each other (abduction). The ventricular folds attach to the same cartilages and can also be adducted and abducted.

Airway Protection

As can be seen from Figure 4-3, the food channel, from the mouth to the esophagus, and the airway, from the nose and mouth to the larynx, cross paths in human beings. This is not true in some animals where the larynx projects upward into the nasopharynx. Such an animal (for instance, a cat)

4-5. *Coronal section of a human fetal larynx.*

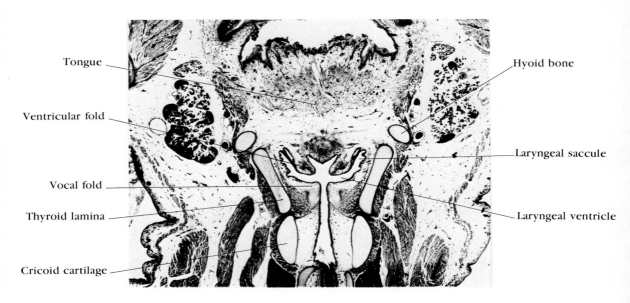

Tongue

Ventricular fold

Vocal fold

Thyroid lamina

Cricoid cartilage

Hyoid bone

Laryngeal saccule

Laryngeal ventricle

can drink and breathe simultaneously. However, human beings must close off the laryngeal airway during swallowing to prevent food from entering the trachea and lungs. When the larynx is closed for swallowing, the ventricular folds and vocal folds are both approximated. At the same time, the larynx is elevated and the laryngopharynx is enlarged. The elevation of the larynx causes much of the liquified food to pass around the epiglottis into the pyriform sinuses and from there into the esophagus (Figure 4-7).

Pressure-Valving

Under certain circumstances, the larynx closes off in order to prevent air from entering or leaving the lungs, a function that will be referred to here as pressure-valving. In the preceding chapter it was learned that the abdominal muscles contract to increase abdominal pressure during forceful urina-

tion, defecation, vomiting, and while "pushing" during childbirth. When high levels of abdominal pressure are required, the larynx closes both to prevent elevation of the diaphragm and to stabilize the rib cage against the pull of the abdominal muscles. (Of course, the larynx must also close during vomiting to prevent stomach contents from entering the lungs.) The larynx also closes to fix the rib cage during heavy lifting, since muscles such as pectoralis major and serratus anterior attach to the rib cage.

Pressure-valving is also used to build up high levels of subglottic pressure prior to coughing. Sudden opening of the larynx coincident with high subglottic pressure results in a rapid forceful expulsion of air in an attempt to remove foreign material from the larynx. Pressure-valving involves approximation of both the ventricular folds and the vocal folds.

4-6. Superior view of the vocal folds. A, Open position (abduction); B, Closed position (adduction).

4-7. Posterior view of the oropharyngeal food passage via the pyriform sinuses and laryngopharynx to the esophagus.

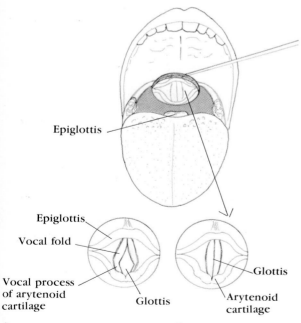

Epiglottis

Epiglottis

Vocal fold

Vocal process of arytenoid cartilage

Glottis

Glottis

Arytenoid cartilage

A   B

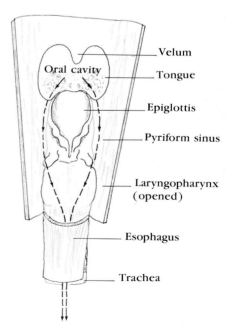

Velum

Oral cavity

Tongue

Epiglottis

Pyriform sinus

Laryngopharynx (opened)

Esophagus

Trachea

Phonation

As discussed in Chapter 1, the larynx acts as a sound generator by rapidly opening and closing the airway, thus interrupting the breath stream. This activity is a function of the vocal folds. During respiration, the laryngeal airway is open (Figure 4-8). At the initiation of phonation, the vocal folds are adducted, or nearly so, and exhalation begins. The obstruction to airflow caused by the approximated vocal folds creates an increase in subglottic pressure. Subglottic pressure increases until it is sufficient to overcome the muscular and elastic

---

4-8. *Coronal view of vocal fold activity in phonation.*

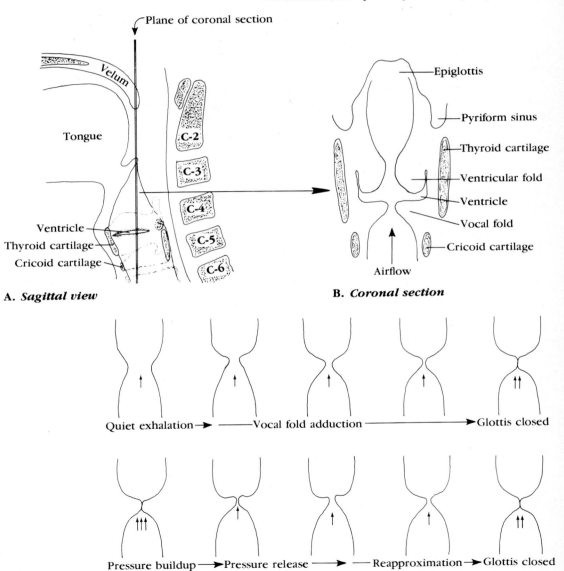

forces holding the vocal folds in approximation. When subglottic pressure is sufficient, the vocal folds are "blown" apart. The subglottic pressure is thus released, and the vocal folds reapproximate owing to the original adductory force, which is maintained, and to aerodynamic factors. This begins the same cycle again. Each cycle of activity takes less than 10 msec.

Two aerodynamic forces operate on the vocal folds during phonation. One of these is the subglottic pressure referred to above [43]. The other is the law of energy conservation, which states that velocity and pressure of an airstream are inversely related. That is, as the velocity of an airstream increases, its pressure drops. This is important to laryngeal function because of the configuration of the subglottic airway. The airway narrows as it approaches the partially approximated vocal folds; thus the velocity of the airstream increases and is greatest at the glottis. Air pressure drops as the airstream approaches and traverses the glottis. The negative pressure within the glottis draws the vocal folds toward one another. This relationship between velocity and pressure is called the **Bernoulli effect.**

The response of the vocal folds to the aerodynamic events is controlled, in large part, by their elasticity. The elasticity of the vocal folds can be modified by two means: either by stretching the vocal folds, or by increasing or decreasing the stiffness of the folds by varying the degree of contraction of the vocal muscles. The stiffness of the vocal folds will increase if the vocal folds are stretched and/or if the vocalis muscles increase their contraction. An increase in stiffness of the vocal folds also changes the nature of their motion.

Radiological studies of the larynx have shown that at low pitch the vocal folds are relatively thick, have a larger area of approximation than at high pitch, and their motion suggests a low level of stiffness [16]. As can be seen in Figure 4-9, during the opening phase of their motion, the vocal folds begin to separate inferiorly while their upper parts are still in approximation. In the closing phase, the inferior part begins medial motion first. Another way of describing this activity is that there is a vertical phase difference in vocal fold motion.

As pitch rises, a number of changes take place. The vocal folds become longer and thinner (Figure 4-10), and motion suggests greater stiffness.

4-9. *Vocal fold motion during low pitch phonation.*

4-10. *Vocal fold motion during high pitch phonation.*

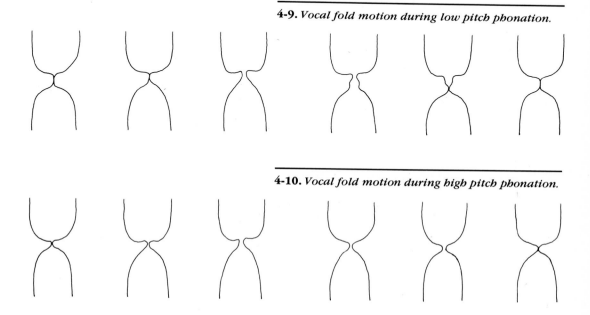

While at low pitch the entire fold seems to undulate during motion, at high pitch motion is limited to the medial parts of the folds and is more shutter-like. Ultraslow motion films of the larynx have shown that at very high pitch (falsetto) the anterior parts of the vocal folds vibrate while the posterior glottis remains closed [10] and only the medial edges of the anterior portions undergo motion.

There is also a longitudinal phase difference in vocal fold motion. During the opening phase, the posterior glottis typically opens first, with opening proceeding anteriorly. In the closing phase the posterior glottis typically closes last. However, there is a good deal of variability in the opening and closing pattern.

Phonation can be initiated with the glottis open or closed. In the first case, exhalation may begin as the vocal folds are in the process of being adducted. As the folds approach midline, the airflow through the glottis will gradually set the folds into vibration. Exhalation may not begin until the vocal folds are nearly adducted, with the folds separated by a few millimeters. In either of these cases, the initial movement of the vocal folds will be toward midline due to the Bernoulli effect. On the other hand, the vocal folds may be adducted into firm contact prior to initiation of the breath stream. In this case the initial motion will be away from midline as the folds are blown apart [30].

The activity of the larynx in producing sound as described thus far is called the **myoelastic aerodynamic theory** of voice production, since it involves the airstream setting the muscular vocal folds into vibration, while control of vibration frequency is by changes in length, mass, and stiffness of the vocal folds brought about by muscular activity. This theory, put forth by Müller in 1843, has been challenged only once since it was proposed. In 1950, Husson [22] claimed that the subglottic airstream was not necessary for vocal fold vibration and that vibration was caused, cycle by cycle, by muscular contractions. Husson's **neurochronaxic theory** has been disproven on two grounds. First, the musculature to provide the movement patterns seen during vocal fold vibra-

tion are not present [38]. Second, it has been demonstrated that vocal fold vibration does not occur in the absence of subglottic pressure [32]. In addition, extremely rapid trains of muscular contractions would be required over long periods of time to explain active vocal fold vibration, and even if this were possible, it would require enormous levels of energy.

Changes in subglottic pressure are responsible for changes in the amplitude of vocal fold vibration. It has been suggested that changes in subglottic pressure may also influence the frequency of vocal fold vibration [4,24]. However, the evidence obtained thus far is inconclusive [33].

It is perceptually apparent that there are voice quality differences across the pitch range of an individual. Such a difference exists, for example, between a "normal" voice and a falsetto voice. There has been considerable controversy in the literature with regard to the definition of those parts of the pitch range that are different from one another. These different "voices" are called **registers** and have been variably named as, for example, chest voice, head voice, falsetto, vocal fry, and modal register. There is also disagreement on how many registers there are. One definition of the boundary of two registers of the voice is that point in the pitch range at which a smooth transition of pitch is not possible. Hollien [17] suggested that ". . . before the existence of a particular register can be established, it must be operationally defined: (1) perceptually, (2) acoustically, (3) physiologically and (4) aerodynamically." On that basis he proposed that three registers can be identified. In order of ascending pitch, he called these "pulse," "modal," and "loft." His **pulse register** is what has frequently been called **glottal fry.** This is the lowest pitch range and is characterized by popping or pulsing as opposed to the smooth tone produced at higher frequencies. The typical pitch range a person uses is what Hollien calls **modal register. Loft** is his term for what is more commonly called **falsetto.**

Sonninen [40], Hollien [16], Hollien and Moore [21], and others have shown that in the modal register, vocal fold length within an individual is systematically and directly related to pitch. However, this does not seem to be the case in either pulse register [18] or in loft register [20,21]. Vocal fold thickness is inversely related to pitch in modal register [17] but is not consistently related to pitch outside of modal register [19].

It has been noted above that pitch rise is associated with vocal fold lengthening. This relationship can be demonstrated by plucking a rubber band while it is being stretched. Its rate of vibration will increase *even though* it is longer, because stretching causes an increase in its elasticity. On the other hand, if we compare two larynges, and one is larger and has longer vocal folds than the other, the larger larynx will be characterized by a lower pitch range than the smaller larynx. Thus, children have higher pitched voices than adults, and women typically have higher pitched voices than men.

CARTILAGINOUS FRAMEWORK

The major cartilages of the larynx are the thyroid cartilage, the cricoid cartilage, the paired arytenoid cartilages, and the epiglottic cartilage (Figure 4-11). Other small bits of cartilage, the corniculate and cuneiform cartilages, will also be examined.

Thyroid Cartilage

The thyroid cartilage is composed of two roughly quadrilateral plates of hyaline cartilage that are fused anteriorly (Figure 4-12). Each of the quadrilateral plates is called a **lamina,** and the line of fusion between the two laminae is called the **angle.** The fusion is incomplete superiorly, producing a **notch** superior to the angle. Immediately below the notch the angle is quite prominent, particularly in adult males, and can be felt and usually seen externally as the Adam's apple. From the angle, the two laminae diverge posteriorly so that their posterior borders are widely separated. The posterior border of each lamina extends into a relatively long **superior horn** and a relatively short **inferior horn.** The inferior horns are twisted so that their deep surfaces face anteromedially rather than posteromedially as do the deep surfaces of the laminae. An articular facet is located on the anteromedial surface of each inferior horn. These articular facets articulate with the cricoid cartilage and so are called **cricothyroid articular facets.** On the superficial surface of each lamina is a ridge called the **oblique line.** It extends from the superior border of the lamina near the root of the superior horn to the midpoint of the inferior border.

Many of the dimensions of the thyroid cartilage

4-11. *Laryngeal cartilages, midsagittal section.*

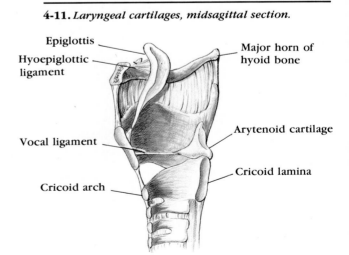

Epiglottis

Hyoepiglottic ligament

Major horn of hyoid bone

Vocal ligament

Arytenoid cartilage

Cricoid lamina

Cricoid arch

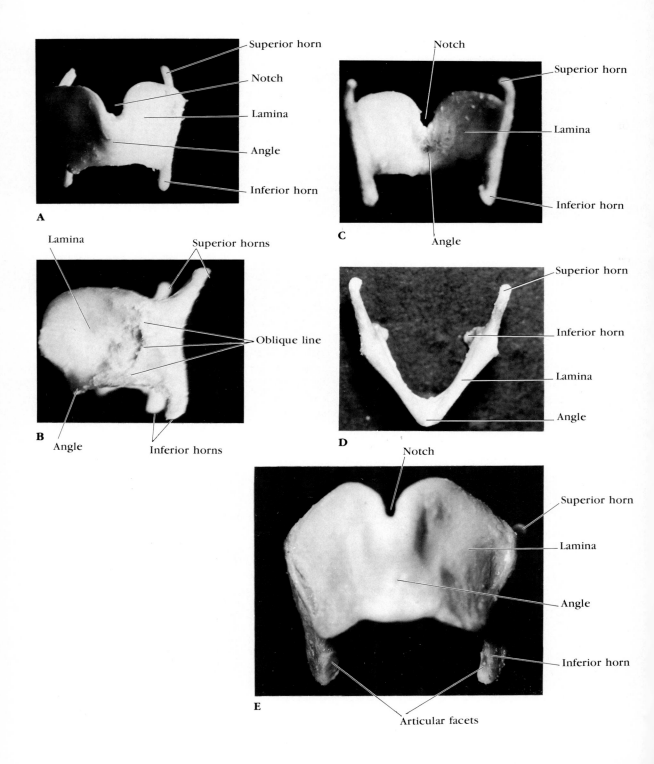

4-12. *Thyroid cartilage. A, Anterior view; B, Anterolateral view of the left side; C, Posterior view; D, Superior view; E, Anterior view showing the cricothyroid articular facets on the inferior horns; F, Inferior view showing the cricothyroid articular facets on the inferior horns; G, Lateral view of the left side showing articulation with the cricoid cartilage.*

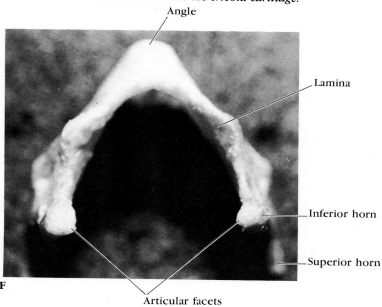

Angle

Lamina

Inferior horn

Superior horn

Articular facets

F

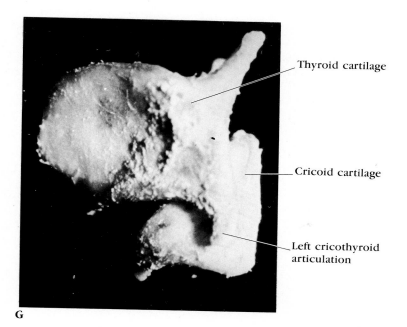

Thyroid cartilage

Cricoid cartilage

Left cricothyroid articulation

G

are extremely variable, including: the anterior height of the laminae; the distance between the left and right horns, both superior and inferior, measured at their distal points; and the anteroposterior dimension of the laminae. The length of the superior horns and the degree of separation of the laminae posteriorly are far less variable [27,29]. Maue [27] found obvious sex differences in the majority of her measurements of adult larynges, with those of the male larynx larger in all cases. In differentiating the male and female thyroid cartilages, the overall size, prominence of the angle, and weight of the cartilage were most notable. Also, the anterior angle formed by the laminae was rounded in the female in contrast to the male (Figure 4-13).

The average height of the thyroid cartilage from the tip of the superior horn to the tip of the inferior horn averages approximately 44 mm in the adult male and 38 mm in the female. The anteroposterior dimension of the thyroid cartilage averages 37 mm in the male and 29 mm in the female. The male thyroid cartilage is approximately double the weight of the female thyroid cartilage (8 g and 4 g, respectively) according to Maue and Dickson [29].

Cricoid Cartilage

The cricoid (Figure 4-14) is a ring of hyaline cartilage located at the top of the trachea, to which it attaches. The cricoid is frequently found to be fused with the first tracheal ring on one or both sides. The posterior aspect of the cricoid is enlarged into a **lamina** that is roughly hexagonal in shape when viewed from behind. The more anterior part of the ring is called the **arch.** The width, length, and laminar height of the cricoid are almost identical. Viewed from the side, the lateral surface of the cricoid cartilage on each side is marked by the **cricothyroid articular facet** near the junction of the arch and the lamina. These articular facets serve for articulation with the inferior horns of the thyroid cartilage. The superior rim of the lamina of the cricoid cartilage is rather short and ends on each side at the medial margin of the **cricoarytenoid articular facet.** The cricoarytenoid articular facets are angled downward laterally and anteriorly at approximately a 45-degree angle to the horizontal. These facets articulate with the arytenoid cartilages.

From the back, a vertical midline ridge is seen to separate the cricoid lamina into left and right halves. Inferiorly, this **posterior ridge** broadens and extends across the lamina from side to side, creating concavities on each side of the posterior aspect of the lamina.

Cricoid measurements in general are less variable within sexes than thyroid cartilage measurements. All measures taken by Maue [27,29] were larger in the male than in the female. The average laminar height was 25 mm for the male and 19 mm for the female. As with the thyroid cartilage, male cricoid weight (5.8 g) was double female cricoid weight (2.89 g).

4-13. *Differences in contour of male and female thyroid cartilages, superior view.*

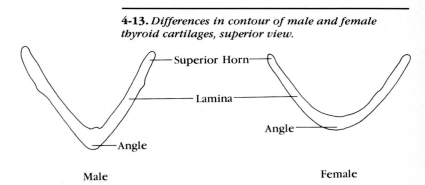

Male   Female

4-14. *Cricoid cartilage. A, Lateral view of the left side; B, Posterior view showing the lamina; C, Superior view; D, Posterior view showing articulations with the thyroid cartilage and the arytenoid cartilages.*

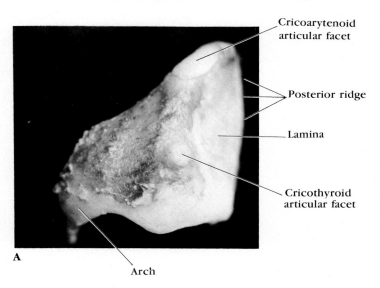

Cricoarytenoid
articular facet

Posterior ridge

Lamina

Cricothyroid
articular facet

A

Arch

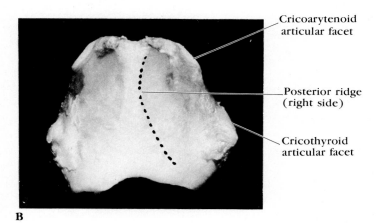

Cricoarytenoid
articular facet

Posterior ridge
(right side)

Cricothyroid
articular facet

B

4-14. *(continued)*

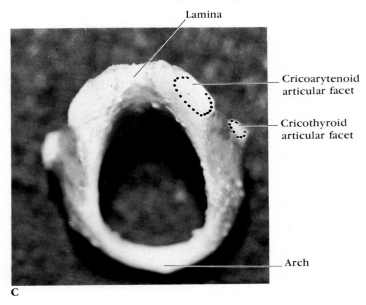

C

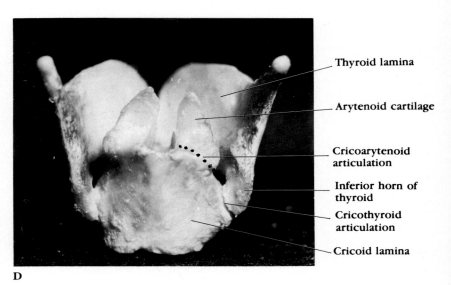

D

Arytenoid Cartilages

The two very small arytenoid cartilages (Figure 4-15) articulate with the cricoid cartilage. Each arytenoid is shaped roughly in the form of a pyramid with its **apex** located superiorly. Each has a flat **medial surface** that ends anteriorly in the **anterior ridge.** Posteriorly, each medial surface curves into the **dorsal surface,** which is concave from superior to inferior and which ends laterally in the **posterior ridge.** The third surface, called the **anterolateral surface,** extends from the posterior ridge to the anterior ridge. It contains a superior rounded depression called the **superior fossa** (also called the **triangular fossa**), and an

inferior depression called the **inferior fossa** (also called the **oval fossa**). The long axis of the oval lies in a horizontal plane. The anterior and posterior ridges meet superiorly at the apex. Anteriorly, the base of the arytenoid is elongated into the **vocal process.** The anterior ridge forms the superior border of the vocal process. The anterolateral surface of the vocal process forms the anteriormost part of the inferior fossa. The dorsolateral part of the base of the arytenoid is expanded into a large rounded **muscular process,** the dorsal surface of which is bisected by the posterior ridge. The **cricoarytenoid articular facet** is located on the inferior surface of the muscular process.

4-15. *Arytenoid cartilages. A, Anterior view showing the anterolateral surface of each cartilage; B, Inferomedial view of the left arytenoid; C, Posteromedial view of the right arytenoid; D, Posterior view of the right arytenoid; E, Superior view showing articulation with the cricoid cartilage; F, Lateral view of the left arytenoid showing articulation with the cricoid cartilage.*

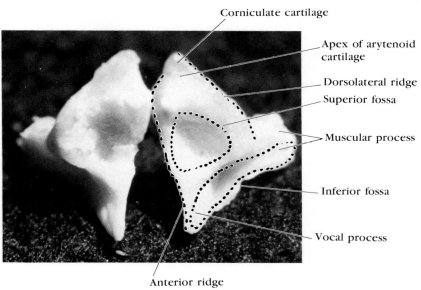

Corniculate cartilage

Apex of arytenoid cartilage

Dorsolateral ridge

Superior fossa

Muscular process

Inferior fossa

Vocal process

Anterior ridge

A

4-15. *(continued)*

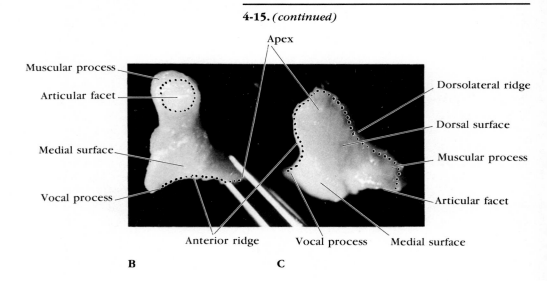

Apex

Muscular process

Articular facet

Medial surface

Vocal process

Dorsolateral ridge

Dorsal surface

Muscular process

Articular facet

Anterior ridge   Vocal process   Medial surface

B   C

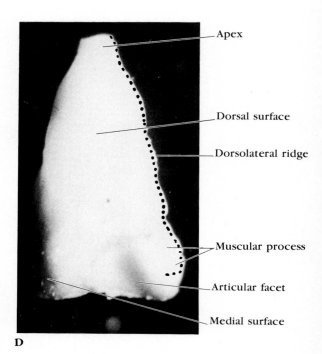

Apex

Dorsal surface

Dorsolateral ridge

Muscular process

Articular facet

Medial surface

D

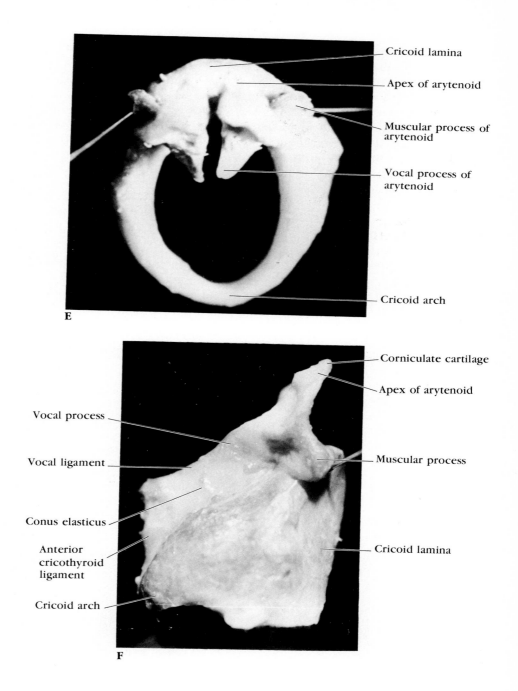

E

Cricoid lamina

Apex of arytenoid

Muscular process of arytenoid

Vocal process of arytenoid

Cricoid arch

F

Corniculate cartilage

Apex of arytenoid

Vocal process

Vocal ligament

Muscular process

Conus elasticus

Anterior cricothyroid ligament

Cricoid lamina

Cricoid arch

Maue [27] reported an extraordinary degree of similarity among all of the arytenoid cartilages she examined from 20 male and 20 female adult larynges. However, the male arytenoid was larger in all dimensions than the female. The average height of the arytenoid was 18 mm in the male and 13 mm in the female. The average anteroposterior measure was 14 mm in the male and 10 mm in the female. The male-female arytenoid weights showed a 2:1 ratio; 0.39 g in the male and 0.20 g in the female.

Corniculate Cartilages

The corniculate cartilages are two small roughly cone-shaped bits of elastic cartilage which lie on the apices of the arytenoid cartilages (see Figure 4-15). They extend the apex dorsomedially, and may be fused to it.

Cuneiform Cartilages

The cuneiform cartilages are small rod-shaped bits of cartilage that vary in number and lie in the aryepiglottic fold that extends from the apex of the arytenoid to the epiglottis.

Epiglottis

The epiglottis (Figure 4-16) is shaped like an inverted and flattened teardrop. It is composed of one or more pieces of elastic cartilage and lies with its flattened surfaces facing anteriorly and posteriorly. Its inferior point is attached by a ligament to the deep surface of the angle of the thyroid cartilage below the thyroid notch. This

---

4-16. *Epiglottis. A, Posterior surface; B, Midsagittal section.*

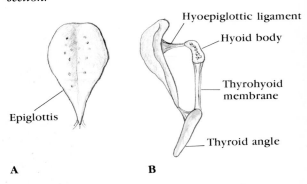

4-17. *Cricothyroid joint. A, Asymmetry of the cricothyroid articular facets (arrows) on the left and right sides of the same cricoid cartilage; B, absence of cricothyroid articular facet unilaterally; C, Posterior cricothyroid ligament, left side; D, Lateral cricothyroid ligament, right side. (B and C from Maue WM and Dickson DR: Cartilages and ligaments of the adult human larynx.* Arch Otolaryngol *94:432, 1971. Copyright 1971, American Medical Association.)*

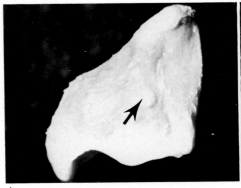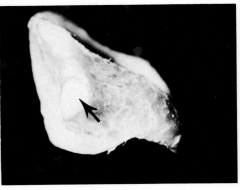

A

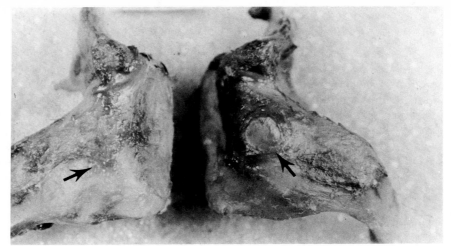

B

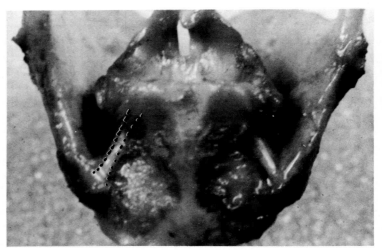

C

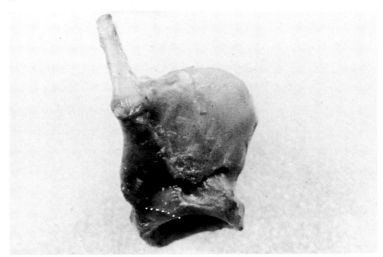

D

149

ligament is called the **thyroepiglottic ligament.** Superiorly, the epiglottis extends behind the body of the hyoid and between its major horns. Its superior curvature lies posterior to the root of the tongue. The anterior surface of the epiglottis is attached to the body of the hyoid bone by the **hyoepiglottic ligament.**

Cricothyroid Joints

The cricothyroid joints are plane synovial joints formed between articular surfaces on each side of the cricoid arch near its junction with the lamina and the articular surfaces found on the anteromedial aspects of the inferior horns of the thyroid cartilage. The articular facets on the thyroid cartilage vary considerably in size, shape, and definition. They may be round, oval, or irregular. The surfaces of these facets may be concave, flat, or convex. They are not typically bilaterally symmetrical (Figure 4-17). The cricothyroid facets on the cricoid cartilage are frequently composed of soft tissue only; when the connective tissue which in-

vests the cartilage is stripped away, no evidence of a facet is visible. Bilateral asymmetry of these facets can be extreme. These facets, or their soft tissue equivalents, consistently face dorsolaterally and slightly superiorly. When a hard tissue facet is present, its shape tends to mirror that of the opposing facet of the thyroid cartilage.

In addition to the joint capsule, there are two ligaments that bind this joint. The **posterior cricothyroid ligament** lies on the dorsal surface of the cricoid lamina. It attaches to the inferior thyroid horn and extends superomedially to end just below the cricoarytenoid joint. The ligament is attached over most of its length to the cricoid lamina. Thus its potential functional length is very short. The **lateral cricothyroid ligament** also attaches to the inferior horn of the thyroid cartilage. It extends anteroinferiorly from the anterior surface of the inferior thyroid horn and attaches to the lateral surface of the cricoid arch.

The functional potential of the cricothyroid joint is limited by the plane of the joint and by its

4-18. *Functional potential of the cricothyroid joint. A and B, Configuration of the articular facets. C and D, Ligaments of the joint. E and G, rotary motion. F and H, Sliding motion. Note change in position of the vocal ligaments in G and H.*

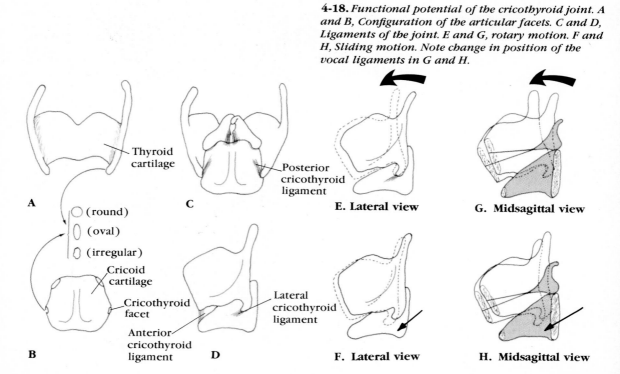

A

(round)
(oval)
(irregular)

Thyroid cartilage

Posterior cricothyroid ligament

Cricoid cartilage

Cricothyroid facet

Anterior cricothyroid ligament

Lateral cricothyroid ligament

B

C

D

E. Lateral view

F. Lateral view

G. Midsagittal view

H. Midsagittal view

ligaments (Figure 4-18). The obliquity of the joint precludes sliding motion of the cricoid cartilage in a posterosuperior to anteroinferior direction. In order for this motion to occur, the inferior horns of the thyroid cartilage would have to be spread apart. The position of the two ligaments also opposes sliding at this joint. However, rotation at this joint is freely permitted and results in adduction and abduction of the two cartilages anteriorly. Anterior abduction is limited by the **anterior cricothyroid ligament,** which extends from the deep surface of the thyroid angle to the anterior cricoid arch. Anterior adduction increases the distance from the thyroid angle to the superior rim of the cricoid lamina, while abduction shortens that distance. This action changes the length of the vocal folds. Dickson and Dickson [4] reported that "in manipulating fresh human larynges taken at autopsy, it has been found that by rotating the cricothyroid joint to its maximum degree, vocal fold length changes of approximately 25 per cent can be demonstrated. This degree of change would seem to be consistent with that observed in the living larynx via cineradiography, photography, and indirect laryngoscopy during pitch change" (Figure 4-19).

4-19. *Motion resulting from rotation at the cricothyroid joint. A, Lateral view; B, Anterior view.*

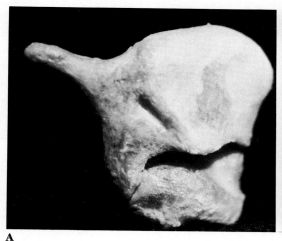
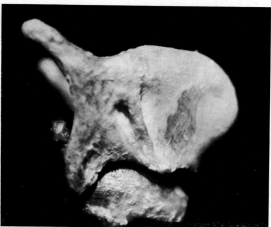

A

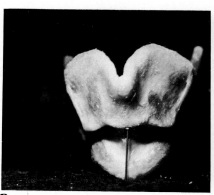
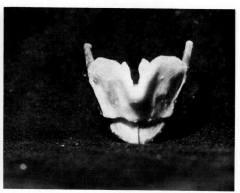

B

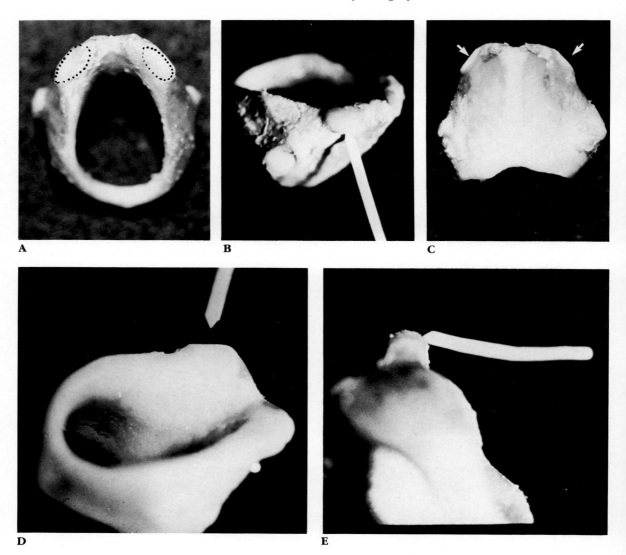

4-20. *Cricoarytenoid articular facets on the cricoid cartilage. A, Superior view; B, Face of the left facet; C, Posterior view; D, Long axis of the right facet; E, Short axis of the right facet.*

Cricoarytenoid Joints

These joints have received considerable attention in the research literature since they are the fulcrum of motion of the posterior ends of the vocal folds, which attach to the arytenoid cartilages. Investigations of the structure and functional potential of these joints have been reported by Snell [37], Sonesson [39], von Leden and Moore [44], Frable [12], Maue and Dickson [29], and Dickson and Dickson [4].

The cricoarytenoid joints are synovial saddle joints. The articular facets on the cricoid cartilage (Figure 4-20) are extremely uniform among larynges and show a high degree of bilateral symmetry. These facets are located on the most lateral portion of the superior border of the cricoid lamina. Each is oval in shape, with its long axis extending from posteromedial to anterolateral. The long axis is ordinarily flat, occasionally saddle-shaped, and, on rare occasions, slightly convex. The width of the facet is approximately half of its length. The two facets are separated by a variable distance equal to about two facet lengths. From a posterior view, each facet is inclined from superomedial to inferolateral at an angle of about 45 degrees from the horizontal. Examined from a superior view, the two facets form an angle with each other that varies extremely from one larynx to another, sometimes being quite acute and sometimes quite obtuse.

The facets on the arytenoid cartilage are uniform in size and shape among larynges and within any one larynx. The articular facet is located on the inferior surface of the muscular process. This facet is round in shape, flat from dorsomedial to anterolateral, and concave from dorsolateral to anteromedial. The concavity opposes the convexity of the cricoid facet, and its flat dimension opposes the flat dimension of the cricoid facet (Figure 4-21).

Two ligaments affect motion of the cricoarytenoid joint. One of these, the **posterior cricoarytenoid ligament** (Figure 4-22) is contiguous with the joint. It attaches to the superior rim of the cricoid lamina between the two cricoarytenoid facets and extends anteriorly to the medial surface of the arytenoid cartilage. The **vocal ligament** attaches to the vocal process of the arytenoid cartilage and extends anteriorly to the deep surface of the thyroid angle.

The functional potential of the cricoarytenoid joint is limited by the shapes of the opposing articular facets, by the position of its two ligaments, and by the presence of a tight fibrous articular capsule that encloses the joint. Motion at this joint has traditionally been described (Figure 4-23) as rotatory about a vertical axis [2,3,41], sliding along the long axis of the cricoid facet [11], or a combination of rotation and sliding [31]. However, the investigations of this joint cited previously have all demonstrated that rotation of the arytenoid about a vertical axis is not possible and that sliding of the arytenoid along the longitudinal axis of the cricoid facet is extremely limited.

4-21. Cricoarytenoid joint, posterior view.

Arytenoid facet removed

Arytenoid cartilage

Arytenoid facet

Cricoid facet removed

Cricoid facet

Cricoid cartilage

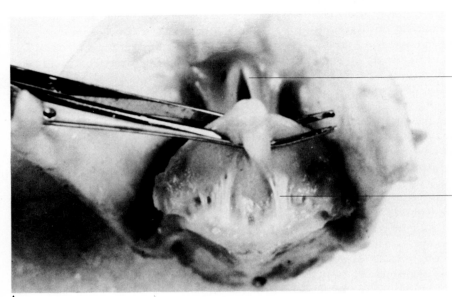

Right vocal ligament

Right posterior
cricoarytenoid ligament

A

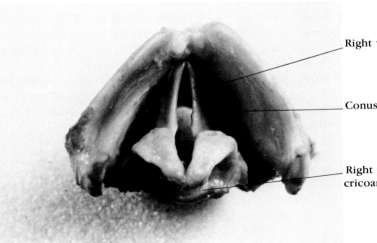

Right vocal ligament

Conus elasticus

Right posterior
cricoarytenoid ligament

B

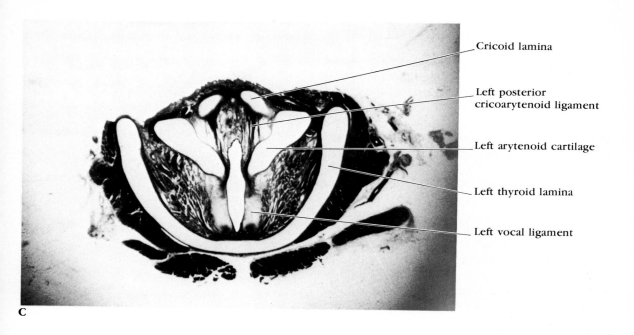

Cricoid lamina

Left posterior
cricoarytenoid ligament

Left arytenoid cartilage

Left thyroid lamina

Left vocal ligament

C

4-23. *Hypothesized motions at the cricoarytenoid joint. A, Rotary motion; B, Sliding motion. Superior views.*

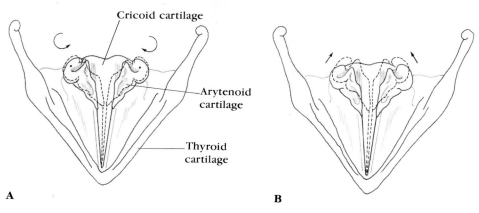

Cricoid cartilage

Arytenoid
cartilage

Thyroid
cartilage

A   B

As illustrated in Figure 4-24, the shapes of the articular facets permit two types of motion at a 90-degree angle to each other, as is typical of saddle joints. One is sliding of the arytenoid cartilage along the long flat axis of the cricoid facet. The other is a rocking action of the arytenoid over the short convex axis of the cricoid facet. The sliding motion of the arytenoid cartilage on the cricoid is severely limited by the tight joint capsule. In fresh autopsy specimens, only a few millimeters of sliding motion are possible. The rocking motion, on the other hand, is quite free (Figure 4-25). During rocking motion, the vocal ligament and posterior cricoarytenoid ligaments act as guy wires. An analogy may help here. Imagine a tall beam erected vertically and held by two guy wires opposite each other, one to the north and the other to the south (Figure 4-26). The beam would be free to tilt from east to west but could not tilt from north to south. The east-west tilt is analogous to the rocking motion of the arytenoid. The north-south tilt, which is prevented, or at least highly restricted, is analogous to the sliding motion of the arytenoid.

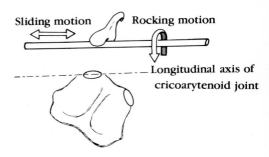

4-24. *Functional potential at the cricoarytenoid joint.*

4-25. *Motion resulting from rocking at the cricoarytenoid joint. A, Lateral view; B, Posterior view; C, Superior view.*

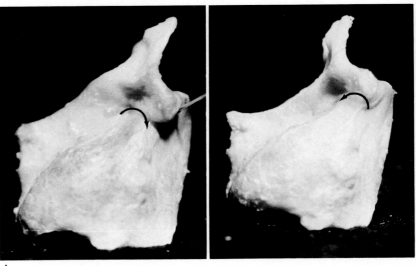

A

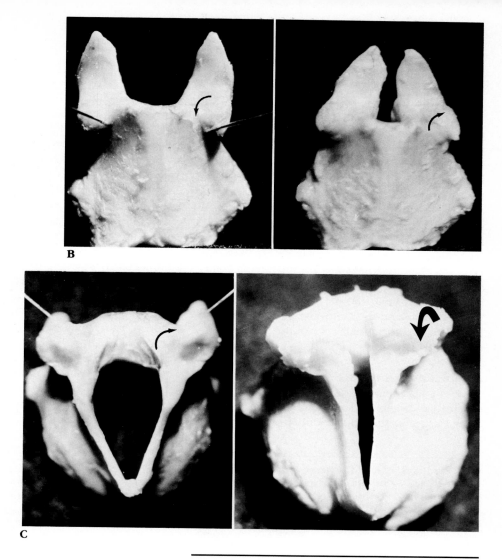

B

C

4-26. *Guy-wire function of the cricoarytenoid ligaments.*

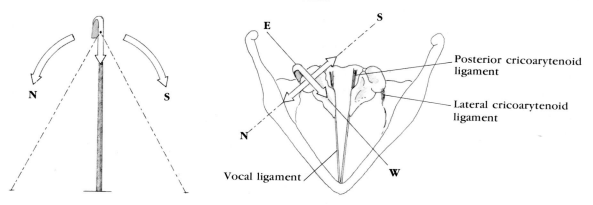

Posterior cricoarytenoid ligament

Lateral cricoarytenoid ligament

Vocal ligament

An important consideration at this point is that the vocal ligament forms the medial edge of the vocal fold. Thus motion of the vocal folds is reflected by motion of these ligaments. The actions of the vocal folds and, therefore, the vocal ligaments, has been the subject of extensive radiological and cinephotographic study. The vocal ligaments are separated posteriorly during respiration, more widely during inhalation than during exhalation. If all of the laryngeal muscles are paralyzed, the vocal ligaments assume a paramedian position. In this position, the posterior cricoarytenoid ligament and vocal ligament form a straight line with the arytenoid cartilage suspended between them (Figure 4-27). This paramedian position of the vocal ligaments (and, therefore, the vocal folds) is also the position they commonly assume at the initiation of phonation.

Membranes of the Larynx

Two membranes serve as internal supporting structures for the larynx. These are the quadrangular membrane and the cricothyroid membrane.

4-27. Relationship of the arytenoid cartilage to its ligaments. (Short arrow, posterior cricoarytenoid ligament; long arrow, vocal ligament.)

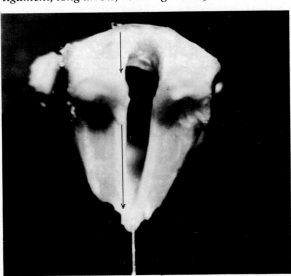

QUADRANGULAR MEMBRANE. The quadrangular membrane (Figure 4-28) is a bilateral structure that lies within the lateral walls of the laryngeal vestibule. Its superior border lies within the aryepiglottic fold. Posteriorly, it attaches to the apex and superior fossa of the arytenoid cartilage. Anteriorly, it attaches to the lateral border of the epiglottis. Its inferior border lies within the ventricular fold. The lower border is slightly thickened and is called the **ventricular ligament.** The quadrangular membrane and ventricular ligament are not well defined anatomically. They are difficult to isolate in dissection and are usually not obvious in laryngeal sections.

CRICOTHYROID MEMBRANE. The cricothyroid membrane is also a bilateral structure and lies within the lateral walls of the inferior division of the larynx (Figure 4-29). Its superior border is the vocal ligament, and its anterior border is the anterior cricothyroid ligament. Its inferior border attaches to the superior rim of the cricoid arch back to the cricoarytenoid facet. Its posterior border is the posterior end of the vocal ligament, which attaches to the vocal process and inferior fossa of the arytenoid cartilage. The body of the cricothyroid membrane is called the **conus elasticus,** which forms the supporting structure for the deep surfaces of the vocal folds at and below the vocal

4-28. Quadrangular membrane, posterior view.

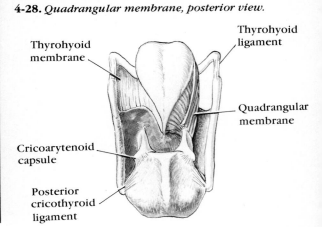

Thyrohyoid membrane

Thyrohyoid ligament

Quadrangular membrane

Cricoarytenoid capsule

Posterior cricothyroid ligament

4-29. *Cricothyroid membrane and its parts. A, Dissection with the thyroid cartilage removed; B, Artist's rendering.*

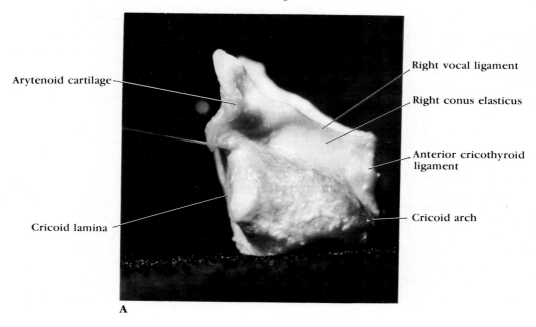

Arytenoid cartilage

Right vocal ligament

Right conus elasticus

Anterior cricothyroid ligament

Cricoid arch

Cricoid lamina

A

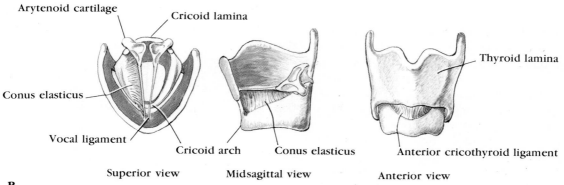

Arytenoid cartilage

Cricoid lamina

Conus elasticus

Vocal ligament

Cricoid arch

Conus elasticus

Thyroid lamina

Anterior cricothyroid ligament

Superior view

Midsagittal view

Anterior view

B

ligaments. Unlike the quadrangular membrane, the cricothyroid membrane is well defined anatomically.

MUSCLES OF PHONATION

It might be helpful at this point to review some of the internal adjustments known to take place within the larynx that must be accounted for in the function of the intrinsic muscles, including opening the larynx for respiration, closing the vocal folds for phonation, varying the length and stiffness of the vocal folds for pitch change, closing the larynx firmly against pressure, and rapidly opening and closing the vocal folds with the changes from voiced to voiceless to voiced sounds during connected speech. With these functions in mind, we will examine the intrinsic muscles from superficial to deep.

It is important to note that the larynx is a midline structure and that all of its muscles except the transverse arytenoid are paired both anatomically *and functionally.* That is, paired muscles of the larynx always function bilaterally; one side (in the normal larynx) never functions independently.

Cricothyroid

This muscle arises from the superficial surface of the anterior and lateral parts of the cricoid arch by two muscular bellies that lie next to each other (Figure 4-30). The more anterior belly, called the **erect portion,** rises to insert into the inferior border of the anterior half of the thyroid lamina. The more posterior belly, called the **oblique portion,** inserts into the inferior border of the posterior half of the thyroid lamina and onto the superficial and deep surfaces of the inferior thyroid horn. Contraction of the cricothyroid muscle would adduct the cricoid and thyroid cartilages anteriorly, acting as a class 3 lever (Figure 4-31). Thus, contraction of the cricothyroid muscle would lengthen the vocal folds. In addition, if the arytenoid cartilages are in the abducted position, contraction of this muscle would result in adduction of the arytenoids. This would occur either if tipping of the cricoid lamina placed un-

opposed stretch on the vocal ligaments, or if muscles extending between the arytenoids and the thyroid angle were to contract. In either case, the arytenoid cartilages would be prevented from moving posteriorly with the cricoid lamina, but instead would be moved anteromedially (the motion permitted by the cricoarytenoid joint) into adduction.

Posterior Cricoarytenoid

A large, fan-shaped muscle located on the dorsal surface of the cricoid lamina (Figure 4-32), the posterior cricoarytenoid has a broad area of origin from the concavity that covers the lateral half of the cricoid lamina. Its fibers converge to insert onto the arytenoid cartilage by a short tendon that covers the entire superior surface of the muscular process of the arytenoid cartilage.

The principal force of this muscle would be along a line that bisects the longitudinal axis of the muscle (Figure 4-33) and extends from the in-

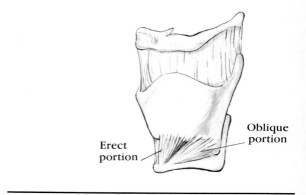

4-30. *Cricothyroid muscle, lateral view.*

Erect portion

Oblique portion

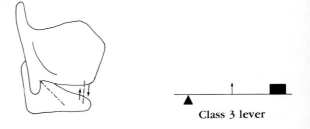

4-31. *Functional potential of the cricothyroid muscle.*

Class 3 lever

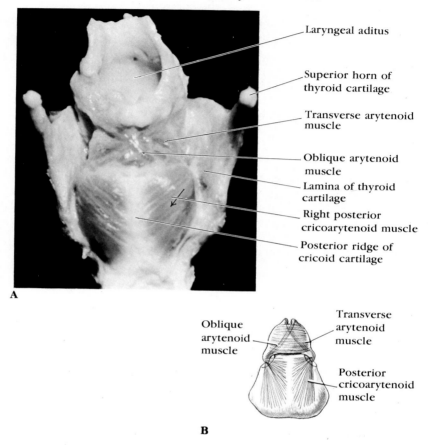

4-32. *A and B, Posterior intrinsic muscles of the larynx. Arrow indicates the direction of pull of the posterior cricoarytenoid muscle.*

Laryngeal aditus

Superior horn of thyroid cartilage

Transverse arytenoid muscle

Oblique arytenoid muscle

Lamina of thyroid cartilage

Right posterior cricoarytenoid muscle

Posterior ridge of cricoid cartilage

A

Oblique arytenoid muscle

Transverse arytenoid muscle

Posterior cricoarytenoid muscle

B

4-33. *Functional potential of the posterior cricoarytenoid muscle.*

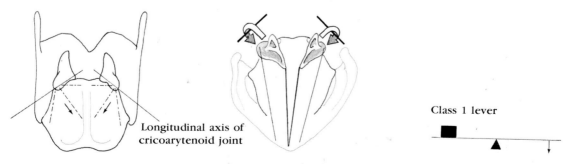

Longitudinal axis of cricoarytenoid joint

Class 1 lever

feromedial cricoid lamina to the muscular process of the arytenoid. The force would be at a right angle to the long axis of the cricoarytenoid facet on the cricoid cartilage. Thus, this muscle is ideally situated to tip the arytenoids dorsolaterally, abducting the vocal folds as a class 1 lever.

Oblique Arytenoid

This is a very small muscle that originates from the medial half of the muscular process of the arytenoid cartilage (see Figure 4-32). The fibers extend superomedially, cross midline, and insert, in part, onto the apex of the contralateral arytenoid cartilage. Some of the fibers bypass the apex and extend anteriorly into the aryepiglottic fold and are called the aryepiglottic muscle. This muscle could be considered an adductor of the vocal folds. As such, its contraction would have greatest potential to move the attachment most distal from the cricoarytenoid joint (the apex) and would function as part of a class 2 lever (Figure 4-34).

Transverse Arytenoid

The transverse arytenoid is an unpaired muscle that extends horizontally across midline deep to the oblique arytenoid muscle. Its attachment, on each side, is to the entire length of the dorsolateral ridge and the dorsomedial surface of the arytenoid cartilage (see Figure 4-32).

This muscle would approximate the two arytenoid cartilages and so would be a vocal fold adductor. The force applied to each arytenoid car-

tilage acts on a class 3 lever (Figure 4-35). The direction of force on the arytenoid cartilages is approximately 25 degrees off the direction of arytenoid cartilage motion. It would appear to operate most efficiently in holding the arytenoid cartilages in an adducted position once adduction is achieved. However, the transverse arytenoid muscle is large and powerful relative to the task to be performed.

Thyroarytenoid

The thyroarytenoid (Figure 4-36) is a large muscle that extends anteroposteriorly and makes up the muscular mass of the vocal fold. Its origin is from the deep surface of the thyroid lamina lateral to the attachment of the vocal ligament. Its fibers extend posteriorly to the arytenoid cartilage. The most medial fibers insert onto the inferior fossa of the arytenoid cartilage and adjacent part of the vocal process and are called the vocalis muscle. The more lateral fibers insert onto the entire length of the dorsolateral ridge of the arytenoid cartilage. This muscle has been the subject of anatomical investigation for over 100 years [25]. Two debates have arisen. One is whether there is an anatomical basis for considering the vocalis and the more lateral part of the thyroarytenoid as separate muscles. The other is whether fibers of the vocalis muscle insert into or mingle with the fibers of the vocal ligament. There is general agreement that no fascial planes separate the two parts of the muscle. There is some evidence that fibers of the two parts intermingle [46] but probably only in

4-34. Functional potential of the oblique arytenoid muscle.

4-35. Functional potential of the transverse arytenoid muscle.

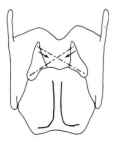

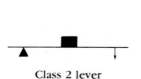

Class 2 lever

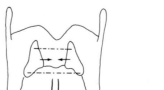

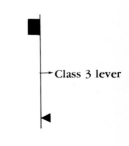

Class 3 lever

the subglottic area. The work of Sonesson [38] and others offers convincing evidence that the vocalis muscle fibers run parallel to and do not insert into the vocal ligament. Some fibers may, however, be interrupted by intermediate tendons [46]. Fibers of this muscle do insert into the conus elasticus.

The thyroarytenoid muscle, acting alone, would approximate the arytenoid cartilages and the thyroid angle, thus shortening the vocal folds. If the arytenoid cartilage were considered the functional origin, the muscle would work at a severe mechanical disadvantage in attempting to elevate the thyroid angle. However, its pull on the arytenoid cartilages would constitute a direct adductory and shortening force on the vocal folds, ventricular folds, and the epiglottic folds as a part of a class 3 lever (Figure 4-37). If contracted isometrically, the vocalis muscle could act to vary vocal fold stiffness. Since the lateral fibers of the thyroarytenoid extend superiorly lateral to the ventricular fold, they could serve as an adductor of those folds. The fibers that insert into the conus elasticus could stiffen that membrane or draw it lateralward.

4-36. *Thyroarytenoid muscle. A, Left lateral view; B, Superior view; C, Coronal section.*

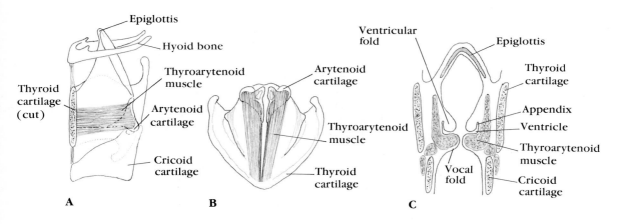

4-37. *Functional potential of the thyroarytenoid muscle. Left, Sagittal section; Right, Superior view.*

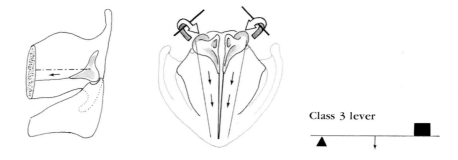

Aryepiglottic

This muscle consists of a few muscle fibers that lie in the aryepiglottic fold and extend from the apex of the arytenoid to the epiglottis (Figure 4-38). Some or all of these fibers may be extensions of the oblique arytenoid muscle. This muscle could move the epiglottis posteroinferiorly and shorten the aryepiglottic folds. It could also have a minor effect on the arytenoid cartilages, moving them toward adduction.

Musculoepiglottic

This muscle lies on the lateral surface of the thyroarytenoid muscle (see Figure 4-38). Its origin

is from the anterior half of the muscular process of the arytenoid cartilage. Its fibers extend anterosuperiorly to insert on the epiglottis near its junction with the aryepiglottic fold. This muscle could lower the epiglottis.

Thyroepiglottic

This muscle is composed of fibers from the deep surface of the thyroid lamina, superior to the fibers of thyroarytenoid, to the aryepiglottic fold (see Figure 4-38). These fibers could pull anteriorly on the apices of the arytenoids.

Lateral Cricoarytenoid

This is a small muscle that originates from the superolateral rim of the cricoid cartilage. Its fibers

4-38. *Lateral musculature of the larynx. Left side of the thyroid cartilage has been removed. Pointer indicates the muscular process of the left arytenoid cartilage.*

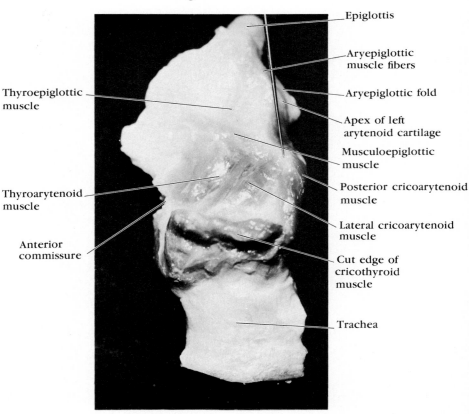

Epiglottis

Aryepiglottic muscle fibers

Aryepiglottic fold

Apex of left arytenoid cartilage

Musculoepiglottic muscle

Posterior cricoarytenoid muscle

Lateral cricoarytenoid muscle

Cut edge of cricothyroid muscle

Trachea

Thyroepiglottic muscle

Thyroarytenoid muscle

Anterior commissure

extend posterosuperiorly to insert onto the lateral half of the muscular process of the arytenoid cartilage (see Figure 4-38). This muscle's apparent potential is to move the arytenoid cartilages toward adduction as part of a class 3 lever. It could also serve to slide the arytenoid cartilages anterolaterally on the cricoid facets. The direction of its pull for adduction is oblique to the direction of motion of the arytenoid cartilages (Figure 4-39). The sliding motion, if any, would tend to abduct the

arytenoid cartilages. Many authors also ascribe "medial compression" (approximation of the vocal processes) to this muscle, though such an action would seem to require at least some degree of rotation of the arytenoid cartilages, which is prevented by the structure of the joint.

Innervation

The innervation of the larynx has received a great deal of attention in the research and clinical literature [5,28]. Motor and sensory innervation of the larynx apparently come from the branch of cranial nerve XI that travels with cranial nerve X. The fibers of XI and X come together at the **nodose ganglion** in the brain stem (Figure 4-40). This ganglion gives rise to two nerves that innervate the larynx: the superior laryngeal nerve and the recurrent laryngeal nerve. The **superior laryngeal nerve** divides into internal and exter-

4-39. *Functional potential of the lateral cricoarytenoid muscle, superior view.*

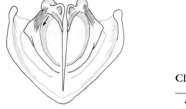

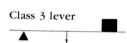

Class 3 lever

4-40. *Innervation of the larynx. Left, Lateral view; Right, Contributions of cranial nerve X and the bulbar portion of cranial nerve XI to the vagus nerve.*

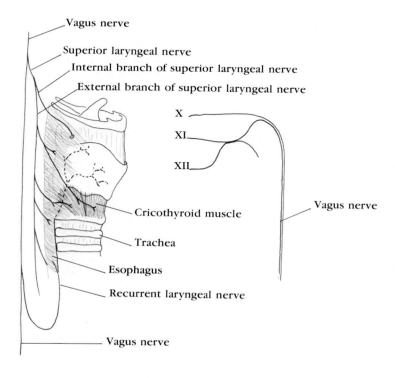

Vagus nerve

Superior laryngeal nerve

Internal branch of superior laryngeal nerve

External branch of superior laryngeal nerve

X

XI

XII

Cricothyroid muscle

Trachea

Esophagus

Recurrent laryngeal nerve

Vagus nerve

Vagus nerve

nal branches. The **internal branch** is sensory and supplies the mucosa of the epiglottis and larynx above the glottis. Some of its branches anastomose with fibers of the recurrent laryngeal nerve to form **Galen's anastomosis.** The **external branch** of the superior laryngeal nerve is motor and supplies the cricothyroid muscle.

Early in development, the **recurrent laryngeal nerve** passes inferior to the aortic arches of the heart before entering the larynx. In the process of growth, the larynx and aortic arches become increasingly separated, and the nerve then descends to loop around the adult form of those arches (the subclavian artery on the right and the aortic arch on the left) before rising to the larynx. The recurrent nerve is primarily motor but probably also contains sensory fibers that supply the mucosa inferior to the glottis. The motor fibers supply all of the intrinsic laryngeal muscles except the cricothyroid. A **posterior branch** leaves the recurrent nerve prior to its entrance into the larynx and supplies Galen's anastomosis.

While the above description of laryngeal innervation represents the typical view, it is by no means agreed with by all investigators. There is disagreement on sensory-motor subdivision of the nerves and about which sensory branches supply specific structures. As pointed out by Dickson and associates [5], the contribution of the sympathetic nervous system to control of the larynx is also a subject of dispute. Apparently, sympathetic fibers enter the larynx as part of the superior laryngeal nerve. The sympathetic system controls secretomotor functions of the larynx.

Most investigators agree that laryngeal muscles are supplied with muscle spindles [1], but there has been little mention of gamma efferent control of the larynx even though such control over the precise adjustments of the larynx would seem inevitable [26,42,45].

Functional Potentials of Laryngeal Structures

From an anatomical standpoint, two functions of the larynx seem to be easily accounted for. The cricothyroid muscle has singular potential for increasing the length of the vocal folds and the posterior cricoarytenoid muscle is uniquely positioned to provide for vocal fold abduction. Adduction, on the other hand, may be a function of more than one muscle. The lateral part of the thyroarytenoid muscle and the transverse arytenoid muscle have a common attachment to the dorsolateral ridge of the arytenoid cartilage. These two muscles together may serve the function of adduction. During adduction, the arytenoid cartilage moves anteromedially at a right angle to the long axis of the cricoid facet (Figure 4-41). The lateral part of the thyroarytenoid pulls anteriorly, while the transverse arytenoid pulls medially. The combined force of the two could provide the motion seen in adduction.

The medial part of the thyroarytenoid (vocalis) muscle may function with the lateral part of

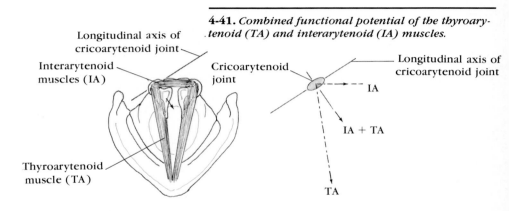

4-41. *Combined functional potential of the thyroarytenoid (TA) and interarytenoid (IA) muscles.*

Longitudinal axis of cricoarytenoid joint

Interarytenoid muscles (IA)

Cricoarytenoid joint

Longitudinal axis of cricoarytenoid joint

IA

IA + TA

Thyroarytenoid muscle (TA)

TA

thyroarytenoid in adduction. However, there is another function for which it is uniquely placed. As pitch rises, the vocal folds increase in length and stiffness. The vocalis muscle could contract to a sufficient degree to increase vocal fold stiffness but not enough to overcome the lengthening effect of the cricothyroid muscle. This would mean that the lateral thyroarytenoid and transverse arytenoid muscles would be antagonistic to the posterior cricoarytenoid during adduction and abduction. The vocalis and cricothyroid muscles could act together to regulate stiffness.

Once the vocal folds are adducted, the lateral thyroarytenoid could be freed to interact with the cricothyroid during vocal fold length changes. The transverse arytenoid would be capable of maintaining adduction once it had occurred. The cricothyroid could also function either to aid adduction or as a synergist during adduction to prevent the contraction of the lateral thyroarytenoid from tipping the cricoid lamina. Other muscles may serve to assist in these functions. The oblique arytenoid muscle may function with the transverse arytenoid. The thyroepiglottic, aryepiglottic, musculoepiglottic, and lateral cricoarytenoid muscles may be functional components of the lateral thyroarytenoid. Leidy [25] stated that from his dissections he considered the thyroepiglottic and the aryepiglottic muscles to be extensions of the thyroarytenoid muscle. Dickson and Dickson [4] found that "In laryngeal dissection it would appear logical to designate as a single muscle the combination of lateral cricoarytenoid, thyroarytenoid, and thyroepiglottic. The lateral cricoarytenoid appears to be an inferior extension of the lateral part of the thyroarytenoid which happens to attach anteriorly to the cricoid cartilage rather than the thyroid cartilage." They found it difficult to distinguish the two muscles along their course.

A factor of medial compression has been postulated to explain the lack of motion of the arytenoids during high-pitched phonation. It has been further postulated that the lateral cricoarytenoid muscle provides the force for medial compression. However, it could be assumed

that all of the intrinsic musculature except the posterior cricoarytenoid increase their degree of contraction with pitch rise. If so, the increasing muscular forces operating on the arytenoid cartilages could account for their decreasing freedom to respond to the aerodynamic events of phonation.

It has also been noted that the vocal folds decrease in cross-sectional area during pitch rise. This would be a natural product of increasing vocal fold length. However, it could also be, at least in part, a function of contraction of those muscle fibers from the vocalis muscle that attach to the conus elasticus.

Since the arytenoids assume a paramedian position when all laryngeal muscles are paralyzed, it could be assumed that the posterior cricoarytenoid muscle maintains the open airway during respiration.

In laryngeal closure for swallowing, coughing, and pressure maintenance, all of the muscles except the posterior cricoarytenoid and possibly the cricothyroid could act together to close the vocal folds, and, by medial pressure from the lateral musculature, approximate the ventricular folds. It is known that the ventricular folds approximate during these maneuvers as a first line of defense against entrance of foreign material from above (for example, during swallowing).

Electromyographic Evidence

Electromyographic investigations have demonstrated a number of consistent findings (Figure 4-42). The posterior cricoarytenoid muscle contracts during respiration. It increases its contraction during the inspiratory phase but is inactive or at a low level of activity during phonation [6,7,15,36]. The cricothyroid, thyroarytenoid, lateral cricoarytenoid, and interarytenoid (transverse and oblique arytenoid) muscles all show a burst of activity at the initiation of phonation followed by reduced but continual activity. During phonation, contractions of the cricothyroid, thyroarytenoid, and lateral cricoarytenoid muscles all correlate with pitch while contraction of the interarytenoids does not. When a voiceless consonant is produced between two voiced phonemes, the posterior cricoarytenoid contracts briefly while the interarytenoids reciprocate with a brief reduction in their level of contraction [13,14,36].

A correlation between subglottic pressure and contraction of the thyroarytenoid and cricothyroid muscles was reported by Shipp and McGlone [36]. They reasoned that the resulting muscular force may be necessary to adjust vocal fold resistance to changing levels of subglottic pressure.

Figure 4-42 illustrates the relationships described. Only those muscles are shown for which there has been consistent evidence across a number of studies. While there is a substantial body of evidence regarding the function of these muscles, electromyographic evidence is lacking or insufficient for the other intrinsic muscles. There are two reasons for this. The vocalis muscle lies within the vocal fold and thus undergoes oscillating motion during phonation. This causes motion artifacts in electromyographic recordings from electrodes placed on or within the muscle. The motion artifacts mask the electrical activity of the muscle. For other muscles, including the oblique arytenoid, aryepiglottic, thyroepiglottic, and musculoepiglottic, no method of electrode insertion has been found that demonstrates validity of place-

4-42. *Extent of activity of the intrinsic laryngeal muscles. PCA, posterior cricoarytenoid muscle; IA, interarytenoid muscles; TA, thyroarytenoid muscle; LCA, lateral cricoarytenoid muscle; CT, cricothyroid muscle. Dashed line indicates rest level.*

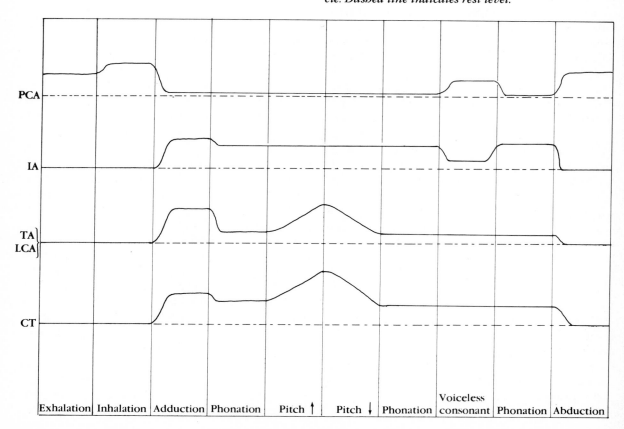

ment within these small deep muscles. Available data on swallowing evidence strong contraction of the thyroarytenoid, interarytenoid, and cricothyroid muscles, while the posterior cricoarytenoid ceases contraction. A number of areas still need study, including exploration of the nerve-muscle fiber ratio, muscle fiber types, and sensory control mechanisms.

EXTRINSIC STRUCTURES
Hyoid Bone

The hyoid bone (Figure 4-43) is suspended in the neck just below the mandible (lower jaw) and lies between the muscles of the tongue above and the larynx below. It is the only bone in the body that does not articulate directly with any other bone or cartilage. In the adult, it is a single horseshoe-shaped bone that lies in the horizontal plane. The closed end of the horseshoe is called the **body,** and the posterior extensions are the **major horns** (also called **major cornua**). Superiorly at the junction of the major horn and body on each side are the small **minor horns.**

The distal ends of the major horns are posi-

tioned immediately superior to the superior horns of the thyroid cartilage. The hyoid and thyroid horns on each side are bound to one another by the **thyrohyoid ligament.** The **thyrohyoid membrane** extends from the lower border of the major horns and body of the hyoid bone to the superior border of the thyroid cartilage. The **hyoepiglottic ligament** extends from the posterior midline of the hyoid body to the anterior surface of the epiglottis. The **stylohyoid ligament** extends from the styloid process of the temporal bone to the minor horn of the hyoid bone.

Radiological studies have shown that the hyoid bone moves anterosuperiorly with increasing pitch and posteroinferiorly with decreasing pitch [8] through an arc determined, in part, by the stylohyoid ligament. The hyoid bone also elevates during swallowing. Its attachment to the larynx via the thyrohyoid membrane indicates that motion of the hyoid bone and larynx are related.

Suprahyoid Muscles

The suprahyoid muscles extend superiorly from the hyoid bone, and form a sling from the mandi-

4-43. *Hyoid bone. A, Superior view; B, Midsagittal section; C, Lateral view with larynx; D, Anterior view with larynx.*

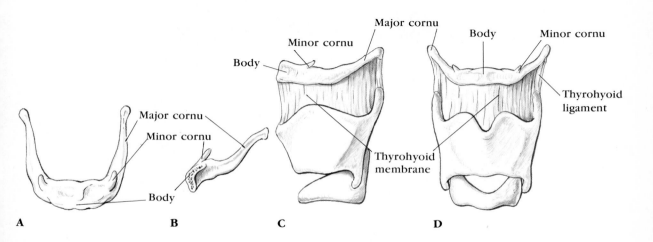

A   B   C   D

ble to the hyoid bone to the posterior base of the cranium.

DIGASTRIC. The digastric muscle (Figure 4-44) is named for its two-bellied form. It is formed by two fusiform muscles joined end to end by an intermediate tendon. The anterior belly of the digastric muscle attaches to the deep surface of the mandible adjacent to the mandibular symphysis. The muscle courses posteriorly and slightly inferiorly to its intermediate tendon. Over its anterior course, the digastric is deep only to the skin and superficial fascia and so can be palpated between

the chin and hyoid bone just off midline on each side (Figure 4-45). The intermediate tendon of the digastric passes through a ligamentous loop attached to the superior surface of the hyoid body near the minor horn. The posterior belly courses superolaterally to attach to the **mastoid process** of the **temporal bone.** The digastric muscle has potential for moving the mandible and/or the hyoid bone (Figure 4-46). If the hyoid bone were stabilized by other muscles, the anterior belly could lower the mandible as a part of a class 2 lever, thereby opening the mouth. Both the anterior and posterior bellies of the digastric muscle

4-44. *A and B, Left lateral view of the suprahyoid and infrahyoid muscles.*

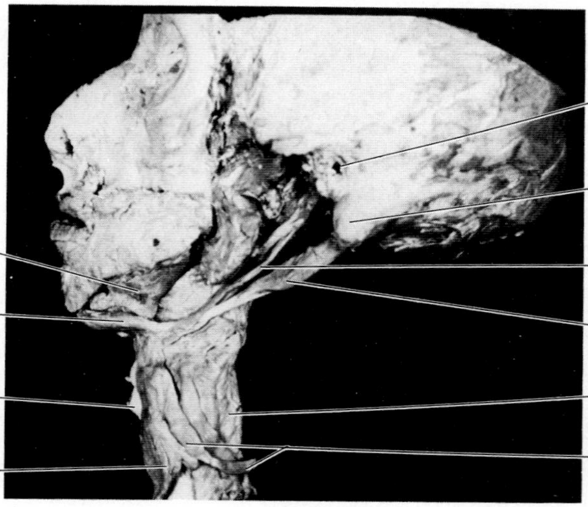

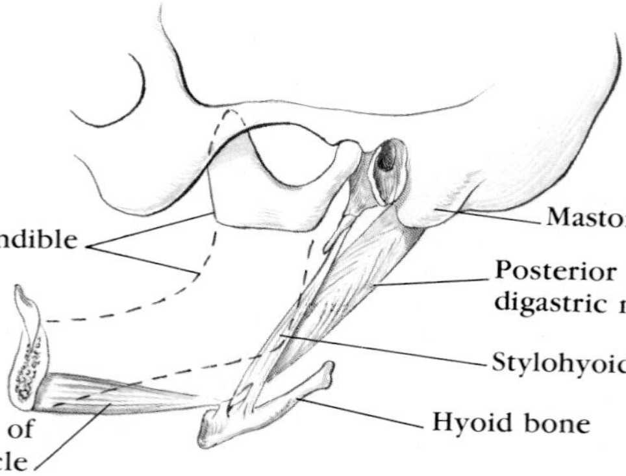

Mylohyoid muscle

Anterior belly of digastric muscle

Angle, thyroid cartilage

Sternohyoid muscle

External auditory meatus

Mastoid process

Stylohyoid muscle

Posterior belly of digastric muscle

Inferior constrictor muscle

Omohyoid muscle

A

Mandible

Anterior belly of digastric muscle

Mastoid process

Posterior belly of digastric muscle

Stylohyoid muscle

Hyoid bone

B

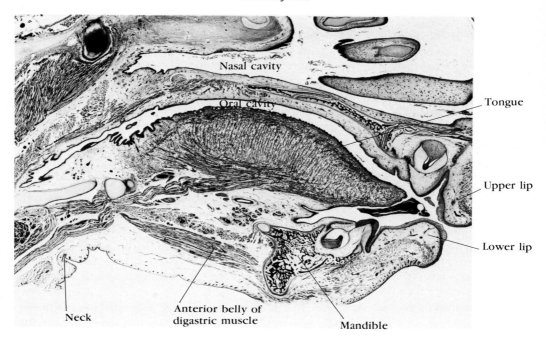

4-45. *Parasagittal section through the oral area of a human fetus.*

Nasal cavity

Oral cavity

Tongue

Upper lip

Lower lip

Neck

Anterior belly of digastric muscle

Mandible

4-46. *Functional potentials of the suprahyoid and infrahyoid muscles. GH, geniohyoid muscle; MH, mylohyoid muscle; AD, anterior belly of the digastric muscle; PD, posterior belly of the digastric muscle; SL, stylohyoid muscle; TH, thyrohyoid muscle; SH, sternohyoid muscle; OH, omohyoid muscle; ST, sternothyroid muscle.*

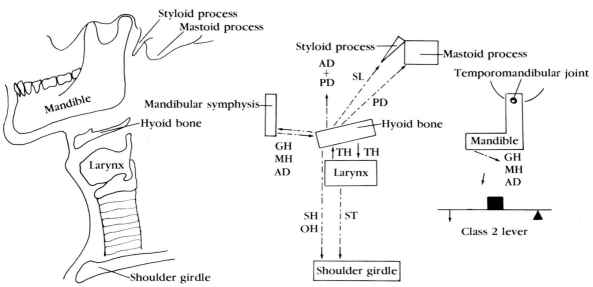

Styloid process
Mastoid process

Mandible

Mandibular symphysis

Hyoid bone

Larynx

Shoulder girdle

Styloid process
AD
+
PD
SL
Mastoid process

PD

GH
MH
AD

Hyoid bone

TH   TH
Larynx

SH   ST
OH

Shoulder girdle

Temporomandibular joint

Mandible

GH
MH
AD

Class 2 lever

are capable of moving the hyoid bone. The anterior belly could move the hyoid anterosuperiorly, and the posterior belly could move it posterosuperiorly. The two bellies together could move the hyoid in any direction from anterosuperior to posterosuperior depending on the relative degree of contraction of the two bellies.

It would be theoretically possible to tip the cranium posteriorly by contracting the posterior belly of the digastric muscle, acting as a class 1 lever with the skull. The jaw-opening function of this and the other suprahyoid muscles will be discussed in the next chapter.

MYLOHYOID. The mylohyoid muscle (Figure 4-47) is paired and forms the muscular floor of the mouth. It originates from a ridge on the deep surface of the body of the mandible that extends from near the symphysis posterosuperiorly to a point near the third molar tooth. This ridge is called the **mylohyoid line.** From this line the muscle fascicles are directed medially and slightly posteriorly and inferiorly. At the midsagittal plane the fibers from the two sides of the mylohyoid attach to a **median raphe** (line or seam of connective tissue), which extends from the mandibular symphysis to the anterior midpoint of the hyoid body. The most posterior fibers of the mylohyoid muscle

attach to the anterior surface of the hyoid body lateral to the midline. The mylohyoid muscle is positioned between the digastric muscle below and the geniohyoid muscle above.

The mylohyoid muscle is capable of elevating the floor of the mouth, lowering the mandible if the hyoid bone is stabilized, and/or drawing the hyoid bone anterosuperiorly if the mandible is stabilized. In its potential for elevation of the floor of the mouth, it could influence tongue position.

GENIOHYOID. The geniohyoid muscle (see Figure 4-47) extends from the deep surface of the mandibular symphysis to the body of the hyoid bone. It is a paired muscle with its left and right bellies lying on either side of midline and in contact with one another. It very nearly parallels the anterior belly of the digastric muscle but lies superior to it. On the deep surface of the symphysis are two pairs of bony elevations called the superior and inferior mental spines. The **inferior mental spines** serve as the anterior attachments for the paired geniohyoid muscle. The functional potential of the geniohyoid muscle is the same as that of the anterior belly of the digastric muscle.

STYLOHYOID. The stylohyoid muscle very nearly parallels the posterior belly of the digastric muscle. It extends from the **styloid process** of the temporal bone to the superior surface of the hyoid body near the minor horn. At its hyoid attachment, the stylohyoid divides into two bundles that pass on either side of the intermediate tendon of the digastric muscle (Figure 4-48). The functional potential of the stylohyoid muscle is the same as for the posterior belly of the digastric muscle. The stylohyoid and geniohyoid together could function as does the entire digastric muscle. It is curious that essentially there are two digastric muscles (the digastric and the stylohyoid-geniohyoid) with apparently identical functional potential. Given more information, this could be explainable on a phylogenetic basis. Structural differences in subhuman species may bring about functional diversity of these muscles. Physiological studies in the human species may also reveal some differences in

4-47. Mylohyoid and geniohyoid muscles, posterosuperior view.

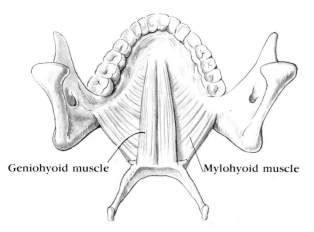

Geniohyoid muscle   Mylohyoid muscle

functional responsibility within their range of potential.

MIDDLE PHARYNGEAL CONSTRICTOR. The middle
pharyngeal constrictor (Figure 4-49) is a sheet of
muscle that originates from the major and minor
horns of the hyoid bone and the stylohyoid ligament. The fibers encircle the lateral and posterior
walls of the pharynx to insert in the **median
pharyngeal raphe** at the midline of the posterior
pharyngeal wall from the level of the hyoid
superiorly to the level of the oral cavity. While this
muscle is not usually classified as a suprahyoid
muscle, it does have the potential to move the
hyoid bone. However, it is generally believed that
its sole action is as a constrictor of the pharynx.
This activity will be discussed in the next chapter.

Infrahyoid Muscles
The infrahyoid muscles extend from the hyoid
bone to the shoulder girdle as well as from either
of those structures to the larynx.

STERNOHYOID. The sternohyoid muscle (Figure
4-50) is a long, flat muscle that originates at the
posterolateral part of the superior border of the
manubrium of the sternum. It passes superficial to
the lamina of the thyroid cartilage and inserts onto
the lower border of the body of the hyoid bone. Its
singular functional potential is to lower the hyoid
bone.

OMOHYOID. The omohyoid muscle ("omo" means
shoulder) originates at the superior border of the
scapula just lateral to its superior angle (see Figure

4-48. *Insertion of the left stylohyoid muscle around
the intermediate tendon of the digastric muscle onto
the hyoid bone.*

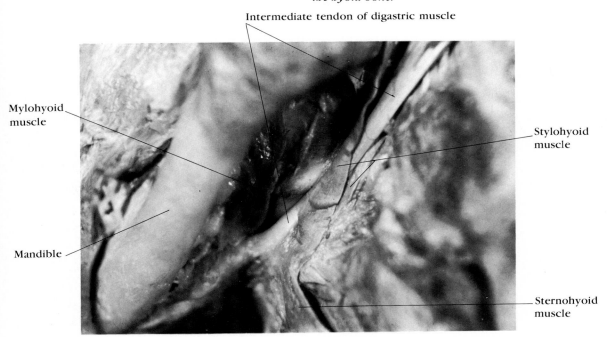

Intermediate tendon of digastric muscle

Mylohyoid
muscle

Stylohyoid
muscle

Mandible

Sternohyoid
muscle

4-50). It extends anterosuperiorly to a position superior to the medial end of the clavicle, where it is bound to cervical fascia. From there it rises superiorly, lateral to the sternohyoid, to insert onto the inferior border of the lateral part of the hyoid body. Its functional potential is similar to that of the sternohyoid except that its pull on the hyoid would be inferior and somewhat posterior. The functional significance of its investment in the cervical fascia is not clear.

STERNOTHYROID. The sternothyroid muscle (see Figure 4-50) takes its origin from the deep surface of the manubrium of the sternum and medial end of the first costal cartilage. It rises deep to the sternohyoid muscle to insert on the oblique line of the thyroid cartilage. Its functional potential is to lower the larynx.

THYROHYOID. The thyrohyoid muscle (see Figure 4-50) takes its origin from the oblique line of the thyroid cartilage. It rises deep to the sternohyoid muscle and inserts onto the lower border of the lateral part of the hyoid body and adjacent part of the major horn of the hyoid. While this muscle has the potential to either lower the hyoid or raise the

4-49. *Pharyngeal constrictor muscles, lateral view.*

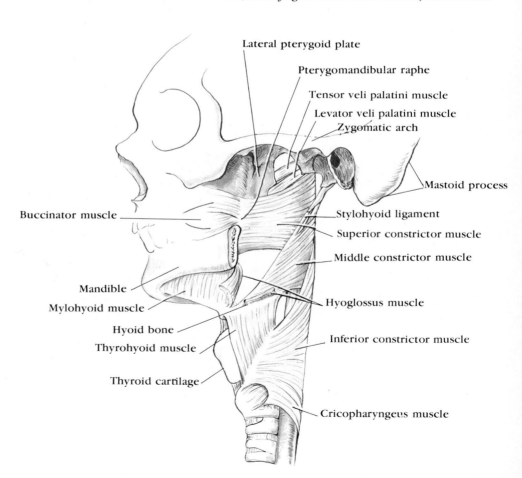

Lateral pterygoid plate

Pterygomandibular raphe

Tensor veli palatini muscle

Levator veli palatini muscle

Zygomatic arch

Mastoid process

Buccinator muscle

Stylohyoid ligament

Superior constrictor muscle

Middle constrictor muscle

Mandible

Mylohyoid muscle

Hyoglossus muscle

Hyoid bone

Inferior constrictor muscle

Thyrohyoid muscle

Thyroid cartilage

Cricopharyngeus muscle

larynx, the latter is more likely, since it is the only muscle that can do so directly (although the larynx can be elevated by raising the hyoid bone); in addition, it would be a logical antagonist to the sternothyroid.

INFERIOR PHARYNGEAL CONSTRICTOR. The inferior pharyngeal constrictor (see Figure 4-49), although not usually classified as an infrahyoid muscle, is an extrinsic muscle of the larynx and should be considered here. This is the most inferior of a group of muscles that form the muscular wall of the pharynx (the entire group will be considered in the next chapter). The inferior constrictor originates from the oblique line of the thyroid cartilage deep to the sternothyroid, and from the lateral part of the cricoid arch between the erect and oblique parts of the cricothyroid muscle. The fibers

pass posteriorly through the lateral wall of the pharynx, turn medially to pass through the posterior pharyngeal wall, and meet the fibers from the opposite side at the median pharyngeal raphe. The raphe is not well defined, and some fibers may cross midline. The most inferior portion of this muscle, that which arises from the cricoid arch, is horizontal and is called the **cricopharyngeus.** The fibers above this assume increasing superior obliquity, with the most superior fibers extending as high as the level of the oral cavity. The principal function of this muscle would seem to be to decrease the size of the pharynx. Its insertion (the pharyngeal raphe) is free to move anteriorly. There is no apparent way to stabilize the raphe in order to use this muscle to move the larynx. The cricopharyngeus muscle could function as a sphincter at the entrance to the esophagus.

4-50. *Extrinsic muscles of the larynx, anterior view, with the sternohyoid muscle removed on the subject's left side.*

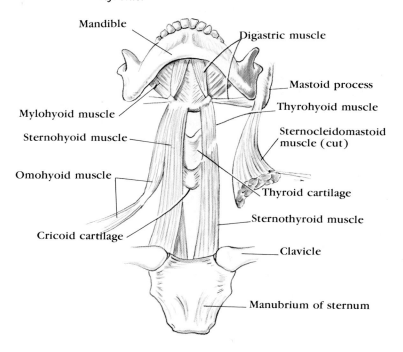

Mandible

Digastric muscle

Mastoid process

Thyrohyoid muscle

Mylohyoid muscle

Sternohyoid muscle

Sternocleidomastoid muscle (cut)

Omohyoid muscle

Thyroid cartilage

Sternothyroid muscle

Cricoid cartilage

Clavicle

Manubrium of sternum

Innervation

The anterior belly of the digastric muscle and the mylohyoid muscle receive their motor innervation from cranial nerve V. The posterior belly of the digastric and the stylohyoid muscles are innervated by cranial nerve VII. The other extrinsic muscles except for the pharyngeal constrictors are innervated by cranial nerve XII and perhaps also by branches from the upper cervical nerves. The middle constrictor receives motor supply from cranial nerves IX and/or X and from the pharyngeal plexus (see Chap. 5, Articulation). The inferior constrictor receives branches from the pharyngeal plexus, the superior laryngeal nerve, and from cranial nerve XI.

Electromyographic Evidence

Electromyographic evidence regarding the extrinsic muscles of the larynx is sparse. In general, it agrees with expectation [8,9], that is, that the sternothyroid muscle contracts during thyroid cartilage descent, the sternohyoid muscle contracts during hyoid descent, and the thyrohyoid muscle contracts during laryngeal elevation. There is also some evidence that the mylohyoid muscle does not contract during elevation of the larynx [8,9], and that the cricopharyngeus muscle is capable of contraction independent of the inferior constrictor muscle [35]. The cricopharyngeus does function as a sphincter at the entrance to the esophagus and is important to the development of esophageal phonation following surgical removal of the larynx.

GROWTH OF THE LARYNX

Sasaki and associates [34] studied the position of the larynx in the neck in the infant period from birth to 18 months of age. They found that in the newborn the epiglottis is in contact with the soft palate, whereas the two structures were widely separated by the age of six months. Even then, the larynx rises into palatal contact during swallowing. By 12 to 18 months such contact was inconsistent.

Our studies and those of Kahane [23] have demonstrated that growth of the laryngeal cartilages is more linear in the female than in the male. Rapid changes in the size of the male cartilages during the pubertal growth spurt account for the adult sex differences found by Maue [27]. Laryngeal growth is linearly related to growth in body height for both sexes. One change in internal laryngeal relationships with growth is the proportion of the vocal fold length into which the vocal processes of the arytenoid cartilages extend. This proportion decreases from the fetal period to the adult. Unfortunately, there have been no comprehensive studies of laryngeal growth.

REFERENCES

1. Baken RJ: Neuromuscular spindles in the intrinsic muscles of a human larynx. *Folia Phoniatr.* (Basel) 23:204, 1971.
2. Cooley RN, et al: Radiology and radiologic examination of the larynx. *Am J Med Sci* 248:601, 1964.
3. DeWeese DD, Saunders WH: *Textbook of Otolaryngology.* St Louis, CV Mosby, 1973.
4. Dickson D, Dickson W: Functional anatomy of the human larynx. *Proc Pa Acad Ophthal Otolaryngol* Spring, 1971, p 29.
5. Dickson DR, Grant JCB, Sicher H, DuBrul EL, Paltan J: Status of research in cleft lip and palate: Anatomy and physiology, Part 2. *Cleft Palate J* 12:131, 1975.
6. Faaborg-Andersen K: Electromyographic investigation of intrinsic laryngeal muscles in humans. *Acta Physiol Scand* 41:7, 1957.
7. Faaborg-Andersen K, Buchthal F: Action potentials from internal laryngeal muscles during phonation. *Nature (Lond)* 177:340, 1956.
8. Faaborg-Andersen K, Sonninen A: Function of the extrinsic laryngeal muscles at different pitches. *Acta Otolaryngol* 51:89, 1960.
9. Faaborg-Andersen K, Vennard W: Electromyography of extrinsic laryngeal muscles during phonation of different vowels. *Ann Otol Rhinol Laryngol* 73:248, 1964.
10. Farnsworth DW: High speed motion pictures of the human vocal folds. *Bell Lab Rec* 18:203, 1940.
11. Fink BR, Basek M, Epanchin V: The mechanism of opening of the human larynx. *Laryngoscope* 66:410, 1956.
12. Frable MA: Computation of motion at the cricoarytenoid joint. *Arch Otolaryngol* 73:551, 1961.
13. Hirose H, Gay T: The activity of the intrinsic

laryngeal muscles in voicing control. *Phonetica* 25:140, 1972.

14. Hirose H, Ushijima T: The function of the posterior cricoarytenoid in speech articulation. *Haskins Lab Status Report on Speech Research* SR 37/38:99, 1974.

15. Hiroto I, et al: Electromyographic investigation of the intrinsic laryngeal muscles related to speech sounds. *Ann Otol Rhinol Laryngol* 76:861, 1967.

16. Hollien H: Some laryngeal correlates of vocal pitch. *J Speech Hear Res* 3:52, 1960.

17. Hollien H: On vocal registers. *J Phonetics* 2:125, 1974.

18. Hollien H, Coleman RF: Laryngeal correlates of frequency change: A STROL study. *J Speech Hear Res* 13:272, 1970.

19. Hollien H, Colton RH: Four laminagraphic studies of vocal fold thickness. *Folia Phoniatr* (Basel) 21:179, 1969.

20. Hollien H, Dew D, Philips P: Phonation frequency ranges of adults. *J Speech Hear Res* 14:755, 1971.

21. Hollien H, Moore P: Measurements of the vocal folds during changes in pitch. *J Speech Hear Res* 3:157, 1960.

22. Husson R: Étude des phénomèmes physiologiques et acoustiques fondamentaux de la voix chantée. Thesis, Paris, 1950.

23. Kahane JC: The developmental anatomy of the human prepubertal and pubertal larynx. University of Pittsburgh, PhD dissertation, 1975.

24. Ladefoged P, McKinney NP: Loudness, sound pressure, and subglottal pressure in speech. *J Acoust Soc Am* 35:454, 1963.

25. Leidy J: On several important points in the anatomy of the human larynx. *Am J Med Sci* 12:141, 1846.

26. Malannino N: Laryngeal neuromuscular spindles and their possible function. *Folia Phoniatr* (Basel) 26:291, 1974.

27. Maue W: Cartilages, lilgaments, and articulations of the adult human larynx. University of Pittsburgh, PhD dissertation, 1970.

28. Maue-Dickson W: Cleft lip and palate research: An updated state of the art. Section II. Anatomy and physiology. *Cleft Palate J* 14:270, 1977.

29. Maue WM, Dickson DR: Cartilages and ligaments of the adult human larynx. *Arch Otolaryngol* 94:432, 1971.

30. Moore P: Discussion of Lieberman P: Vocal cord motion in man. *Ann NY Acad Sci* 155:39, 1968.

31. Pressman JJ: Physiology of the vocal cords in phonation and respiration. *Arch Otolaryngol* 35:355, 1942.

32. Rubin HJ: The neurochronaxic theory of voice production—A refutation. *AMA Arch Otolaryngol* 71:913, 1960.

33. Rubin HJ: Experimental studies on vocal pitch and intensity in phonation. *Laryngoscope* 73:973, 1963.

34. Sasaki CT, Levin PA, Laitman JT, Crelin ES: Postnatal descent of the epiglottis in man. A preliminary report. *Arch Otolaryngol* 103:169, 1977.

35. Shipp T: EMG of pharyngoesophageal musculature during alaryngeal voice production. *J Speech Hear Res* 13:184, 1970.

36. Shipp T, McGlone RE: Laryngeal dynamics associated with voice frequency change. *J Speech Hear Res* 14:761, 1971.

37. Snell C: On the function of the crico-arytenoid joints in the movements of the vocal cords. *Proc Kon Nederl Acad Wet* 50:1370, 1947.

38. Sonesson B: Die funktionelle Anatomie des Cricoarytaenoidgelenkes. *Z Anat Entw* 121:292, 1959.

39. Sonesson B: On the anatomy and vibratory pattern of the human vocal folds with special reference to a photo-electric method for studying the vibratory movements. *Acta Otolaryngol* [Suppl] 156:1, 1960.

40. Sonninen A: Is the length of the vocal cords the same at all different levels of singing? *Acta Otolaryngol* [Suppl] 118:219, 1954.

41. Sullivan WW, Sauer ME, Corssen G: A study of the rotary component of the motion of the arytenoid cartilages in man. *Tex Rep Biol Med* 18:284, 1960.

42. Tanabe M, Kiajima K, Gould WJ: Laryngeal phonatory reflex. The effect of anesthetization of the internal branch of the superior laryngeal nerve: Acoustic aspects. *Ann Otol Rhinol Laryngol* 84:206, 1975.

43. Van den Berg J: Direct and indirect determination of the mean subglottic pressure. *Folia Phoniatr* (Basel) 8:1, 1956.

44. von Leden H, Moore P: The mechanics of the cricoarytenoid joint. *Arch Otolaryngol* 73:541, 1961.

45. Wyke B: Laryngeal myotatic reflexes and phonation. *Folia Phoniatr* (Basel) 26:249, 1974.

46. Zenker W: Vocal muscle fibers and their motor end-plates. In Brewer D (Ed): *Research Potentials in Voice Physiology*. New York, State University of New York, 1964.

Articulation

In speech production, articulation consists of those adjustments of the supraglottic spaces that modify the sounds produced by the larynx into the sounds of speech. Thus we will be concerned with the structures of the pharynx, oral cavity, nasal cavities, and some of the muscles of the face. Before proceeding to an examination of those structures, we need to consider their skeletal framework, the skull.

THE SKULL

The mature skull is composed of two parts, the **mandible** and the **craniofacial complex.** The craniofacial complex contains a large number of bones that, in the adult, are fused to one another. The **cranium** is that portion of the skull surrounding the cranial vault, which contains the brain. The **face** is the portion of the skull that includes the forehead and the bony framework for the eyes, nose, and mouth.

When the skull is viewed from the front (Figure 5-1), we can see that the **mandible** forms the lower jaw. The **maxillary bones,** which extend superiorly between the orbit and nasal cavity on each side, form the upper jaw. The **zygomatic bones** form the prominences of the cheeks as well as the inferior and lateral margins of the orbits. The **nasal bones** form the bridge of the nose. The **frontal bone** underlies the forehead and forms the superior margins of the orbits. A small projection at the junction of the two maxillary bones in midline at the inferior border of the nasal cavities is called the **anterior nasal spine.**

In a lateral view of the skull (Figure 5-2) we can see that the frontal bone articulates with the **parietal bones** at the **coronal suture.** The posterior-inferior portion of the skull is formed by the **occipital bone.** The **temporal bone** forms part of the side of the skull and contains the **external auditory meatus.** The **mastoid process** projects inferiorly from the temporal bone. Anteriorly the **zygomatic process** of the temporal

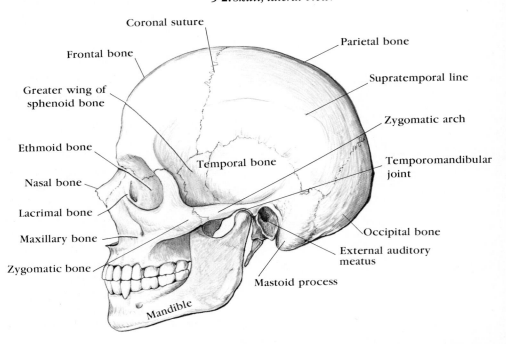

5-1. *Skull, anterior view.*

Frontal bone

Parietal bone

Nasal bone

Temporal bone

Zygomatic bone

Maxillary bone

Anterior nasal spine

Mandible

5-2. *Skull, lateral view.*

Coronal suture

Frontal bone

Parietal bone

Greater wing of
sphenoid bone

Supratemporal line

Ethmoid bone

Zygomatic arch

Nasal bone

Temporomandibular
joint

Lacrimal bone

Temporal bone

Maxillary bone

Zygomatic bone

Occipital bone

External auditory
meatus

Mandible

Mastoid process

180

bone articulates with the **temporal process** of the zygomatic bone to form the **zygomatic arch.** The **greater wing** of the **sphenoid bone** lies between the temporal and zygomatic bones. The joint between the mandible and temporal bone (called the **temporomandibular joint**) can be seen at the temporal root of the zygomatic arch. The **supratemporal line** crosses the frontal and parietal bones and terminates posteriorly at the mastoid process.

In an inferior view of the cranial base (Figure 5-3) we can see the **hard palate,** which is composed of the **palatine processes** of the maxillary and palatine bones. The posterior rim of the hard palate extends posteriorly at midline as the **posterior nasal spine.** Posterior to the hard palate on each side of the posterior nasal openings (**poste-**

rior choanae) are inferior projections of the sphenoid bone called the **pterygoid processes.** Each process gives rise to **medial** and **lateral pterygoid plates.** These are separated by the **pterygoid fossa.** The posterior rim of the medial pterygoid plate bifurcates superiorly to form the **scaphoid fossa.** Inferiorly the medial pterygoid plate ends in a small hook of bone, the **hamulus.** The **foramen magnum,** through which the spinal cord passes, marks the posterior half of the cranial base. Anterior to it, the **basilar portion** of the occipital bone articulates with the **body** of the sphenoid bone. Medial to the temporomandibular joint, the **petrous portion** of the temporal bone extends anteromedially between the sphenoid and occipital bones. Between the temporomandibular joint and petrous portions of the temporal bone

5-3. *Skull, inferior view.*

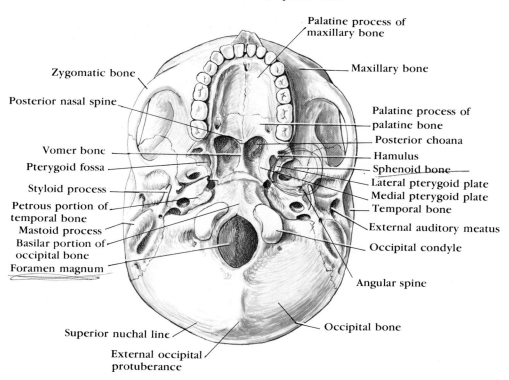

Palatine process of maxillary bone

Maxillary bone

Zygomatic bone

Palatine process of palatine bone

Posterior nasal spine

Posterior choana

Vomer bone

Hamulus

Pterygoid fossa

Sphenoid bone

Styloid process

Lateral pterygoid plate

Medial pterygoid plate

Petrous portion of temporal bone

Temporal bone

Mastoid process

External auditory meatus

Basilar portion of occipital bone

Occipital condyle

Foramen magnum

Angular spine

Occipital bone

Superior nuchal line

External occipital protuberance

the sphenoid bone projects posteriorly. At the posterior limit of this projection is a small bony process, the **angular spine** of the sphenoid, which projects inferiorly. At midline between the medial pterygoid plates, the **vomer bone** forms the posterior and inferior parts of the **nasal septum** (Figure 5-4). On either side of the anterior half of the foramen magnum are the **condyles** (see Figure 5-3), the articular processes for the

first cervical vertebra. Posterior to the foramen magnum is the **superior nuchal line** of the occipital bone. At the midsagittal point of the superior nuchal line is an eminence, the **external occipital protuberance.**

Each of the bones of the skull will now be examined in somewhat more detail. Special attention will be given to landmarks with significance to the function of the speech musculature.

5-4. *Skull, medial view of right half, midsagittal section.*

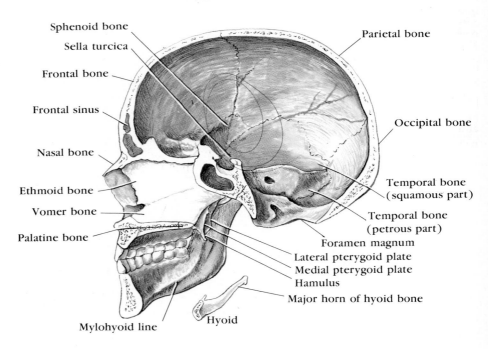

Sphenoid bone
Sella turcica
Frontal bone
Frontal sinus
Nasal bone
Ethmoid bone
Vomer bone
Palatine bone
Mylohyoid line
Hyoid

Parietal bone
Occipital bone
Temporal bone (squamous part)
Temporal bone (petrous part)
Foramen magnum
Lateral pterygoid plate
Medial pterygoid plate
Hamulus
Major horn of hyoid bone

Mandible

The mandible is considered to be an unpaired bone, since there is complete fusion of its anterior **symphysis** early in life. The horseshoe-shaped anterior and lateral parts of the mandible (Figure 5-5) together are called the **body.** The enlarged posterior part of the mandible is the **ramus.** The junction of the inferior border of the body and posterior border of the ramus is the **angle.** Superiorly, the ramus bifurcates into the **coronoid process** anteriorly and the **condyle** posteriorly. The condyle articulates with the temporal bone to form a condyloid joint.

That portion of the mandible containing the roots of the teeth is the **alveolar process.** The alveolar process is composed of spongy bone that forms as the teeth erupt early in life and resorbs when teeth are lost. The deep surface of the mandible reveals the **mylohyoid line,** a ridge that extends from near the symphysis posterosuperiorly to the area inferior to the third molar. On the deep surface of the symphysis are two pairs of small bony processes called the **superior** and **inferior mental spines.**

5-5. *Mandible. A, External surface; B, Internal surface.*

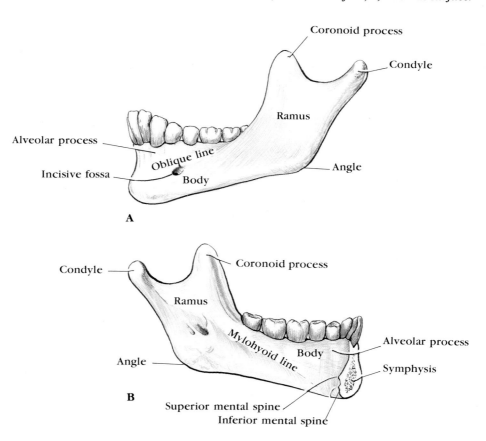

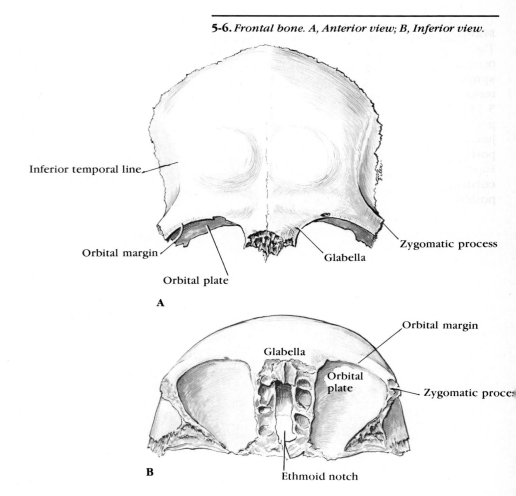

5-6. *Frontal bone. A, Anterior view; B, Inferior view.*

Inferior temporal line

Orbital margin

Orbital plate

Zygomatic process

Glabella

A

Orbital margin

Glabella

Orbital plate

Zygomatic process

Ethmoid notch

B

Frontal Bone

The frontal bone (Figure 5-6) is unpaired. It lies deep to the skin of the forehead and forms the anterior part of the cranium. The inferior margin of the anterior surface on each side forms the **orbital margin.** Posteriorly from the orbital margin the bone projects as the **orbital plate,** which forms part of the vault of the orbital cavity. Between the orbital margins is a bony prominence, the **glabella.** Laterally, the orbital rim terminates in the **zygomatic process,** which articulates with the zygomatic bone. The **inferior temporal line** originates at the posterior border of the zygomatic process and then arches superiorly and then posteriorly. An inferior view of the frontal bone reveals the **ethmoid notch** between the orbital plates; this notch is filled in by the ethmoid bone. Anterior to the ethmoid notch, the frontal bone articulates with the nasal bones, the frontal processes of the maxillary bones, and laterally with the **lacrimal bones.** The posterior rim of the frontal bone articulates with the parietal bones above the level of the orbit and, below that, with the greater wings of the sphenoid bone. The posterior margins of the orbital plates articulate with the lesser wings of the sphenoid bone.

Parietal Bones

The parietal bones (Figure 5-7) are roughly quadrilateral. They articulate superiorly with each other at the sagittal suture. Anteriorly they articulate with the frontal bone, posteriorly with the occipital bone, and inferiorly with the squamous portion of the temporal bone. The **inferior temporal line** traverses the superficial surface of each parietal bone.

5-7. *Left parietal bone, lateral view.*

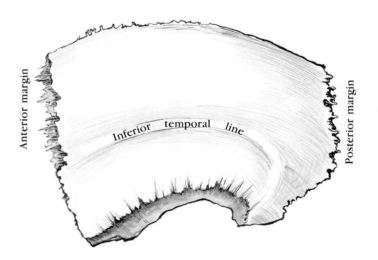

Occipital Bone

The occipital bone (Figure 5-8) is unpaired. The superior part of the occipital bone articulates with the parietal bones anteriorly. Inferolaterally it articulates with the temporal bones. Anteriorly the **basal portion** articulates with the body of the sphenoid bone at the **inferior angle** of the occipital. The condyles, foramen magnum, superior nuchal line, and external occipital protuberance have already been described.

5-8. *Occipital bone. A, Inferior view; B, Lateral view.*

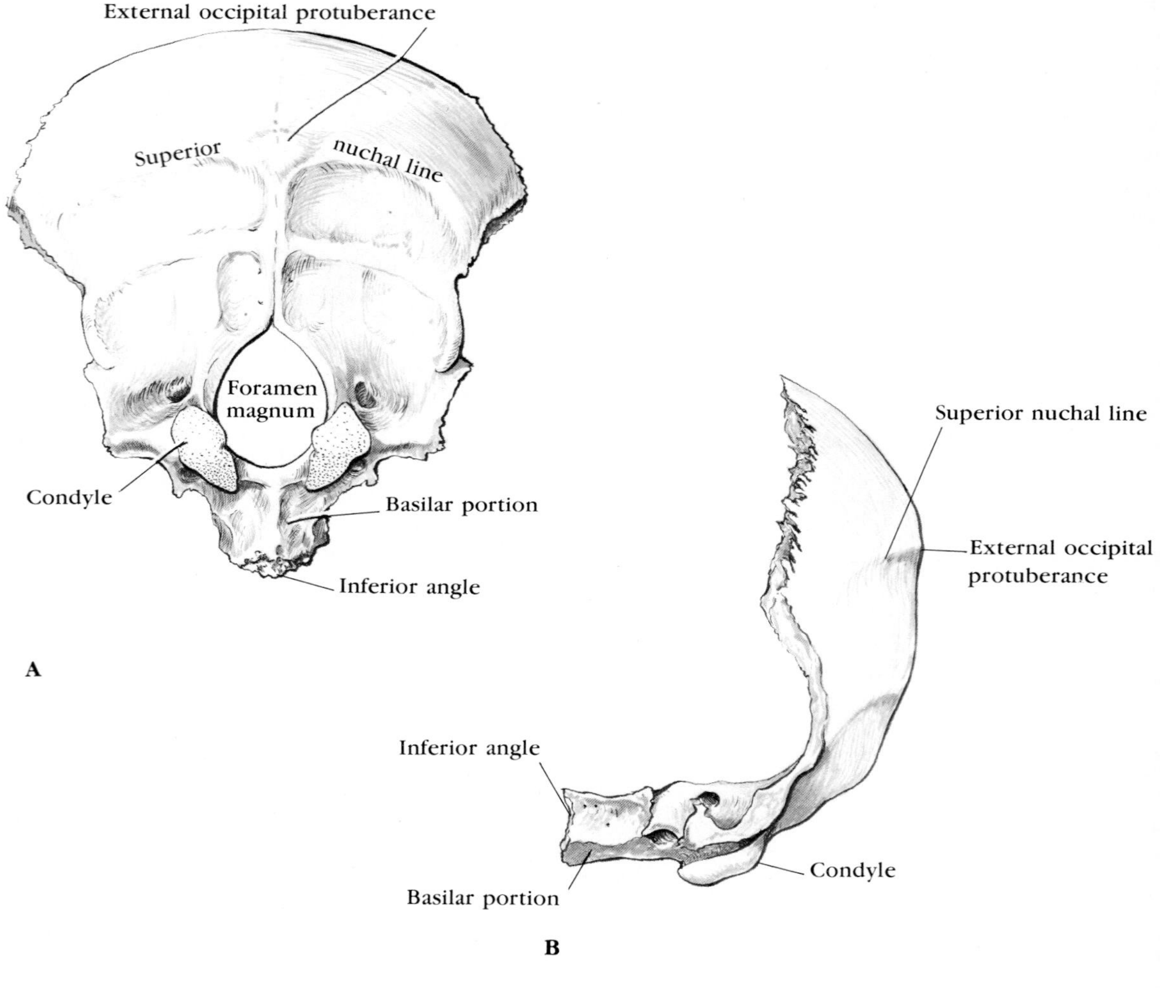

A

B

Temporal Bones

The temporal bones (Figure 5-9) form part of the lateral cranial vault and cranial base. They contain the structures of the auditory and vestibular systems, which will be described in detail in Chapter 6, Audition. The flattened part of the temporal bone superior to the zygomatic process is called the **squamous portion** and is crossed by the **inferior temporal line.** Inferior to the root of the zygomatic process and anterior to the external auditory meatus is the **mandibular fossa,** which, with the mandibular condyle, forms the **tem-** **poromandibular joint.** That part of the temporal bone between the mandibular fossa and mastoid process is called the **tympanic portion.** The **styloid process** projects anteroinferiorly from it. The deep surface of the temporal bone reveals the petrous portion, which contains the auditory and vestibular structures. The temporal bones articulate with the zygomatic bones via the zygomatic processes, with the sphenoid bones anteriorly, the parietal bones superiorly, and the occipital bone medially and posteriorly.

5-9. *Left temporal bone. A, Lateral view; B, Medial view.*

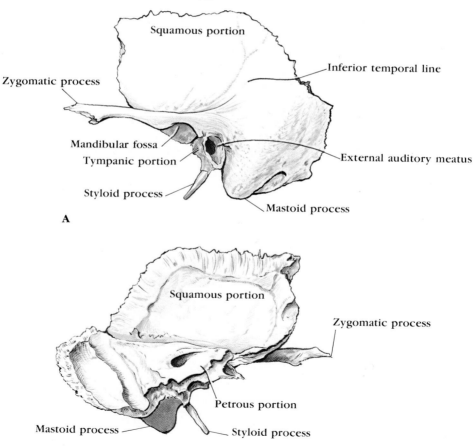

Ethmoid Bone

The ethmoid is unpaired. Located in the anterior cranial base, it forms part of the skeleton of the nasal cavities. Its principal components are two **lateral masses** and a **perpendicular plate,** which forms part of the nasal septum (Figure 5-10). The spaces between the perpendicular plate and the lateral masses on each side form part of the nasal airway. The **crista galli** projects superiorly into the cranial cavity from the anterior part of the perpendicular plate. On either side of the perpendicular plate, forming the roof of the nasal cavities, is the **cribriform plate.** The lateral surface of each lateral mass is called the **lamina papyracea** and forms part of the medial orbital

wall. Two convoluted processes project into the nasal airway from each lateral mass. These are the **superior** and **middle concha.** The **inferior concha** is a separate paired bone that articulates with the **uncinate process,** which projects inferiorly from beneath the superior concha of the ethmoid.

In addition to the articulations described above, the ethmoid articulates with the nasal bones anteriorly, with the lacrimal bones at the anterior borders of the laminae papyraceae, with the maxillary bones at the inferior borders of the laminae papyraceae, with the palatine bones posteriorly, and with the vomer bone at the inferior border of the perpendicular plate.

Sphenoid Bone

This unpaired bone (Figure 5-11) forms part of the cranial base, part of the lateral walls of the cranium, the vault of the pharynx, and the posterior part of the lateral walls of the nasal cavities. The midline mass of the sphenoid is called the **sphenoid body.** The superior surface of the body is concave from anterior to posterior and is called the **sella turcica.** Anterior to the sella turcica are lateral extensions of the superior surface of the body called the **lesser wings** of the sphenoid. The **greater wings** extend laterally from each side of the inferior part of the body. They then expand to form part of the lateral base and lateral wall of the cranial cavity. The inferior surface of each greater wing is called the **infratemporal crest.** The medial surface of each greater wing is the **orbital surface** and forms part of the wall of the orbital cavity. The **petrosal process** extends posteriorly from each greater wing between the squamosal and petrosal portions of the temporal bones. The most posterior extension of each petrosal process extends inferiorly as the **angular spine.**

The **pterygoid processes** of the sphenoid extend inferiorly from the lateral part of the body on each side. Each pterygoid process divides into a **medial** and a **lateral pterygoid plate** separated posteriorly by the **pterygoid** and **scaphoid fossae.** Each medial pterygoid plate terminates inferiorly in the **hamulus.**

5-10. *Ethmoid bone. A, Anterior view; B, Superior view; C, Lateral view, right side.*

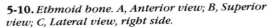

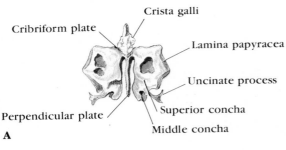

Crista galli
Cribriform plate
Lamina papyracea
Uncinate process
Superior concha
Middle concha
Perpendicular plate

A

Crista galli
Cribriform plate

B

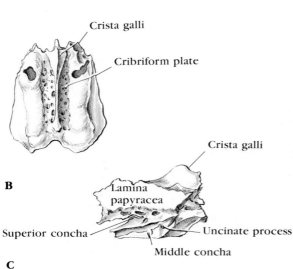

Crista galli
Lamina papyracea
Superior concha
Uncinate process
Middle concha

C

5-11. *Sphenoid bone. A, Superior view; B, Anterior view; C, Posterior view.*

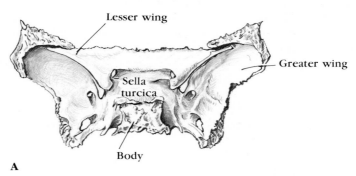

A

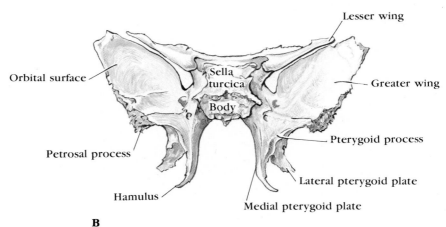

B

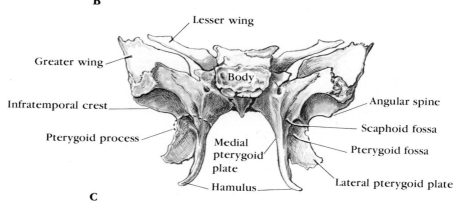

C

The greater wings of the sphenoid articulate anteriorly with the frontal bones, superiorly with the parietal bones, posteriorly with the temporal bones, and laterally with the zygomatic bones. The lesser wings also articulate with the frontal bone anteriorly. The medial part of the petrosal process articulates with the frontal bone. The pterygoid plates articulate with the palatine bones and with the tuberosities of the maxillae anteriorly. The sphenoid body articulates with the ethmoid anteriorly, the vomer bone inferiorly, and the occipital bone posteriorly.

Maxillary Bones

The maxillary bones (Figure 5-12) form the upper jaw, the lateral walls of the nasal cavities, part of the floor of the orbit and the anterior three-fourths of the hard palate. Each maxillary bone has a **facial surface** anteriorly, an **orbital surface** superiorly, a **nasal surface** medially, and an **infratemporal surface** posteriorly. From the **body** of each maxilla, its anterior pyramidal part, the **frontal process** extends superiorly between the nasal cavity and the orbit. The concavity that forms the anterior nasal opening is called the **nasal notch.** The **anterior nasal spine** projects anteriorly from the inferior midline terminus of the nasal notch. The **zygomatic process** extends laterally from the body. There is a small depression, the **canine fossa,** on the facial surface below the orbit. On the nasal surface of the frontal process are two small crests, the superiorly placed

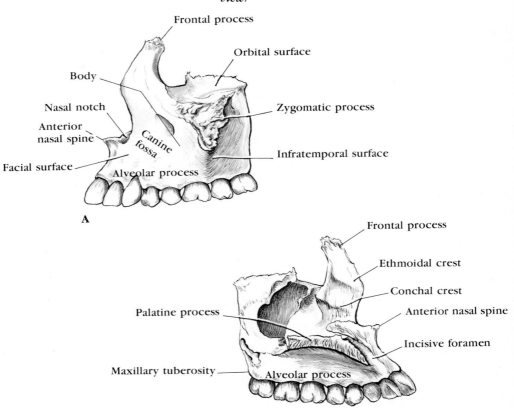

5-12. *Left maxillary bone. A, Lateral view; B, Medial view.*

ethmoid crest and the more inferiorly placed **conchal crest.** At the inferior boundary of the infratemporal surface is the **maxillary tuberosity.** The anterior three-fourths of the hard palate is formed from the **palatine processes** of the maxillae. The **incisive foramen** is a small opening at midline in the anterior hard palate. Surrounding the anterior and lateral margins of the hard palate is the **alveolar process.**

The frontal process of the maxilla articulates with the frontal and nasal bones. The orbital surface articulates with the ethmoid, lacrimal, and zygomatic bones. The zygomatic process of each maxilla also articulates with the corresponding zygomatic bone. The palatine process articulates with the vomer at the superior sagittal midline and with the palatine bone posteriorly. The inferior conchal bone articulates with the conchal crest of the maxilla.

Lacrimal Bones

This is a pair of small bones (Figure 5-13), each of which forms part of the medial wall of the orbit between the frontal process of the maxilla and the lamina papyracea of the ethmoid. It also articulates with the frontal bone superiorly and the inferior conchal bone.

Nasal Bones

This pair of small bones together form the bridge of the nose (Figure 5-14). Medially they articulate with each other; laterally with the frontal processes of the maxillae; and posteriorly with the perpendicular plate of the ethmoid.

Zygomatic Bones

This paired bone (Figure 5-15) forms the prominence of the cheek and the inferolateral part of the orbit. From the central part of each zygomatic

5-13. *Left lacrimal bone. A, Lateral view; B, Anterior view.*

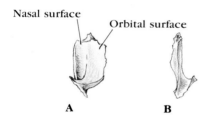

Nasal surface Orbital surface

A			B

5-14. *Left nasal bone. A, External surface; B, Internal surface.*

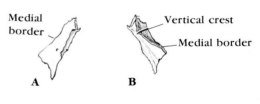

Medial border		Vertical crest Medial border

A			B

5-15. *Left zygomatic bone. A, External surface; B, Internal surface.*

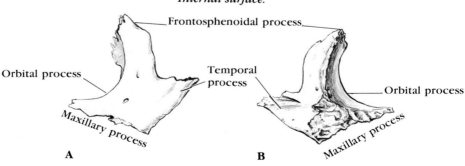

Frontosphenoidal process

Orbital process			Temporal process			Orbital process

Maxillary process			Maxillary process

A						B

bone a **maxillary process** extends inferomedially, a **frontosphenoidal process** extends superiorly, and a **temporal process** extends laterally. Each process articulates with the corresponding bone. In addition, a **posterior orbital process** projects posteriorly to articulate with the sphenoid and maxillary bones.

Vomer Bone

This is a flat plowshare-shaped unpaired bone (Figure 5-16) that makes up the inferior and posterior parts of the nasal septum. It articulates with the inferior border of the perpendicular plate of the ethmoid bone. The inferior border of the vomer articulates with the palatine processes of

the maxillae at the sagittal midline and extends posteriorly to a similar articulation with the horizontal parts of the palatine bones. Posterosuperiorly the vomer articulates with the body of the sphenoid bone.

Palatine Bones

These bones are L-shaped, each with a **vertical part** and a **horizontal part** (Figure 5-17). The vertical part forms part of the lateral wall of the nasal cavity. The horizontal part projects toward midline, where it articulates with the opposite palatine bone and with the maxillary bone to form the posterior fourth of the hard palate. At the posterior midline of the hard palate is a small posterior projection, the **posterior nasal spine.** The posterior surface of each vertical part projects into the **pyramidal process,** which articulates with the pterygoid process of the sphenoid bone. The superior portion of the vertical part gives off a small anterior projection, the **sphenoid process,** which articulates with the vomer bone, and a **lateral orbital process.** The medial surface of each vertical part is marked superiorly by an **ethmoi-**

5-16. *Vomer bone, lateral view, left side.*

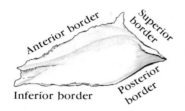

Anterior border
Superior border
Posterior border
Inferior border

5-17. *Left palatine bone. A, Medial view; B, Posterior view.*

← Posterior   Anterior→

Sphenoid process
Orbital process
Ethmoidal surface
Ethmoidal crest
Vertical part
Posterior nasal spine
Conchal crest
Horizontal part

A

←Lateral   Medial→

Orbital process
Sphenoid process
Vertical part
Pyramidal process
Horizontal part

B

dal crest, which articulates with the ethmoid, and inferiorly by a **conchal crest,** which articulates with the inferior conchal bone.

Joints of the Skull

Most of the joints of the skull are sutures and so are immovable. Cartilaginous joints exist only in two places: between the basilar portion of the occipital bone and the body of the sphenoid bone, and between the two halves of the mandible anteriorly at midline. These joints ossify in adult life, precluding any motion.

The only moveable joint of the skull is the temporomandibular joint, which is a synovial condyloid joint (Figure 5-18). A cartilaginous disk called the **meniscus** is interposed between the condyle and the mandibular fossa and lies within the synovial capsule.

Three ligaments are associated with this joint. The **temporomandibular ligament** extends from the superficial surface of the zygomatic arch inferoposteriorly to attach to the lateral and posterior surfaces of the neck of the condyle. The **sphenomandibular ligament** extends from the angular spine of the sphenoid bone inferoposteriorly to the deep surface of the mandibular ramus inferior to the condyle. The **stylomandibular ligament** extends from the styloid process of the temporal bone to the posterior border of the mandibular ramus just superior to the angle.

The movements of the mandible are a combination of hinge action and anterior-posterior gliding when opening and closing the mouth (Figure 5-19), and lateral gliding during side-to-side motion of the mandible during chewing. Small degrees of mouth opening and closing, such as dur-

5-18. *Temporomandibular joint and its ligaments. A, Left lateral view; B, Sagittal section through the joint; C, Medial surface of the mandibular ramus in midsagittally sectioned head.*

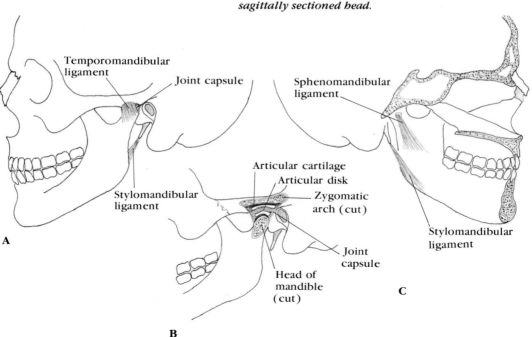

ing quiet speech and most chewing activity, are a function of simple hinge action between the condyle and the meniscus. With more extensive opening, the condyle glides anteriorly as the hinge action continues. The locus of the gliding action is between the meniscus and the mandibular fossa. Both the temporomandibular and sphenoman-

dibular ligaments limit the extent of simple hinge action. These actions of the condyle can be palpated. The mandible can also be moved anteriorly and posteriorly by gliding action alone. Gliding of one side of the mandible swings the symphysis laterally, an activity that occurs commonly during chewing.

5-19. *Functional potential of the temporomandibular joint (TMJ). A, Mandible in occlusal position; B, Maximum opening with hinge motion only; C, Maximum opening with hinge and gliding motion; D, Mandibular protrusion.*

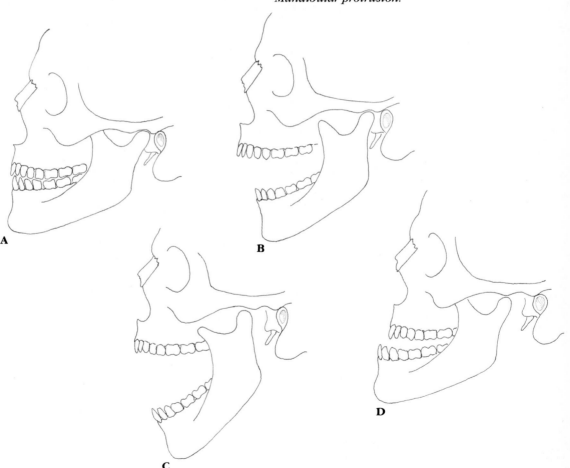

A

B

C

D

PHARYNX AND VELUM
Topographical Anatomy

The adult pharynx is the common pathway for food and air in the human being. It extends from the cranial base posterior to the nasal cavities to the superior end of the esophagus posterior to the larynx (Figure 5-20). The pharynx is widest superiorly and narrows as it descends to the esophagus. The pharynx lies immediately anterior to the vertebral column, separated from it by prevertebral muscles and fascia. Anteriorly, the pharynx communicates with the nasal cavities, oral cavity, and the aditus of the larynx. Inferiorly, the pharynx is continuous with the esophagus. The part of the pharynx that extends superior to

the level of the velum (soft palate) is commonly called the **nasopharynx** (Figure 5-21).

The pharyngeal orifices of the auditory tubes open into the lateral walls of the nasopharynx (Figure 5-22). The **auditory tube** connects the pharynx with the middle ear and serves to maintain air pressure equilibrium between the middle ear and the external atmosphere. The **pharyngeal orifice** of each auditory tube is bounded posteromedially by the enlarged medial end of the auditory tube cartilage, the **torus tubarius.** The torus tubarius projects from the lateral pharyngeal wall, creating a sulcus between itself and the posterior pharyngeal wall called the **Rosenmüller fossa.** The projection of the torus tubarius into the

5-20. The pharynx, posterior view with the posterior wall opened midsagittally.

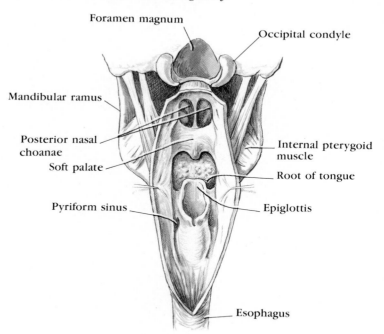

Foramen magnum

Occipital condyle

Mandibular ramus

Posterior nasal choanae

Internal pterygoid muscle

Soft palate

Root of tongue

Pyriform sinus

Epiglottis

Esophagus

lateral pharyngeal wall creates a vertical fold in the lateral wall extending from the level of the torus inferiorly into the oropharynx. The fold, which is largely glandular, is called the **salpingopharyngeal fold.** The superoposterior part of the pharynx contains the **pharyngeal tonsil** (also called the **adenoid**).

The **velum** (**soft palate**) forms the boundary separating the nasopharynx from the oropharynx. Since the velum is mobile, this boundary is arbitrary. The velum is a muscular body that attaches to the posterior rim of the hard palate and the lateral walls of the posterior part of the oral cavity. The posterior free border of the velum hangs into

the oropharynx and ends in a small midline projection, the **uvula.**

The **oropharynx** extends inferiorly to the level of the hyoid bone. The anterior wall of the oropharynx inferior to the opening into the oral cavity is formed by the posterior surface of the root of the tongue.

The **palatopharyngeal fold** (**posterior faucial arch**) extends from the sides of the velum into the lateral walls of the pharynx (Figure 5-23). This muscular fold forms the greatest lateral constriction between the oropharynx and oral cavity. The superior end of the epiglottis extends superiorly from the larynx into the oropharynx

5-21. *Midsagittal computed tomogram of the adult head and neck.*

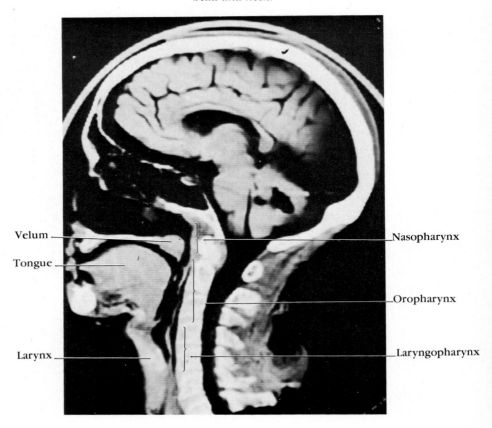

Velum

Tongue

Larynx

Nasopharynx

Oropharynx

Laryngopharynx

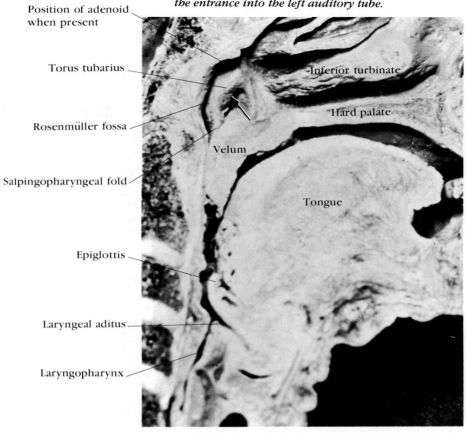

5-22. *Medial view of the lateral pharyngeal wall in a parasagitally sectioned adult head. Arrow indicates the entrance into the left auditory tube.*

Position of adenoid when present

Torus tubarius

Inferior turbinate

Hard palate

Rosenmüller fossa

Velum

Salpingopharyngeal fold

Tongue

Epiglottis

Laryngeal aditus

Laryngopharynx

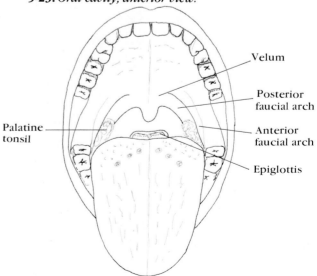

5-23. *Oral cavity, anterior view.*

Velum

Posterior faucial arch

Anterior faucial arch

Palatine tonsil

Epiglottis

immediately posterior to the root of the tongue. Two folds, one on each side, extend from the sides of the epiglottis to the lateral margins of the root of the tongue. These are the **glossoepiglottic folds** (Figure 5-24). The depression between the epiglottis and tongue bounded by the glossoepiglottic folds is the **vallecula,** divided into two parts by a median ridge, the **median glossoepiglottic fold.**

The nasopharynx and auditory tube are lined by ciliated pseudostratified columnar epithelium rich in goblet cells and glands that secrete mucus. The pharynx is lined with stratified squamous epithelium where contact between the pharynx and velum takes place and in the portion that serves as a food channel.

Functions

The pharynx serves as an air passage connecting the mouth and nose to the lungs via the larynx and trachea and as a food passage connecting the mouth to the stomach via the esophagus. Since in human beings these channels are common over part of their length, a sphincter is found at the level of the velum to prevent food from entering the nasal cavities during swallowing.

Constriction of the pharyngeal walls results in changes in the diameter of the pharynx. Such changes are important both to swallowing and to speech. During swallowing the lateral and posterior walls of the pharynx move anteromedially, reducing the cross-sectional area of the pharynx. This results in a wave-like constriction that flows down the pharynx and continues throughout the entire digestive tract. The wave-like motion is called **peristalsis.** In the initial stage of swallowing, the pharynx constricts around the velum while the velum moves somewhat dorsally and superiorly, closing off the nasopharynx from the oropharynx (called **velopharyngeal closure**). The oropharynx expands somewhat, and the larynx moves superiorly and ventrally, opening the pharynx to receive the bolus of food. As the bolus moves into the pharynx, the pharyngeal walls constrict behind it, propelling the bolus toward and into the esophagus.

Oropharyngeal constriction and length changes occur during speech. Such changes affect the resonant frequencies of the vocal tract and thus change the quality of the voice and influence the perception of what phoneme is produced. The lateral walls of the oropharynx move medially on low vowels and laterally on high vowels [45,61].

5-24. *Dorsum of the tongue, superior view.*

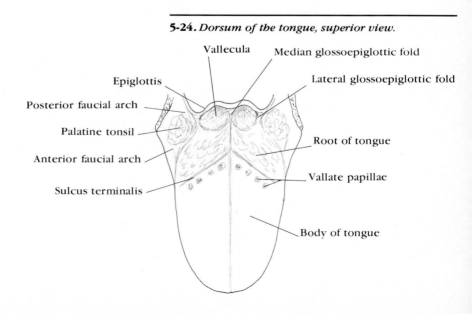

Vallecula

Median glossoepiglottic fold

Epiglottis

Lateral glossoepiglottic fold

Posterior faucial arch

Palatine tonsil

Root of tongue

Anterior faucial arch

Vallate papillae

Sulcus terminalis

Body of tongue

Velopharyngeal closure for speech eliminates the nasal cavities from the resonance system and permits build-up of intraoral breath pressure for the production of fricative and plosive consonants. The nature of velopharyngeal closure for speech is quite different from the activity observed in swallowing. The first reported observation of velopharyngeal closure was by Hilton in 1836 [43]. He described a patient with a large tumor-created defect in the face that permitted an unobstructed view of the nasopharynx. He noted that during speech, the velum moved superiorly and posteriorly against the posterior pharyngeal wall while the lateral pharyngeal walls moved medially against the sides of the velum. By contrast, he reported that velopharyngeal closure for swallowing was primarily pharyngeal. Intensive research since that time has supported his observations.

During speech, the velum elevates and retracts against a stationary posterior pharyngeal wall (Figure 5-25). At the same time, the lateral walls of the nasopharynx move medially, posteriorly, and superiorly against the sides of the velum to complete velopharyngeal closure. Modern investigators who have reported on direct observation of this mechanism in patients with anterior facial defects have agreed that the pharyngeal component of this motion involves the torus tubarius [15,16,20,66]. Radiological investigations that included marking of the torus so that it could be validly identified have provided data demonstrating that the locus of the lateral pharyngeal wall component of velopharyngeal closure is at the level of the torus [44,50] (Figures 5-26, 5-27).

Radiological studies have also demonstrated that during closure for speech, the velum increases in length, particularly in its posterior part [74]. The velum contacts the posterior wall just above the level of the anterior tubercle of the atlas and on a plane with the hard palate [10]. Velar elevation is somewhat greater for males than for females [58], and greatest velar motion is at the

5-25. *Velopharyngeal closure for speech. A, Lateral view; B, Superior view; C, Anterior view.*

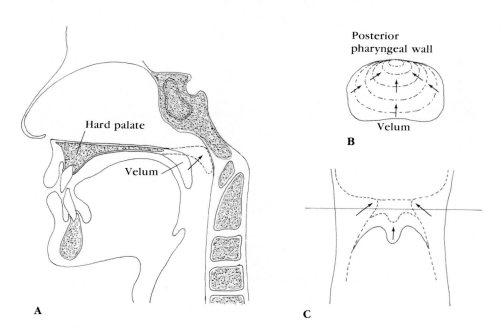

junction of its middle and posterior thirds [75].

It is of interest to note that both velar elevation and the degree of motion of the lateral nasopharyngeal walls during speech are greater for high vowels than for low vowels. This is the reverse of the activity of the lateral walls of the oropharynx. The degree of motion, and, in fact, the degree to which complete closure is achieved is dependent both on the phoneme being produced and its phonemic context. Motion is greatest for fricatives, less for high vowels, and least for low vowels. Velopharyngeal function is greater on vowels in non-nasal context than in nasal consonant context. Finally, the extent of lateral wall motion and the degree of velar motion are synchronized and are directly and highly related to each other [11–13,44,50,51]. Lavorato and Lindholm [51], using nasopharyngoscopy, described the interrelationship as follows: "As the soft palate rises, the lateral margin of its superior surface reaches the level of the inferior tip of the torus tubarius. From that point on, both structures appear to be locked into each other's motion in terms of timing and extent of movement."

5-26. *Frontal radiograph of the pharynx during velopharyngeal closure. Arrow indicates radiopaque marker pasted to the left torus tubarius. (Reproduced, with permission, from Honjo I, Harada H, and Kumazawa T: Role of the levator veli palatini muscle in movement of the lateral pharyngeal wall.* Arch Otorhinolaryngol *212:93, 1976. Copyright by Springer-Verlag, Heidelberg, West Germany.)*

5-27. *Submentovertex cineradiographic frames of the pharynx showing horizontal view through the velopharyngeal port. Arrow indicates marker attached to the left torus tubarius. Frames 11, 23, and 25 approach velopharyngeal closure. Frames 57 and 59 show opening phase. A, Frame 11; B, Frame 23; C, Frame 25; D, Frame 57; E, Frame 59.*

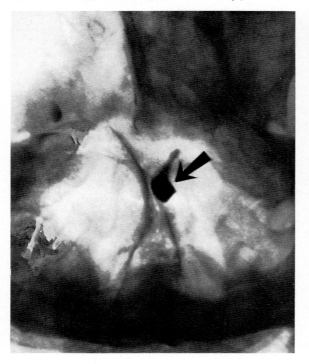

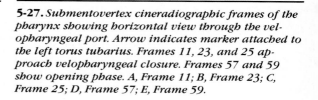
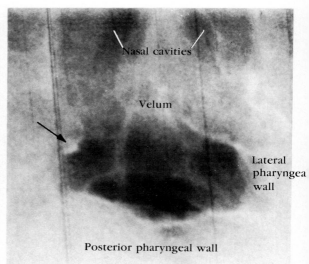

A. Frame 11

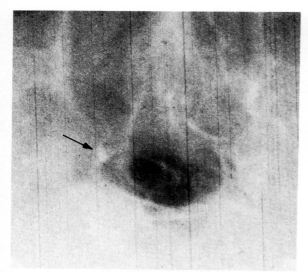

B. Frame 23

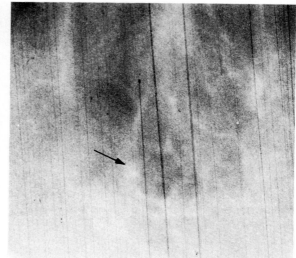

C. Frame 25

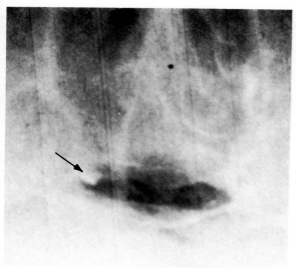

D. Frame 57

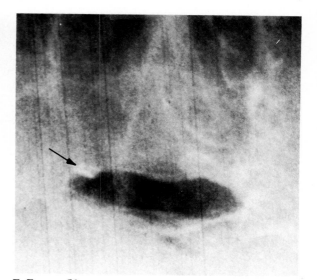

E. Frame 59

Muscles

PHARYNGEAL CONSTRICTORS. The anatomy and function of the middle and inferior constrictors were considered in Chapter 4, Phonation. Thus, only the superior constrictor will be described here. Its anatomy is similar to that of the middle and inferior constrictors (Figure 5-28). Its most superior fibers originate from the soft palate and pterygoid hamulus. Inferior to the hamulus the superior constrictor arises from the pterygomandibular raphe and the posterior end of the mylohyoid line of the mandible. The pterygomandibular raphe is a line of connective tissue between the hamulus and the posterior terminus of the mylohyoid line. The fibers of the superior constrictor extend posteriorly and then medially to insert into the median pharyngeal raphe. The most superior muscle fibers are nearly horizontal and arise from the side of the velum. Laterally the superior fibers are at or below the level of the anterior tubercle of the atlas and typically lie well below the level of the torus tubarius. The more inferior fibers descend from their anterior origin to their posterior insertion. The median pharyngeal raphe extends superiorly beyond the constrictors to attach to the cranial base at the inferior surface of the sphenoid body.

The functional potential of the pharyngeal constrictors is reduction of the pharyngeal cross-

5-28. *Superior constrictor muscle. A, Lateral view of the pharyngeal constrictors; B, Transverse section through the nasopharynx of a human fetus. (B from Dickson DR: Anatomy of the normal velopharyngeal mechanism.* Clin Plastic Surg *2:235, 1975. Copyright W. B. Saunders Co., Philadelphia.)*

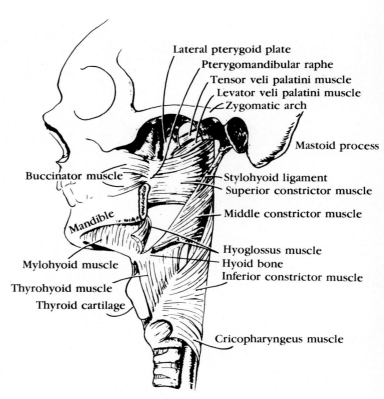

Lateral pterygoid plate
Pterygomandibular raphe
Tensor veli palatini muscle
Levator veli palatini muscle
Zygomatic arch
Mastoid process
Buccinator muscle
Stylohyoid ligament
Superior constrictor muscle
Middle constrictor muscle
Mandible
Hyoglossus muscle
Hyoid bone
Inferior constrictor muscle
Mylohyoid muscle
Thyrohyoid muscle
Thyroid cartilage
Cricopharyngeus muscle

A

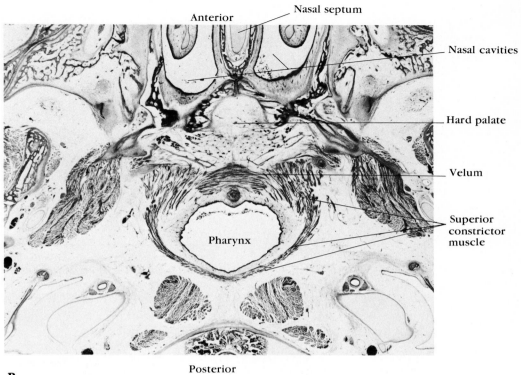

B

Posterior

5-29. *Functional potential of the superior constrictor muscle. LPW, lateral pharyngeal wall; PPW, posterior pharyngeal wall.*

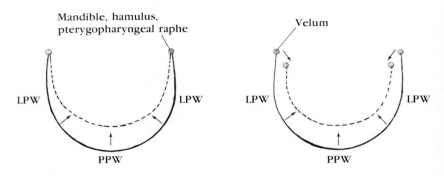

5-30. *Transverse section through the oropharynx of a human fetus. (From Dickson DR: Anatomy of the normal velopharyngeal mechanism.* Clin Plastic Surg 2:235, 1975. Copyright W. B. Saunders Co., Philadelphia.)

Anterior

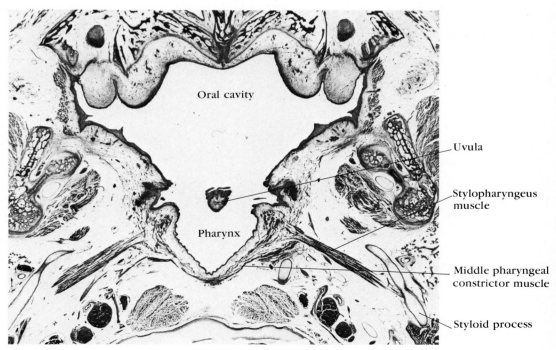

Posterior

sectional area by motion of the lateral pharyngeal walls medially and anteriorly, and movement of the posterior wall anteriorly. It is also possible that the constrictors could, at the same time, move the larynx, hyoid bone, tongue, and velum posteriorly (Figure 5-29).

STYLOPHARYNGEUS. This muscle (Figure 5-30) originates at the styloid process of the temporal bone. Its fibers course inferomedially to the deep surface of the lateral pharyngeal wall at the junction of the superior and middle constrictors. It inserts into the lateral pharyngeal wall between the two constrictors and extends inferiorly as a longitudinal muscle that terminates in the lateral wall. Some of its fibers may extend to the thyroid cartilage. The stylopharyngeus could elevate and widen the pharynx.

PALATOPHARYNGEUS. The palatopharyngeus muscle (Figure 5-31) originates in the velum and passes out of the velum via the posterior faucial pillars. Its most superior fibers are directed horizontally through the lateral and posterior pharyngeal wall, where they intermix with fibers of the superior constrictor. The more inferior fibers arch inferiorly and course down the pharyngeal wall superficial to the constrictors. Some fibers reach the lamina of the thyroid cartilage. The upper fibers of the palatopharyngeus could act as a sphincter with the superior constrictor. The more vertical fibers could lower the velum or elevate the pharynx (Figure 5-32).

SALPINGOPHARYNGEUS. This muscle originates at the torus tubarius (hence, salpingo) and descends within the salpingopharyngeal fold to insert into the lower pharyngeal wall (Figure 5-33). Since this muscle consists of only a few fibers when present and is frequently absent, it probably represents a few fibers of the palatopharyngeus that occasionally bypass the velum and attach to the torus. The salpingopharyngeal fold is essentially glandular [18,33,59,69].

5-31. *Palatopharyngeus muscle.*

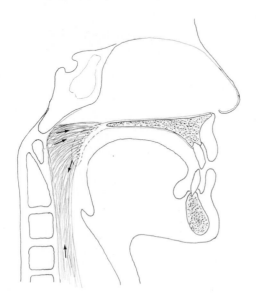

5-32. *Functional potential of the palatopharyngeus muscle (a) as a pharyngeal constrictor; (b) as a velar depressor; (c), as a pharyngeal elevator.*

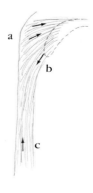

5-33. *Medial view of the lateral pharyngeal wall in a hemisected adult head. Anterior is to the right. A, Undissected. Arrow indicates entrance into the left auditory tube. B, Dissected to show musculature. C, Photomicrograph of salpingopharyngeal fascia from A. Only two or three muscle fibers were identifiable. D, Dissection of a second head to show salpingopharyngeus muscle fibers attaching to the torus tubarius. (B from Dickson DR: Anatomy of the normal velopharyngeal mechanism.* Clin Plastic Surg *2:235, 1975. Copyright W. B. Saunders Co., Philadelphia.)*

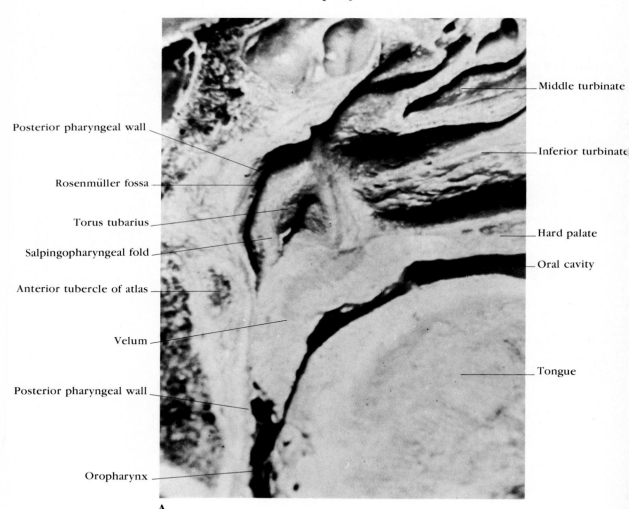

Posterior pharyngeal wall

Rosenmüller fossa

Torus tubarius

Salpingopharyngeal fold

Anterior tubercle of atlas

Velum

Posterior pharyngeal wall

Oropharynx

Middle turbinate

Inferior turbinate

Hard palate

Oral cavity

Tongue

A

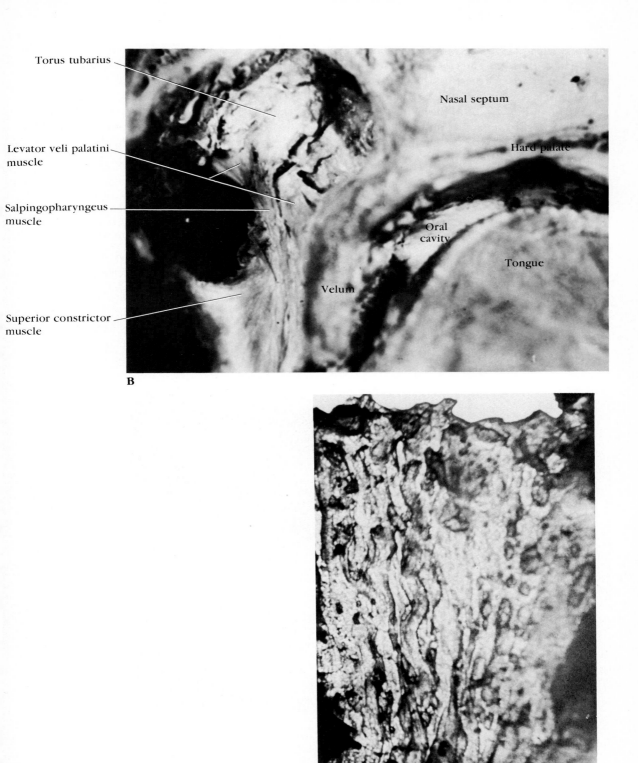

Torus tubarius

Levator veli palatini
muscle

Salpingopharyngeus
muscle

Superior constrictor
muscle

Nasal septum

Hard palate

Oral
cavity

Velum

Tongue

B

C

TENSOR VELI PALATINI. This bipenniform muscle has its origin within the anterior velum. Its long inferior tendon arises from the posterior rim of the hard palate and from the anterior part of the sagittal midline of the velum (Figure 5-34). At midline it joins the tensor tendon from the opposite side. Its fibers pass laterally to the hamulus. Within the velum the tensor veli palatini muscle's tendon is called the **velar aponeurosis.** Laterally, the tendon passes inferior to the hamulus. The musculotendinous junction is immediately lateral to the hamulus. Here the muscle fibers turn superiorly and somewhat dorsolaterally and rise immediately lateral to the auditory tube. The lateral side of the muscle attaches to the pterygoid and scapular fossae and to the angular spine of the sphenoid bone. The medial side attaches to the auditory tube. There has been considerable debate over the exact nature of this attachment. The interaction of the tensor veli palatini muscle, the auditory tube, and middle ear will be discussed in Chapter 6, Audition. Suffice it to say here that on anatomical grounds, the tensor could tense the anterior velum by tension placed on the velar aponeurosis, or it could open the auditory tube.

5-34. *Tensor veli palatini muscle. A, Posterior view; B,▶ Left lateral pharyngeal wall, lateral view; C, Same view, with lateral pterygoid plate removed; D, Same view, with tensor veli palatini muscle sectioned to show attachment of the muscle to the lateral membranous wall of the auditory tube. The auditory tube has been slit to enter the pharynx. (B, C, and D from Dickson DR and Dickson WM: Velopharyngeal anatomy. J Speech Hearing Res 15:377, 1972. Copyright, American Speech-Language-Hearing Association, Rockville, Maryland.)*

5-33 (*continued*)

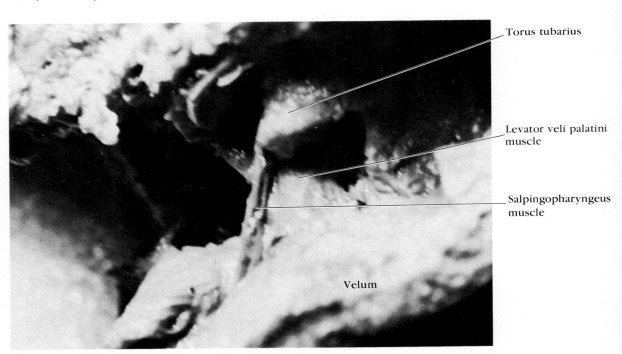

Torus tubarius

Levator veli palatini muscle

Salpingopharyngeus muscle

Velum

D

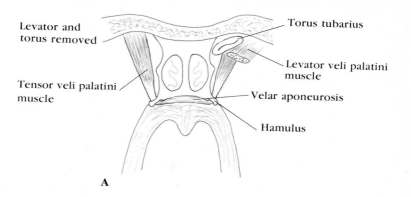

Levator and torus removed

Tensor veli palatini muscle

Torus tubarius

Levator veli palatini muscle

Velar aponeurosis

Hamulus

A

Anterior

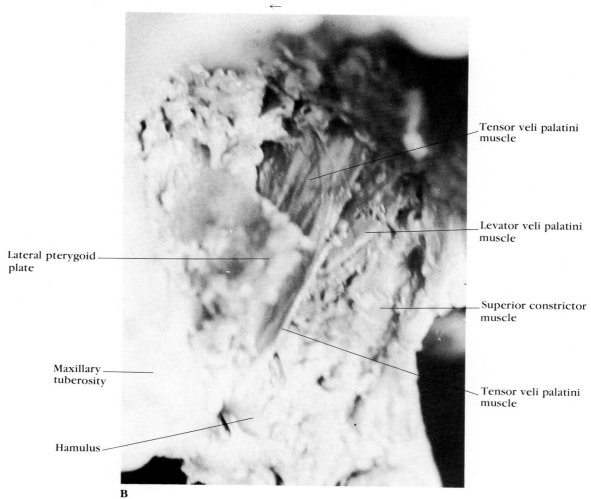

Tensor veli palatini muscle

Levator veli palatini muscle

Lateral pterygoid plate

Superior constrictor muscle

Maxillary tuberosity

Tensor veli palatini muscle

Hamulus

B

5-34 *(continued)*

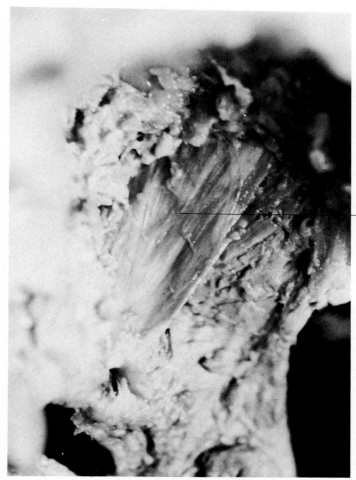

Tensor veli palatini muscle

C

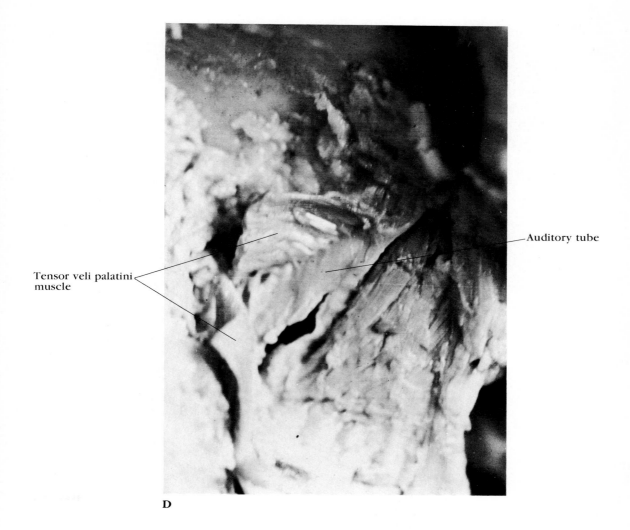

Tensor veli palatini
muscle

Auditory tube

D

LEVATOR VELI PALATINI. The levator muscle has its origin at the apex of the petrous portion of the temporal bone. From its origin it courses inferiorly, medially, and anteriorly to the lateral wall of the pharynx (Figure 5-35). It enters the pharynx above the superior constrictor muscle and immediately inferior to the auditory tube. Just before it passes under the pharyngeal orifice of the audi-tory tube, it lies lateral to the torus tubarius. It then enters the side of the velum where it fans out as it approaches the sagittal midline, extending from just posterior to the hard palate almost to the uvula. At midline, the fibers from the two sides of the levator interconnect. Thus, this paired muscle forms a sling through the velum from the cranial base.

5-35. *Levator veli palatini muscle. A, Medial view. (From Dickson DR: Anatomy of the normal velopharyngeal mechanism.* Clin Plastic Surg *2:237, 1975. Copyright, W. B. Saunders Co., Philadelphia.) B, Posterior view. (From Dickson DR: Normal and cleft palate anatomy.* Cleft Palate J *9:280, 1972. Copyright, American Cleft Palate Association, Pittsburg, Pennsylvania.) C, Coronal section through the velum of a human fetus.*

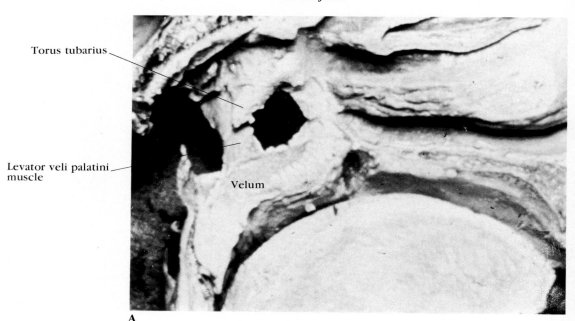

Torus tubarius

Levator veli palatini muscle

Velum

A

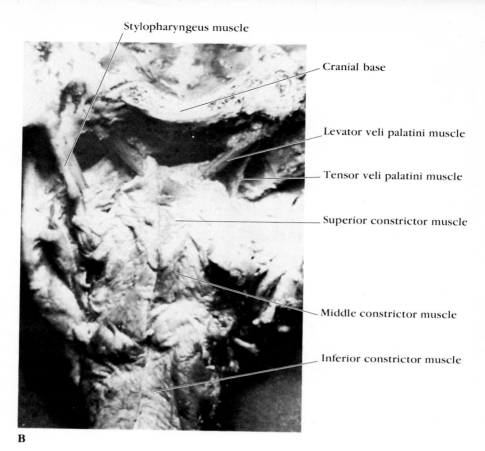

Stylopharyngeus muscle

Cranial base

Levator veli palatini muscle

Tensor veli palatini muscle

Superior constrictor muscle

Middle constrictor muscle

Inferior constrictor muscle

B

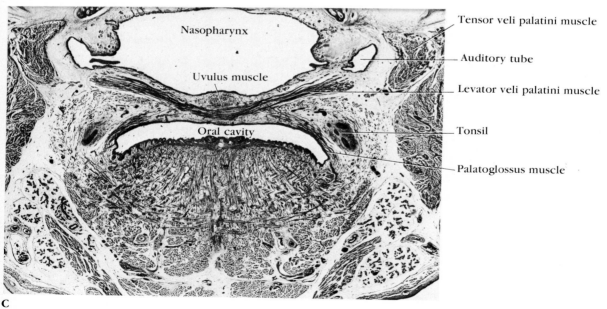

Nasopharynx

Tensor veli palatini muscle

Auditory tube

Uvulus muscle

Levator veli palatini muscle

Oral cavity

Tonsil

Palatoglossus muscle

C

The functional potential of the levator veli palatini is to elevate and retract the velum (Figure 5-36). In doing so, it could also displace the tori tubarius superomedially and posteriorly.

UVULUS. Anatomical studies of the uvulus muscle, conducted only recently, reveal a paired muscle (see Figures 5-35C, 5-37) with the left and right muscles lying in contact with each other in the longitudinal midline of the velum [4]. Anteriorly its fibers attach by a short tendon into the poste-

rior nasal spine. Posteriorly the uvulus muscle inserts into the uvula. It is the most superior muscle of the velum and is thickest in the mid posterior velum, where it passes superior to the middle of the levator veli palatini muscle. The uvulus muscle forms the midline longitudinal convexity of the dorsal surface of the velum.

The uvulus muscle appears to have the potential to shorten the velum, and increase the thickness of the third quadrant of the velum during velopharyngeal closure for speech (Figure 5-38).

5-36. *Functional potential of the levator veli palatini muscle. A, Lateral view; B, Anterior view; C, Superior view.*

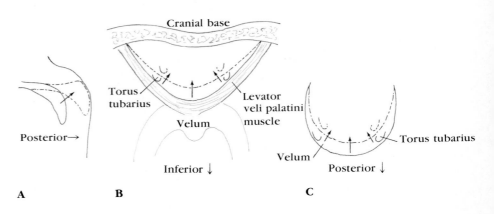

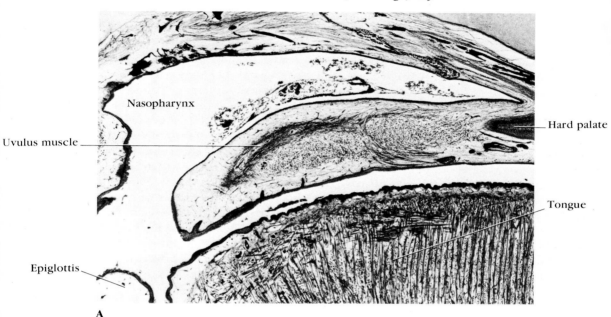

5-37. *Uvulus muscle. A, Parasagittal section of the velum of a human fetus; B, Superior view of dissection of adult velum. MU, Uvulus muscle; LVP, levator veli palatini. (B from Azzam NA and Kuehn DP: The morphology of the musculus uvulae.* Cleft Palate J *41:78, 1977. Copyright, American Cleft Palate Association, Pittsburgh, Pa.)*

Nasopharynx

Uvulus muscle

Hard palate

Tongue

Epiglottis

A

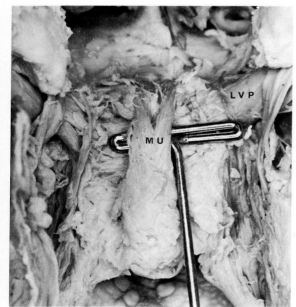

B

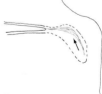

5-38. *Functional potential of the uvulus muscle.*

Uvulus muscle

Posterior

PALATOGLOSSUS. There have been no detailed studies of the insertions of the palatoglossus muscle. It extends from the inferior velum anteriorly and inferiorly through the anterior pillar of fauces to the side of the tongue (see Figures 5-35C and 5-39). It has potential for lowering of the velum, for elevation and retraction of the tongue, and for narrowing the distance between the left and right faucial pillars.

INNERVATION. The innervation of the pharyngeal muscles is not completely agreed upon. All of these muscles are probably supplied from a network of anastomosing fibers from cranial nerves IX, X, and XI called the **pharyngeal plexus.** The middle constrictor may also receive direct fibers from IX, and the inferior constrictor may receive fibers from the recurrent laryngeal nerve.

All of the muscles of the velum except the tensor veli palatini receive their innervation via the pharyngeal plexus. The tensor veli palatini muscle receives its innervation from cranial nerve V.

ELECTROMYOGRAPHIC EVIDENCE. A number of electromyographic studies of the pharyngeal musculature have been conducted. It is apparent that the constrictors are active during swallowing. However, during speech, the middle constrictor is more active than the superior constrictor. Superior constrictor activity is apparently phoneme contingent. For example, Minifie and associates [60] found that the superior constrictor ceased to function during production of plosive consonants. They found no difference, however, in the level of superior or middle constrictor activity for high and low vowels. Based on that finding, they speculated that the vowel-related motion of the lateral walls of the oropharynx referred to earlier may be passive motion in response to pharyngeal pressure. That pressure is higher on high vowels than on low vowels owing to higher oral impedance and therefore may be responsible for the lateral displacement of the pharyngeal walls. Bell-Berti [9], on the other hand, found the superior constrictor to be more active on low vowels than on high vowels, the reverse of the relationship between vowel height and degree of velopharyngeal activity.

There is some evidence that the palatopharyngeus is active during velar lowering; however, its level of activity is also vowel dependent. Thus its role in speech is unclear [8]. The

5-39. *Palatoglossus muscle. A, Lateral view; B, Anterior view.*

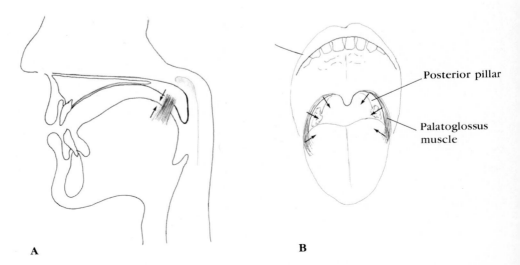

A   B

palatopharyngeus muscle is active during swallowing. The specific result of its activity during swallowing is related to pharyngeal motion but is otherwise unclear. The function of the stylopharyngeus muscle has not been studied.

Velopharyngeal closure during speech has received considerable attention. It is evident that the tensor veli palatini muscle is not active in velopharyngeal function [37]. The palatopharyngeus is active during velar lowering but its activity is inconsistent and vowel dependent. Palatoglossus activity relates more to tongue motion than to velar activity [8]. The superior constrictor and levator veli palatini muscles are the only two velar muscles studied (the uvulus muscle has not been studied) that are active during velopharyngeal function for speech. However, the data of Bell-Berti [9] and Minifie and associates [60] provide support for the conclusion that the superior constrictor is not involved in the process of velopharyngeal function. All investigators agree that levator veli palatini activity is synchronized with velar height.

Indirect evidence indicates that the uvulus muscle plays an essential role in velopharyngeal function. Nasopharyngoscopy has revealed a patient population with hypernasality, a midline longitudinal concavity rather than convexity of the dorsal velar surface, translucency of the longitudinal velar midline, and a small midsagittal gap between the velum and posterior pharyngeal wall during velopharyngeal closure for speech [27,57,73]. This lends presumptive evidence that what has been called the levator eminence (Figure 5-40) is actually a function of the uvulus muscle.

Thus, velopharyngeal closure for swallowing is

5-40. *Lateral cephalometric x-ray during phonation showing velopharyngeal closure.*

Posterior pharyngeal wall

Levator eminence

Hard palate

Anterior tubercle of atlas

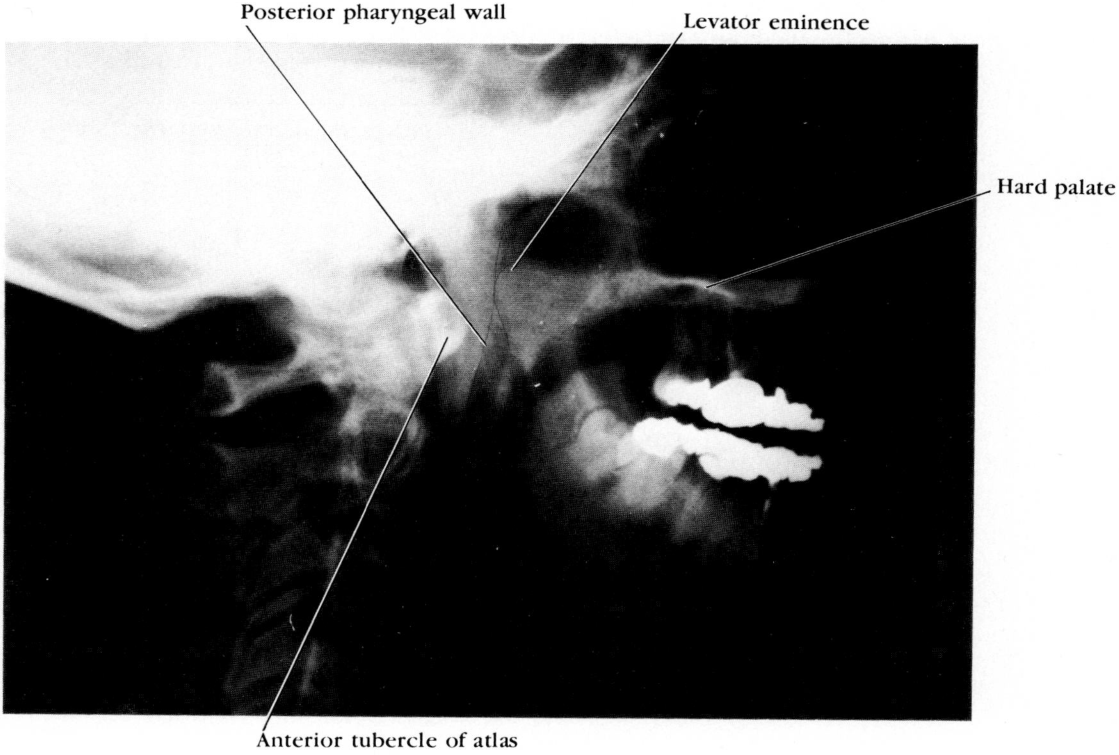

accomplished by the superior constrictor, levator veli palatini, and uvulus. Closure for speech is accomplished by the levator veli palatini and uvulus. The swallowing-speech difference in function is also apparent among persons with velopharyngeal insufficiency due to congenital disproportion between pharyngeal depth and velar length or disproportion following surgery for cleft palate. In our experience, most individuals in this group who are unable to achieve velopharyngeal closure for speech, do so consistently during swallowing.

NASAL CAVITIES

The nasal cavities are the first points of entry and the last points of exit of airflow to and from the lungs. They serve to filter the air as it enters the airway and to control air temperature and humidity. They also serve as resonators for nasal sounds that are produced with the velopharyngeal valve open. The two nasal cavities are separated from each other by the nasal septum (Figure 5-41) in the midsagittal plane. The nasal septum is composed of three parts. The superior part is the perpendicular plate of the ethmoid bone. The inferior

and posterior part is composed of the vomer bone. The anterior part is composed of the **cartilage of the nasal septum.**

The roof of the nasal cavities is formed by the cribriform plate of the ethmoid bone, which is penetrated by the olfactory nerves. Immediately posterior to the perpendicular plate of the ethmoid is the body of the sphenoid, which contains the sphenoid sinus. The floor of the nasal cavities is formed by the hard palate. Anteriorly, the nasal cavities are bounded by the external nose. The framework of the external nose (Figure 5-42) includes the nasal bones and the nasal cartilages. The bridge of the nose is formed by the nasal bones. Inferiorly, the nasal bones articulate with the **lateral nasal cartilages.** The tip of the nose is supported by the **greater alar cartilages.** Small **lesser alar cartilages** support the lateral walls of the anterior nasal openings.

The lateral wall of each nasal cavity is convoluted owing to the presence of the superior, middle, and inferior nasal conchae (Figure 5-43). The conchae have an extremely rich blood supply and provide a large surface area for humidity and tem-

---

5-41. *Nasal septum. A, Anterior view; B, Lateral view.*

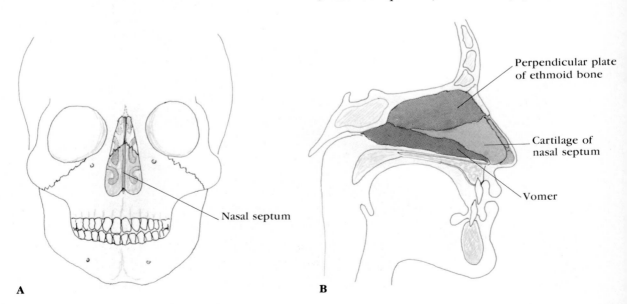

A   B

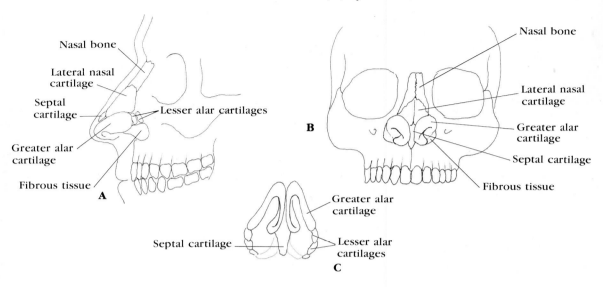

5-42. *Nasal cartilages. A, Left lateral view; B, Anterior view; C, Inferior view.*

Nasal bone

Lateral nasal cartilage

Septal cartilage

Lesser alar cartilages

Greater alar cartilage

Fibrous tissue

A

Nasal bone

Lateral nasal cartilage

Greater alar cartilage

Septal cartilage

Fibrous tissue

B

Greater alar cartilage

Septal cartilage

Lesser alar cartilages

C

5-43. *Medial view of the left lateral wall of the nasal cavity showing the superior (S), middle (M), and inferior (I) nasal conchae.*

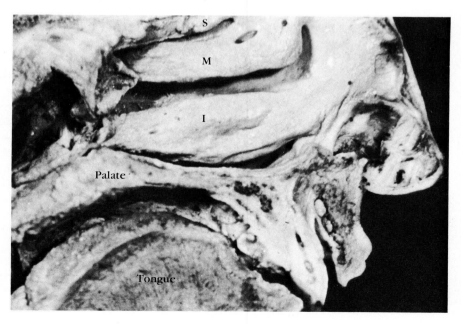

S

M

I

Palate

Tongue

perature control of the air passing over them. Each nasal cavity communicates with the **paranasal sinuses** and other structures through openings in the lateral wall. These include the **sphenoid, frontal,** and **maxillary sinuses** and the **lacrimal gland,** which secretes tears. Anteriorly the nasal cavities communicate with the exterior via the **nostrils** (also called the **anterior nares**). Posteriorly, the nasal cavities communicate with the nasopharynx via the **choanae** (also called the **posterior nares**).

ORAL CAVITY

The oral cavity is composed of two parts. The **vestibule** of the oral cavity is bounded by the lips and cheeks superficially and by the teeth and alveolar arches. The oral cavity proper is bounded by the teeth and alveolar arches anteriorly and laterally, by the hard and soft palate superiorly, by the floor of the mouth inferiorly, and by the anterior faucial pillars posteriorly. The area between the anterior and posterior pillars on each side is the **tonsillar fossa** and contains the **palatine tonsils** (Figure 5-44).

5-44. *Oral surface of the palate.*

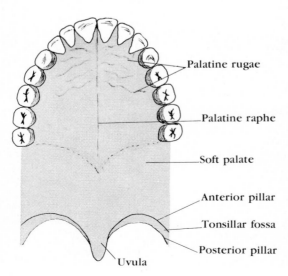

Palatine rugae

Palatine raphe

Soft palate

Anterior pillar

Tonsillar fossa

Posterior pillar

Uvula

The anterior palate is marked by transverse ridges called the **palatine rugae.** A median ridge, the **palatine raphe** extends the length of the midline of the palate. The floor of the mouth is formed principally by the tongue.

The functions of the oral cavity include biting, mastication (chewing), digestion, swallowing, resonance, and speech articulation. All of these except digestion involve movements of the mandible in opening or closing the mouth and movements of the tongue. The teeth are involved in biting, mastication, and speech articulation, and the muscles of the lips and cheeks are involved in mastication and speech articulation. The preliminary part of the digestive process, which takes place in the mouth, is a function of saliva secreted into the oral cavity.

DENTITION

Two sets of teeth make their appearance during infancy and childhood. The **deciduous teeth** appear during the first 2½ years of life. Subsequently they are lost and are replaced by the **permanent teeth** between 6 and 25 years of age. Each tooth consists of three parts (Figure 5-45). The **crown** is that portion of the tooth that projects above the gum line. The **root** of the tooth is embedded within the alveolar bone. The constricted portion of the tooth between the crown and root is the **neck** of the tooth.

The crown of the tooth is covered by **enamel,** which is the hardest substance of the body. The root of the tooth is covered with a thin layer of bone called the **cementum.** Deep to the enamel and the cementum is the ivory part of the tooth called the **dentin.** The dentin surrounds the **pulp chamber,** which contains loose connective tissue richly supplied with vessels and nerves. The vessels and nerves enter the pulp chamber through the **apical foramen** of the root.

The teeth are named for their form (Figure 5-46). The **incisor** teeth are the most anteromedial and have sharp cutting edges. Lateral to the incisors are the **canine** teeth. Canines are characterized by long tapered roots and a biting edge that is somewhat pointed. Posterior to the canines

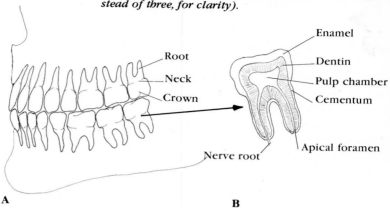

5-45. *Parts of a tooth. A, External structure. B, Sagittal section through a molar (shown with two roots instead of three, for clarity).*

Root

Neck

Crown

Enamel

Dentin

Pulp chamber

Cementum

Apical foramen

Nerve root

A

B

5-46. *Deciduous (A) and permanent (B) teeth. The age at which each tooth type erupts is shown in months or years. The sequence of eruption is indicated numerically.*

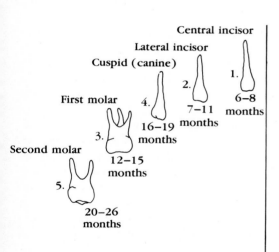

Central incisor

Lateral incisor

Cuspid (canine)

First molar

Second molar

1.

6–8 months

2.

7–11 months

4.

16–19 months

3.

12–15 months

5.

20–26 months

A. Deciduous teeth

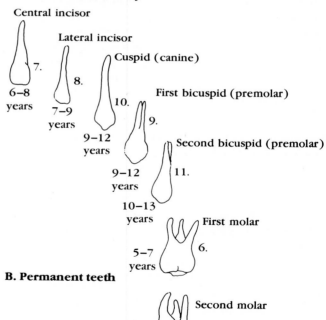

Central incisor

Lateral incisor

Cuspid (canine)

First bicuspid (premolar)

Second bicuspid (premolar)

First molar

Second molar

Third molar (wisdom tooth)

7.

6–8 years

8.

7–9 years

10.

9–12 years

9.

9–12 years

11.

10–13 years

6.

5–7 years

12.

11–14 years

13.

18–40 years

B. Permanent teeth

221

are the **premolar** teeth. Premolars have crowns with two elevations called **cusps** on their biting surface and a bifurcated root. The most posterior teeth are the **molars,** which are marked by three or four cusps on their biting surface and usually three root projections.

The deciduous dentition is composed of 20 teeth and includes two central incisors, two lateral incisors, two canines, and two molars in each jaw. The permanent dentition is composed of 32 teeth and includes, in addition to replacements for the deciduous teeth, four premolars and two molars in each jaw. The ages at which these teeth erupt is quite variable; typical ages are given in Figure 5-46.

In the normal relationship between the upper and lower permanent teeth, the upper incisors overlap the labial surface of the lower incisors, and the upper premolars and molars are approximately one-half space posterior to their lower counterparts. At rest, the upper and lower teeth are slightly separated.

TONGUE
Topographical Anatomy
The tongue is a muscular organ covered by mucous membrane (see Figure 5-24). Its anterior and lateral margins are free. Inferiorly, it attaches to the floor of the mouth and to the hyoid bone. Posterolaterally, it attaches to the lateral walls of the oral cavity. Posteroinferiorly, it attaches to the epiglottis. The anterior tip of the tongue is called the **apex.** The superior surface is the **dorsum.** The dorsum is divided into left and right halves by a shallow depression, the **median lingual sulcus.** The dorsum terminates posteriorly at a V-shaped depression, the **sulcus terminalis,** which divides the tongue into the anterior **body** and posteroinferior **root.** At the midline of the sulcus terminalis is a pit called the **foramen cecum.** Posteriorly, the **lateral** and **medial glossoepiglottic folds** extend from the root of the tongue to the epiglottis. Laterally, the **palatoglossal fold** extends from the side of the body of the tongue to the soft palate. Anteriorly and inferiorly another

fold called the **frenulum** extends from the inferior surface of the body of the tongue to the floor of the mouth.

The structure of the mucous membrane of the tongue varies from one region to another. The mucous membrane of the inferior surface is smooth. On the dorsal surface of the body of the tongue, it is irregular and contains elevations called **papillae,** many of which contain taste buds. Immediately anterior to the sulcus terminalis is a row of large **circumvallate papillae,** which contain taste buds and also excrete serous fluid which bathes the taste buds. The surface of the root of the tongue is covered by many small lymphatic aggregates and also contains the **lingual tonsils.**

Functions
The mass of the tongue is composed of a complex network of striated muscles. Its surface is richly supplied with sensory endings and is exquisitely sensitive to touch, including very fine two-point discrimination. The arrangement of muscles within the tongue and its rich nerve supply make it possible to produce complex motions and shaping of the tongue.

The tongue is involved in a variety of activities, including taste, mastication, swallowing, and articulation of speech sounds. During mastication, the tongue moves food about the mouth with extreme adroitness. It then forms a food bolus and propels it into the pharynx during the first stage of swallowing. During speech, the tongue changes the shape and size of the oral and pharyngeal cavities, thus affecting resonance. The tongue stops or impedes air flow in various parts of the oral cavity for the production of many of the consonant sounds. It is primarily by virtue of this remarkably versatile organ that we are able to produce the wide variety of sounds that characterize human speech.

During the period of infancy, the tongue serves for expression of milk from the nipple during suckling as well as for swallowing. The typical posture of the tongue when not at rest is cup-shaped with the rim of the tongue raised and the center depressed. The principal motion of the tongue is extension and retraction. The cupping of the tongue places the perimeter of the dorsum in contact with the maxillary alveolar arch (and with the nipple during suckling), providing a closed cavity for suction. With maturation of the neuromuscular system, the child learns more complex motions of the tongue.

Connective Tissue Skeleton

The mass of the tongue is composed of several intrinsic and extrinsic muscles separated, in part, by connective tissue. The connective-tissue skeleton of the tongue serves both to surround and separate muscle bundles and as sites of muscle fiber attachment. The structure of the connective-tissue skeleton has not been thoroughly documented; thus, information is incomplete and sometimes conflicting. The connective tissue immediately deep to the mucous membrane covering the tongue penetrates into the spaces among muscle fibers. Thus the mucous membrane is strongly adherent to the underlying musculature [46]. A connective-tissue **median septum** separates the left and right halves of the tongue (Figure 5-47). The septum is incomplete anteriorly and does not extend into the tongue tip. It is reportedly thickest inferiorly and posteriorly and becomes cribriform superiorly, where it permits passage of muscle fibers across the midline [70]. A **paramedian septum** parallels the median septum on either side of the tongue. It, too, terminates anteriorly short of the tongue tip. Posteriorly, it is continuous with the **hyoglossal membrane,** which arises from the major horn of the hyoid bone on either side of the tongue [2].

5-47. *Representative horizontal sections through the tongue of a human fetus from superior (A) to inferior (I).*

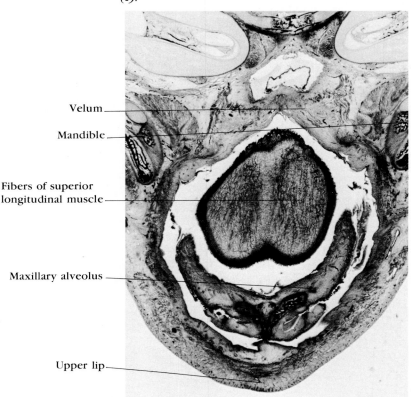

Velum

Mandible

Fibers of superior longitudinal muscle

Maxillary alveolus

Upper lip

A

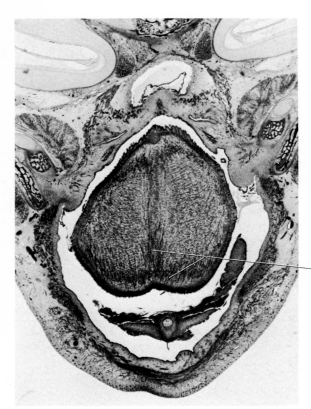

5-47 *(continued)*

—Superior longitudinal muscle

B

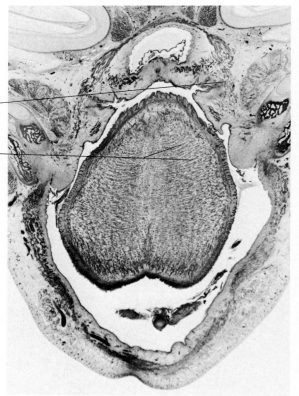

Palatoglossus muscle.

Transverse muscle fibers
separated by bundles
of vertical muscle

C

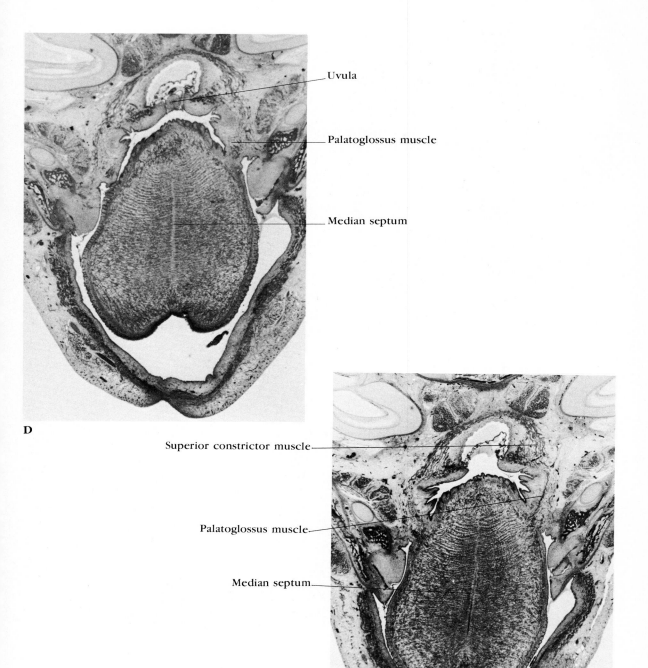

Uvula

Palatoglossus muscle

Median septum

D

Superior constrictor muscle

Palatoglossus muscle

Median septum

E

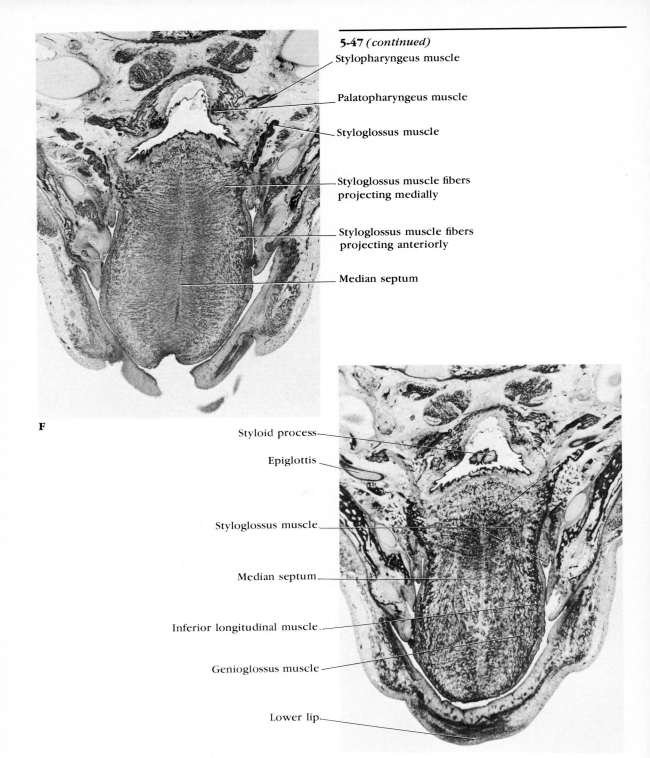

Stylopharyngeus muscle

Palatopharyngeus muscle

Styloglossus muscle

Styloglossus muscle fibers projecting medially

Styloglossus muscle fibers projecting anteriorly

Median septum

F

Styloid process

Epiglottis

Styloglossus muscle

Median septum

Inferior longitudinal muscle

Genioglossus muscle

Lower lip

G

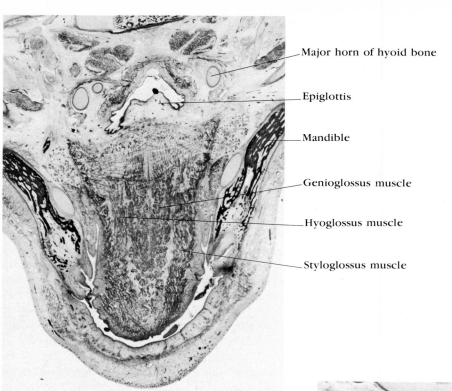

Major horn of hyoid bone

Epiglottis

Mandible

Genioglossus muscle

Hyoglossus muscle

Styloglossus muscle

H

Superior horn of thyroid cartilage

Hyoid bone

Genioglossus muscle

Mandible

I

Muscles

The four intrinsic muscles of the tongue are the **superior longitudinal, inferior longitudinal, verticalis,** and **transversus.** The principal mass of the tongue is composed of fibers of the verticalis and transversus muscles, which form an interlocking network of fibers throughout most of the tongue. It is believed that these two muscles are of primary importance in complex shaping of the tongue. However, it is difficult to distinguish the functional capacities of the intrinsic muscles and the extrinsic muscles that course through the tongue. The extrinsic muscles are named for their external attachment and include the **styloglossus, palatoglossus, hyoglossus,** and **genioglossus.** The intrinsic and extrinsic muscles of the tongue are illustrated in Figures 5-47, 5-48, 5-49, 5-50.

There have been relatively few studies of the anatomy of the lingual musculature [34]. Early work by Sommering [76], Cruveilheir [28], Salter [70], and Hesse [41] as well as more modern reports by Abd-El-Malek [2], Dabelow [30], De Paula Assis [31], Strong [78], Bell [7], Doran and Baggett [35], and Miyawaki [62] describe one or more muscles but give no indication of variability in their findings. Barnwell [5], Langdon and associates [48] and Barnwell and associates [6] do give information on variability of the muscles they studied but still leave us with incomplete information on the highly complicated structure of the musculature within the tongue. Because these muscles both interweave and blend as they course through the tongue, it is extremely difficult either with gross dissection or with serial histological reconstruction to be certain which fiber bundles belong to which muscles. When all these reports are put together with our own detailed studies, however, a fairly clear picture of the muscular arrangements emerges. Nevertheless, the complexity of the muscle bundles of the tongue is so great that it is not at all clear which muscles are responsible for which actions of the tongue. Except for the very large extrinsic muscles, the complex interweaving also makes it impossible to conduct electromyographic experiments within the body of the tongue that would clearly distinguish recordings from individual muscles.

Auditory tube

Superior longitudinal muscle

Nasal cavity

Levator veli palatini muscle

Superior constrictor muscle

Palatoglossus muscle

Hyoglossus muscle

Minor horn of hyoid bone

Major horn of hyoid bone

Anterior tooth bud

Verticalis muscle fibers

Lower lip

Anterior digastric muscle

Mandible

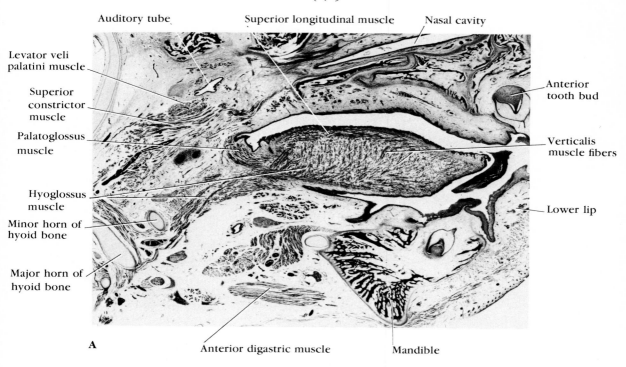

A

Inferior concha

Palatine and maxillary parts of hard palate

Hyoglossus muscle

Superior longitudinal muscle

Inferior longitudinal muscle

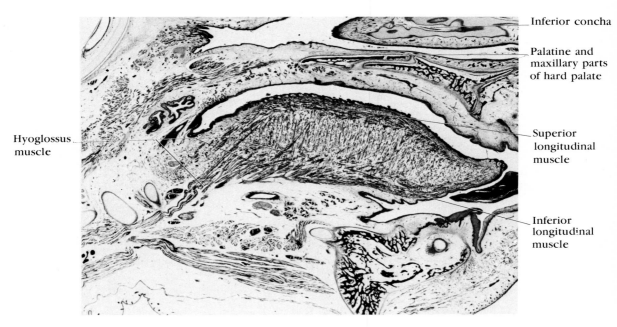

B

5-48 *(continued)*

Fibers of verticalis muscle separated by
bundles of transversus muscle fibers

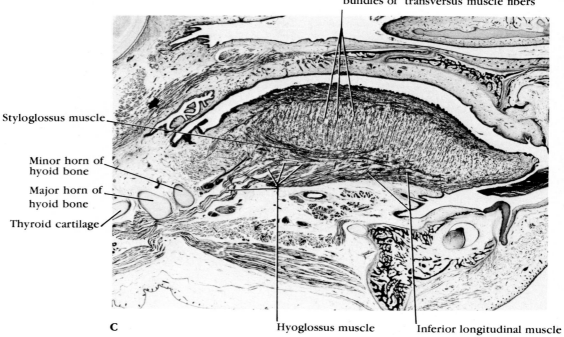

Styloglossus muscle

Minor horn of
hyoid bone

Major horn of
hyoid bone

Thyroid cartilage

C

Hyoglossus muscle   Inferior longitudinal muscle

Superior longitudinal muscle   Inferior longitudinal muscle

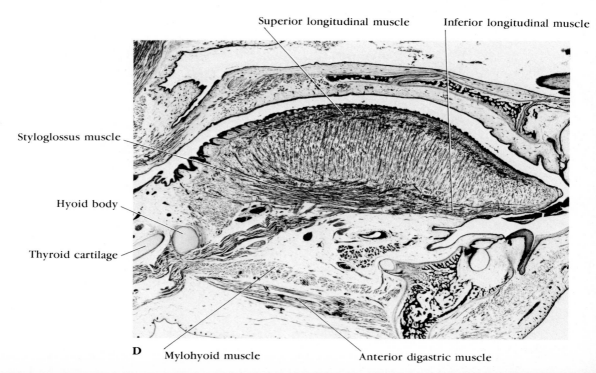

Styloglossus muscle

Hyoid body

Thyroid cartilage

D   Mylohyoid muscle   Anterior digastric muscle

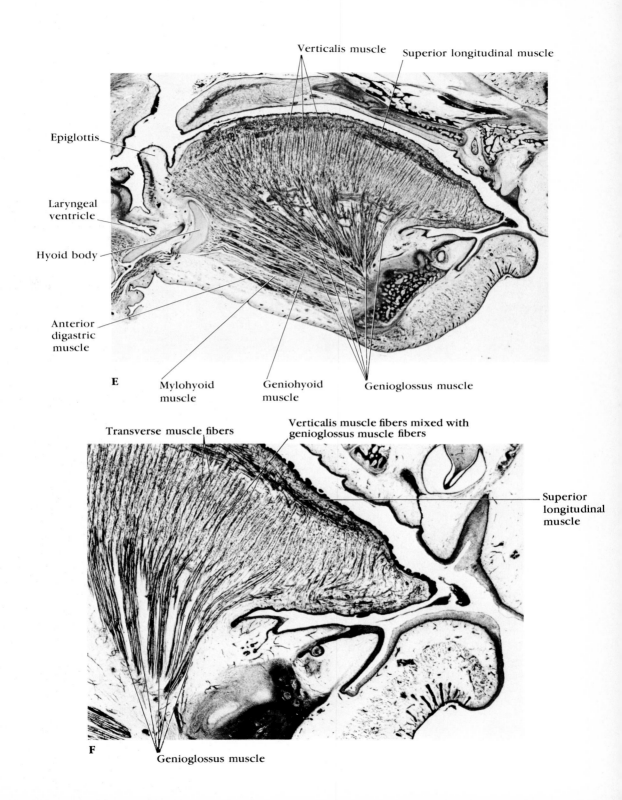

Verticalis muscle   Superior longitudinal muscle

Epiglottis

Laryngeal
ventricle

Hyoid body

Anterior
digastric
muscle

E   Mylohyoid
    muscle

Geniohyoid
muscle

Genioglossus muscle

Transverse muscle fibers   Verticalis muscle fibers mixed with
                           genioglossus muscle fibers

Superior
longitudinal
muscle

F   Genioglossus muscle

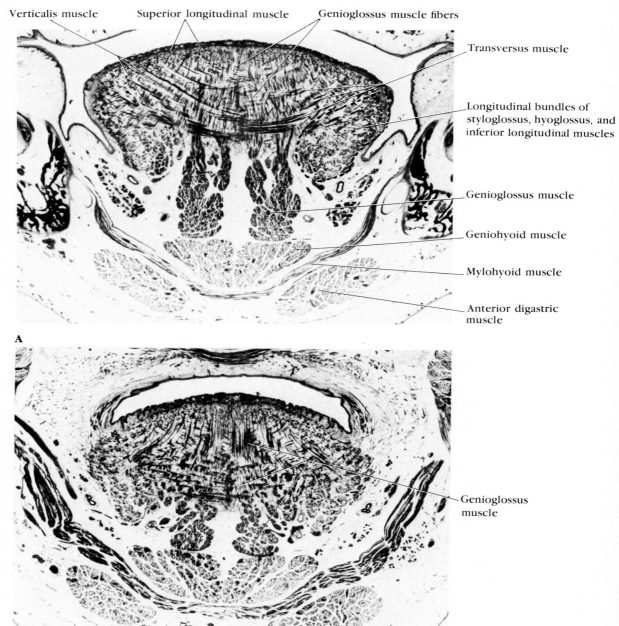

Verticalis muscle   Superior longitudinal muscle   Genioglossus muscle fibers

Transversus muscle

Longitudinal bundles of styloglossus, hyoglossus, and inferior longitudinal muscles

Genioglossus muscle

Geniohyoid muscle

Mylohyoid muscle

Anterior digastric muscle

A

Genioglossus muscle

B

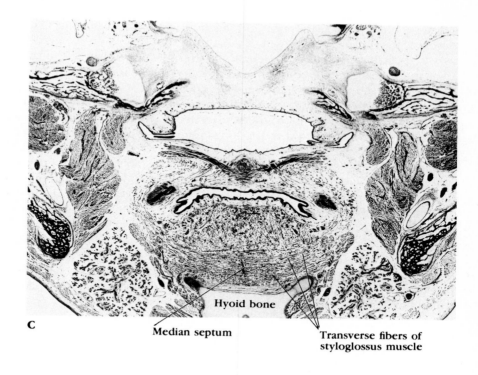

C

Hyoid bone

Median septum

Transverse fibers of
styloglossus muscle

5-50. *Extrinsic muscles of the tongue, lateral dissection.*

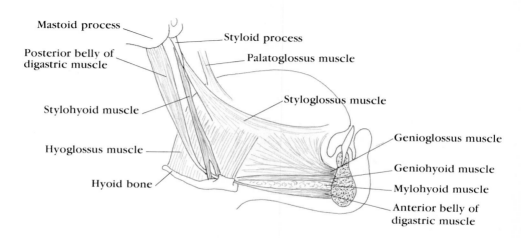

Mastoid process

Styloid process

Posterior belly of
digastric muscle

Palatoglossus muscle

Stylohyoid muscle

Styloglossus muscle

Hyoglossus muscle

Genioglossus muscle

Geniohyoid muscle

Hyoid bone

Mylohyoid muscle

Anterior belly of
digastric muscle

SUPERIOR LONGITUDINAL. The superior longitudinal muscle of the tongue is composed of short, imbricated muscle fibers arranged in a longitudinal (anterior to posterior) orientation to cover the dorsum of the tongue. The fibers lie immediately deep to the connective tissue underlying the mucous membrane of the dorsum (called the **lamina propria**). The muscle is thickest at the longitudinal midline of the tongue and is thicker posteriorly than anteriorly. The fibers extend posteriorly as far as the lower part of the epiglottis and hyoglossal membrane [2]. Anteriorly, the fibers are separated at midline by the insertion of the genioglossus muscle to the dorsal lamina propria. The most anterior fibers of the superior longitudinal have two sites of attachment. The more medial fibers course inferiorly to attach to the median septum, while the more lateral fibers course more anteriorly to end on the lateral part of the lamina propria of the tongue tip [2,6].

The functional potential of this muscle is not clear. Presumably, contraction of one side could result in deviation of the tongue tip to that side. Contraction of the entire muscle would shorten the dorsum and might result in convexity of the dorsum from anterior to posterior (Figure 5-51). The fact that the muscle is composed of short rather than long fibers suggests a capability for contraction of specific parts of the muscle, thus differentially affecting the shape of segments of the dorsum.

INFERIOR LONGITUDINAL. Although the inferior longitudinal has not been identified reliably, the most definitive description of this muscle is presented by Abd-El-Malek [2]. The inferior longitudinal is a penniform muscle that arises from the body of the hyoid bone and from the root of the major cornua and passes into the body of the tongue, where it blends with fibers of other muscles, including the hyoglossus, genioglossus, and styloglossus. It probably inserts into the lamina propria of the inferior surface of the tongue tip.

The functional potential of the inferior longitudinal muscle would be to retract and lower the tongue tip or, by contraction of one side, to deviate the tip to the same side (Figure 5-52).

VERTICALIS. The verticalis muscle is composed of fiber bundles that extend throughout most of the mass of the body of the tongue. They arise from the lamina propria of the dorsum and extend vertically to end within the body of the tongue or to insert into the inferior lamina propria in the lateral

5-51. *Functional potential of the superior longitudinal muscle. A, Lateral view; B, Superior view.*

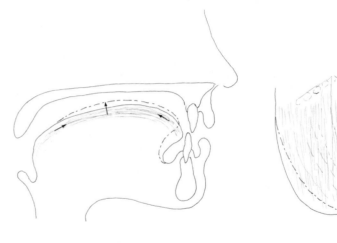

parts of the tongue. There is some question as to whether these fibers reach the tip or extreme posterior limit of the tongue. Observations of Salter [70] and Abd-El-Malek [2] agree with our own that in the median and paramedian portions of the tongue, the fibers of the verticalis arise from the dorsal lamina propria and descend vertically to end on the septa of other muscles in the inferior portion of the tongue. In the lateral parts of the tongue, the fibers descend and arch somewhat laterally from the dorsal lamina propria and insert into the lamina propria of the inferior surface of the tongue. Miyawaki [62] disagrees with this description. From his histological studies he concluded that the verticalis muscle is found only in the superior half of the tongue, at least in the median and paramedian parts of the tongue body. Abd-El-Malek [2] reported that some of the fibers of the verticalis muscle are short and do not reach the lower part of the tongue, while others do so.

The functional potential of the verticalis muscle would be to flatten the tongue, at least in its lateral parts, and perhaps to aid in lowering the median and paramedian parts of the dorsum (Figure 5-53).

TRANSVERSUS. There is general agreement in the literature regarding the anatomy of the transversus muscle. Its fibers arise from the midsagittal plane, either from the median septum or, penetrating the septum, from fibers of the opposite side. The fibers course laterally to insert into the lamina propria of the sides of the tongue. The more superior fibers fan out in a superolateral direction, while the more inferior fibers fan out in an inferolateral direction. Fiber bundles of the transversus muscle extend from immediately beneath the dorsal lamina propria inferiorly to the level of the inferior longitudinal muscle. Some of the fibers may be short and may not extend to the extreme lateral margin of the tongue [2]. In the tongue tip, fibers of the transversus may decussate with fibers of the verticalis, and interdigitate with fibers of superior longitudinal, inferior longitudinal, styloglossus, and hyoglossus [62]. The posterior extent of the muscle is open to question, since transverse fibers of the styloglossus occupy the root of the tongue and may be confused with the transversus muscle.

The functional potential of the transversus would be to narrow the tongue (Figure 5-54).

5-52. *Functional potential of the inferior longitudinal muscle. A, Lateral view; B, Superior view.*

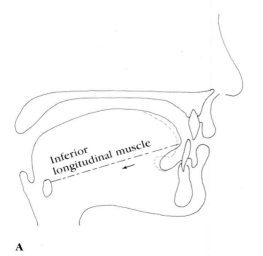

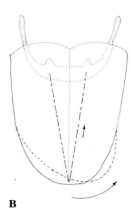

A   B

5-53. *Functional potential of the verticalis muscle. GG, genioglossus muscle; GH, geniohyoid muscle; MH, myohyoid muscle; AD, anterior belly of digastric muscle.*

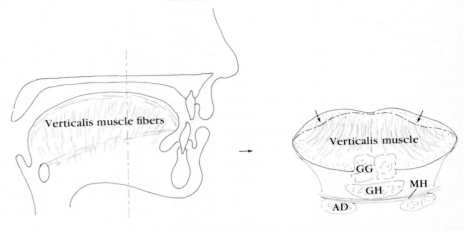

5-54. *Functional potential of the transversus muscle. Coronal view. GG, genioglossus muscle; GH, geniohyoid muscle; MH, mylohyoid muscle; AD, anterior belly of digastric muscle.*

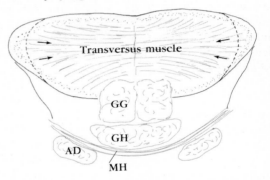

5-55. *Functional potential of the styloglossus muscle. A, Lateral view; B, Superior view, with one side contracting; C, Superior view, with both sides contracting.*

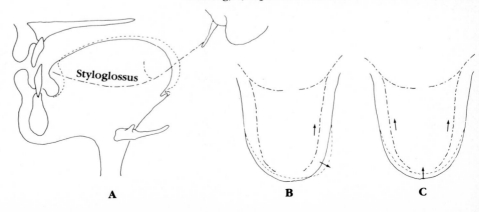

STYLOGLOSSUS. The styloglossus muscle originates from the styloid process of the temporal bone, courses anteriorly, inferiorly, and medially to insert into the sides of the root of the tongue, and then bifurcates. Approximately 75% of the muscle fibers turn medially within the root, penetrate the hyoglossus muscle, and course transversely at least as far as the lateral border of the genioglossus muscle [5]. The more lateral fibers (the remaining 25%) course anteriorly through the lateral margins of the tongue. According to Barnwell [5], "As m. styloglossus coursed forward through the anterior third of the tongue toward the tip, its fibers merged with, were overlapped by, and became indistinguishable from, the more medial fibers of the musculi hyoglossus and longitudinalis inferior and more lateral oblique fibers arising from the lamina propria."

The most apparent functional potential of the styloglossus is to retract the tongue. One side acting alone could deviate the tongue tip toward the same side. Contraction of the fibers that extend anteriorly could also result in shortening of the tongue (Figure 5-55).

PALATOGLOSSUS. The palatoglossus muscle extends from the anterior velum through the anterior pillar of fauces to insert into the side of the root of the tongue. Some authors consider this a muscle of the palate, and others as a muscle of the tongue. The specifics of this muscle's attachment to the velum and tongue have not been studied.

The functional potentials of this muscle are to lower the anterior velum and/or to raise and retract the root of the tongue. However, the anterior velum is relatively immobile, which might suggest a lingual function for this muscle. Medial displacement of the anterior pillars during swallowing would also be possible as a result of contraction of this muscle (Figure 5-56).

HYOGLOSSUS. The hyoglossus is a quadrilateral sheet of muscle that arises from the superolateral part of the hyoid body and the entire superior surface of the major cornua of the hyoid bone. It courses anteriorly and superiorly to insert into the side of the tongue between the styloglossus and the inferior longitudinal muscles. Within the tongue, its more anterior fibers extend anteriorly along the inferior surface of the lateral part of the tongue and blend with the other longitudinal muscles of the tongue tip. The middle part of the muscle extends superiorly and somewhat anteriorly, while the more posterior fibers course superiorly and somewhat posteriorly to the lamina propria of the root of the tongue [62].

The functional potential of the hyoglossus muscle is to draw the tongue posteroinferiorly, particularly at the lateral margins (Figure 5-57).

5-57. *Functional potential of the hyoglossus muscle, lateral view.*

5-56. *Functional potential of the palatoglossus muscle, lateral view.*

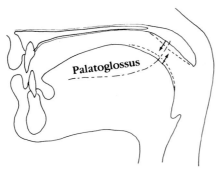

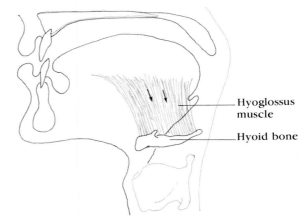

Hyoglossus muscle

Hyoid bone

GENIOGLOSSUS. The genioglossus muscle is a paired, flat, fan-shaped muscle that lies on either side of midline with the left and right muscles separated only by the incomplete median lingual septum. The muscle arises as three groups of fibers from the superior mental spine on the deep surface of the mandibular symphysis. The most inferior segment of the genioglossus projects posteriorly and inserts into the lamina propria of the root of the tongue from immediately superior to the hyoid bone to the level of the foramen cecum. The middle, and largest, of the bundles radiates through an angle of almost 90 degrees, with its inferior fibers inserting in the area of the foramen cecum and its superior fibers inserting at the junction of the body and apex of the tongue. The most superior bundle is the smallest. Its fibers rise almost vertically with the most superior fibers arching anteriorly. It inserts into the lamina propria of the apex and also into the anterior part of the median septum. Doran and Baggett [35] and Miyawaki [62] reported that the fibers of the genioglossus stop short of the tongue tip. However, Langdon and associates [48] and our own studies indicate that the fibers do reach the tip.

In sagittal section it can be seen that the fibers of the genioglossus segregate into bundles that rise through the body of the tongue between layers of fibers of the verticalis and transversus muscles. In coronal section it can be seen that fibers of the genioglossus also project upward between layers of the superior longitudinal muscle. They then radiate to insert into the lamina propria. Decussations of fibers between the left and right genioglossus muscles can be seen both inferior and superior to the median septum.

The functional potential of the genioglossus is to depress the median portion of the tongue and to draw the root of the tongue anteriorly (Figure 5-58).

INNERVATION. Sensory innervation of the tongue provides for the special sense of taste as well as general sensation, including touch and proprioception. Taste is mediated by cranial nerve IX from the root of the tongue and by cranial nerve VII from the body and tip of the tongue. General sensation is provided by cranial nerve IX from the root of the tongue and by cranial nerve V from the body and tip of the tongue. Motor supply to the muscles of the tongue is by cranial nerve XII except for the palatoglossus muscle, which receives its motor innervation from cranial nerve XI along with the other velopharyngeal musculature.

Detailed studies of the innervation of the muscles of the tongue are lacking [34]. Cooper [26] found muscle spindles in a number of muscles of the tongue but reported finding few spindles in the

5-58. *Functional potential of the genioglossus muscle. A, Lateral view; B, Coronal view.*

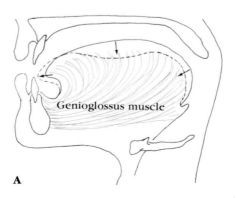

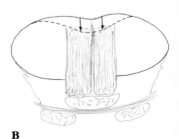

A   B

anterior third of the tongue. She also reported finding ganglia on the lingual nerve in the base of the tongue as well as on the glossopharyngeal nerve. Evidence from a study by Rakhawy [67] suggests that these ganglia are parasympathetic.

The exquisite control that human beings have over complex shaping and motion of the tongue suggests an intricate sensory control system and also a means for fine gradations of contraction of small groups of muscle fibers. The muscles of the tongue possess the highest ratio of nerve fibers to muscle fibers of any muscles of the body with the exception of the muscles of the eye. There may be sensory components within cranial nerve XII that form part of the control mechanism for tongue function; however, thus far they have been reported only in the cat. This is an important consideration, since the pathway for the afferent fibers of XII in the cat is via the posterior branch of that nerve. The human hypoglossal nerve (XII) does not contain a posterior branch [14].

FUNCTIONAL POTENTIALS. A number of authors, most notably Strong [78], have speculated on how various muscle bundles of the tongue could work together to provide for the variety of shapes and positions known to occur during speech. It is probable that small units of muscles of the tongue can function independently. However, our knowledge of specific muscle function remains speculative. Due to the intricate nature of interweaving of the muscle fibers within the tongue, speculations on specific muscle functions for tongue shaping would seem limited largely by one's imagination. Gross actions of the tongue may be easier to hypothesize. For example, extension of the tongue is probably a function of the genioglossus, once the tongue is shaped for extension by the intrinsic muscles. Retraction of the tongue could be a function of the styloglossus, hyoglossus, or both. Lateralization could be a function of the styloglossus, and/or the superior and inferior longitudinals. Elevation of the tongue tip could be accomplished by the superior longitudinal, while depression of the tip could be accomplished by the inferior longitudinal. Verification of the function of individual

muscles and muscle groups and components will be difficult given the complexity of the lingual morphology.

ELECTROMYOGRAPHIC EVIDENCE. Four electromyographic studies of the lingual musculature have been reported. The findings of three of these [17,29,71] were limited to the genioglossus muscle, which was found to be active during inhalation. MacNeilage and Sholes [55] presented conclusions related to the functions of each of the intrinsic and extrinsic lingual muscles during speech production; however, their data was derived from surface electrodes placed on the dorsum of the tongue of one subject and along a straight line off the median from tip to root. They give no evidence for the validity of their conclusions.

MASTICATION

The muscles of mastication are those which influence the position of the mandible (there is one exception, the buccinator muscle, which will be described with muscles of the face). Certain of the suprahyoid muscles (anterior belly of digastric, mylohyoid, and geniohyoid) may subserve depression of the mandible. The anatomy of these three muscles was presented in Chapter 4 (Suprahyoid Muscles) and will not be repeated here. The other muscles of mastication are the **masseter, temporalis,** and the **external** and **internal pterygoid** muscles, all of which attach to the ramus of the mandible and its superior extensions.

Functions

The motions of the mandible have already been described (see Joints of the Skull). Mandibular motion in speech is restricted to opening and closing. Under conditions of conversational speech, this motion is probably largely a hinge action. Since the tongue is attached to the mandible, elevation and depression of the tongue and mandible are not independent. Mandibular position will also influence position of the lower lip.

Gibbs and Messerman [39], comparing the mo-

5-59. *Lateral view of the superficial muscles of the head and neck, A, The skin and superficial fascia have been removed. B, The sternocleidomastoid, platysma, and superficial layer of the masseter muscles have been removed.*

Deep layer of masseter muscle

Temporalis muscle

External auditory meatus

Sternocleidomastoid muscle

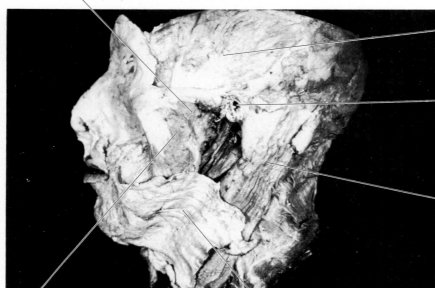

A   Superficial layer of masseter muscle   Platysma muscle

Deep layer of masseter muscle

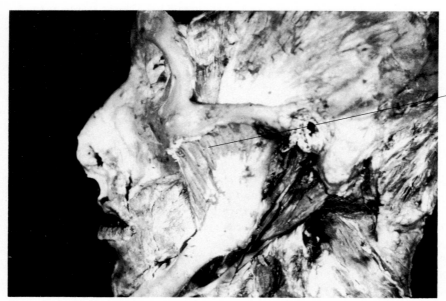

B

tions of the mandible in chewing and in speech, found that during speech the mandible undergoes very little lateral motion. In addition, while the motion of the symphysis of the mandible describes an ellipse during chewing, speech motions are more nearly characterized by simple elevation and depression (see Figure 5-19). While in chewing both the condyles and the symphysis undergo considerable vertical movement, such motion during speech is largely restricted to the symphysis. The maximum velocity of mandibular movement is much greater for chewing than for speech. In speech, velocity varies directly as a function of the degree of opening. Thus both the degree of mandibular motion and the velocity of motion is greater for low vowels than for high vowels, with values for consonants intermediate [79]. The absolute degree of jaw lowering during speech was found to be on the order of 11 to 13 mm for syllable production, in contrast to motion on the order of 25 to 35 mm found during chewing [39].

Muscles

MASSETER. The masseter muscle is composed of a superficial and a deep part and lies superficial to the ramus of the mandible (Figure 5-59). The **superficial part** of the muscle has its origin from the anterior two-thirds of the zygomatic arch. Its fibers course inferiorly and slightly posteriorly to insert onto the superficial surface of the angle of the mandible. The **deep part** takes its origin from the entire length of the zygomatic arch. Its fibers extend inferiorly to attach to the lateral surface of the ramus and part of the coronoid process. The deep fibers parallel the fibers of the superficial part except posteriorly, where they are vertical.

The most obvious functional potential of the masseter muscle is to elevate the mandible, acting as a class 3 lever (Figure 5-60). Roche [68] estimated that the mean strength of the masseter is on the order of 46 kg based on the data of Carlsoo [21]. This would make it second in strength only to the temporalis muscle among the muscles of mastication.

TEMPORALIS. The temporalis is a broad, fan-shaped muscle located on the lateral surface of the cranium (Figure 5-61). Its origin is from the length of the inferior temporal line and the lateral surface of the greater wing of the sphenoid bone. The fibers converge to insert onto the medial surface and anterior border of the coronoid process and the anterior border of the mandibular ramus.

The functional potential of the temporalis muscle is to elevate and retract the mandible in a class

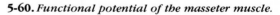

5-60. *Functional potential of the masseter muscle.*

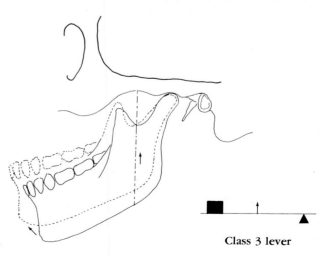

Class 3 lever

3 lever action (Figure 5-62). Retraction of one side of the mandible could assist in moving the symphysis toward the ipsilateral side.

EXTERNAL PTERYGOID. The external pterygoid is a two-bellied muscle (Figure 5-63). Its superior belly arises from the infratemporal crest and lower margin of the greater wing of the sphenoid bone. Its inferior belly arises from the lateral surface of the lateral pterygoid plate. The two bellies converge as they pass posteriorly to insert onto the neck of the condyle of the mandible.

The external pterygoid is capable of moving the condyle in an anterior direction. Contraction of

5-61. *Temporalis muscle, lateral view.*

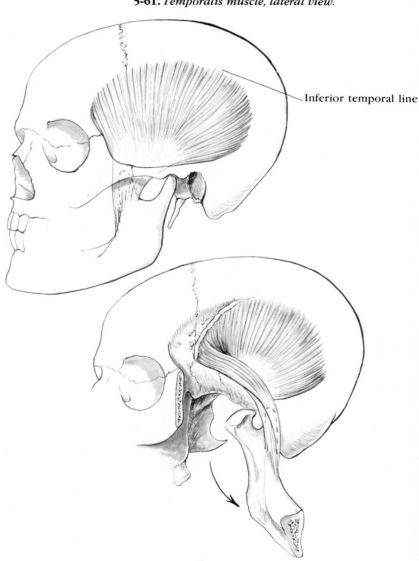

Inferior temporal line

5-62. *Functional potential of the temporalis muscle.*

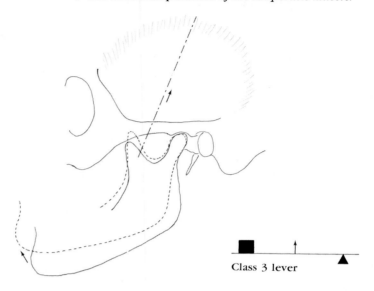

Class 3 lever

5-63. *Pterygoid muscles, mandible removed (indicated by dotted lines).*

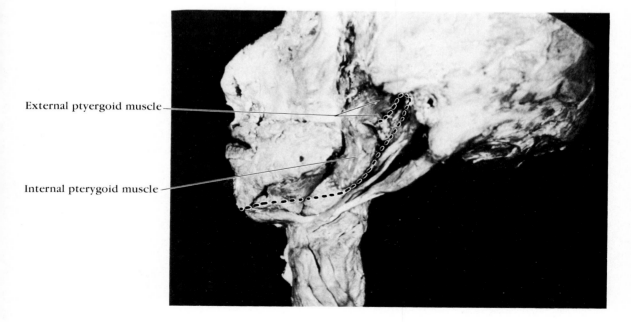

External ptyergoid muscle

Internal pterygoid muscle

one side could assist in moving the symphysis of the mandible toward the contralateral side (Figure 5-64).

INTERNAL PTERYGOID. The internal pterygoid muscle parallels the masseter muscle on the deep surface of the mandibular condyle (see Figure 5-63). Thus the two muscles form a sling around the angle of the mandible. The origin of the internal pterygoid is from the medial surface of the lateral pterygoid plate and from the pyramidal process of the palatine bone. Its fibers course inferiorly, posteriorly, and slightly laterally and insert onto the angle of the mandible.

The functional capacity of the internal pterygoid is the same as for the masseter, that is, to elevate the mandible. Contraction of one side could cause deviation of the condyle toward the contralateral side. However, lateralization would be slight, since the angle of pull of the internal pterygoid is nearly vertical (Figure 5-65).

SUPRAHYOID MUSCLES. The anterior belly of the digastric muscle, the geniohyoid muscle, and, to a lesser extent, the mylohyoid muscle have functional potential for lowering the mandible as part of a class 2 lever (Figure 5-66). While these muscles would be working at a mechanical advantage, a part of their strength would be dissipated by the difference in the direction of motion of the symphysis and the direction of pull of these muscles. Also, since these muscles all attach to the hyoid bone, that bone would need to be stabilized by the synergistic action of other suprahyoid and infrahyoid muscles.

INNERVATION. The muscles of mastication are innervated by the mandibular branch of the trigeminal nerve (cranial nerve V) except for the geniohyoid, which is innervated by cranial nerve XII. Presumably these muscles receive both their motor and sensory supply from the source indicated. Abbs [1] reported that blockade of the gamma efferents of the mandibular branch of the trigeminal by anesthesia reduced jaw acceleration, velocity, and degree of displacement. Further, the degree of reduction increased with increased demand on the system. Muscle spindles have been found in the muscles of mastication, though there

5-64. *Functional potential of the external pterygoid muscle.*

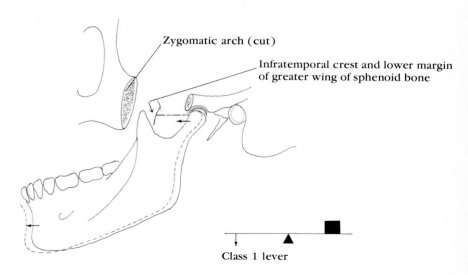

Zygomatic arch (cut)

Infratemporal crest and lower margin of greater wing of sphenoid bone

Class 1 lever

5-65. *Functional potential of the internal pterygoid muscle.*

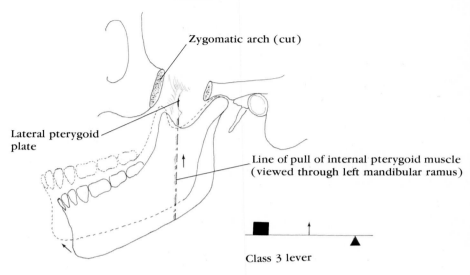

Zygomatic arch (cut)

Lateral pterygoid plate

Line of pull of internal pterygoid muscle (viewed through left mandibular ramus)

Class 3 lever

5-66. *Functional potential of the anterior belly of the digastric, geniohyoid, and mylohyoid muscles. A, Anteroinferior view; B, Midsagittal section. The fulcrum of the lever is the temporomandibular joint.*

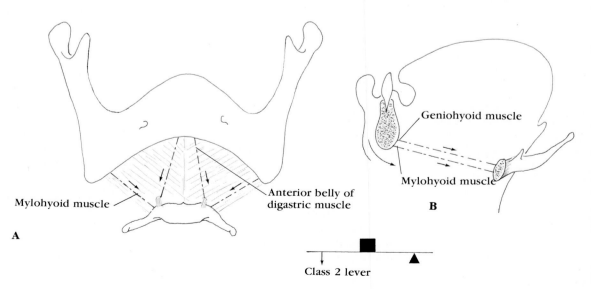

Geniohyoid muscle

Mylohyoid muscle

B

Mylohyoid muscle

Anterior belly of digastric muscle

A

Class 2 lever

is some evidence that the mandibular elevators are more richly supplied with spindles than are the mandibular depressors. However, at least in some of these muscles, the size and complexity of the muscle spindles varies to a considerable degree [36, 80].

The innervation ratio of the muscles of mastication is low and varies from muscle to muscle. Carlsoo [24] has estimated the innervation ratio for the temporal muscle at 1 : 936, and for the masseter at 1 : 640. This is consistent with the findings of Carlsoo and Werner [25] that both the masseter and temporalis muscle have long duration action potentials. Thus, these muscles would not be expected to be capable of fine degrees of contraction based on the independent contraction of small groups of muscle fibers.

ELECTROMYOGRAPHIC EVIDENCE. A large number of studies of the muscles of mastication have been reported in the dental literature with particular emphasis on the process of chewing (the reader is referred to the excellent review of research pertaining to biomechanics and function of the muscles of mastication by Roche [68] and the report of the workshop on Oral Motor Behavior edited by Bryant and others [19]). There is ample evidence that the masseter and internal pterygoid function as mandibular elevators and that the temporalis muscle acts as an elevator and retractor of the mandible [3,21,23,40,49,54,63–65]. However, Sussman and associates [79] found only a low level of activity of the masseter during jaw elevation for speech and little contribution from the internal pterygoid. Lowering of the mandible is at least in part a function of the anterior belly of the digastric muscle [22,42,63–65,79]. The possible function of the other suprahyoid muscles in jaw lowering has not been adequately studied.

Anterior displacement of the mandible has been found to be associated with contraction of the external pterygoid [23]. There is convincing evidence that in posterior motion of the mandible, the temporalis muscle plays the dominant role, while anterior motion is a function of the external pterygoid [21,22,23,40,49,54]. There is some evidence that the two heads of the lateral pterygoid may act independently and perhaps reciprocally [53]. Schaerer and associates [72] and others [38,77] have suggested that action of the mandibular elevators is inhibited by tooth contact and, therefore, may be under control of nerves supplying the teeth. However, Matthews and Vemm [56] found such inhibition in edentulous patients wearing full dentures.

In summary, mandibular elevation is a function of the masseter, internal pterygoid, and also the temporalis muscle, which provides both elevation and retraction. Lowering of the mandible is a function of the anterior belly of digastric (and possibly other suprahyoids) with the external pterygoid providing the anterior motion component. Lateralization of the mandible is a function of the posterior part of the temporalis muscle pulling posteriorly on one side, and the external pterygoid muscle pulling anteriorly on the other side [21,23,42,49,54].

FACE
The muscles of the face and scalp are usually considered together (Figure 5-67). These include the perioral muscles; the muscles of the external nares; the periocular muscles; the muscles that attach to and move the skin of the posterior scalp, forehead, and neck; and the muscles of the pinna (external part of the ear). Our principal concern here will be for the perioral muscles, since they are associated with lip movements and so with speech activities. Muscles of the pinna will be considered in the next chapter.

The **perioral muscles** surround and insert into the lips. While most anatomy texts and atlases describe these muscles, there has been little careful research reported regarding their detailed morphology and variability [47]. In spite of that, there is general agreement on the form and attachments of these superficial muscles.

Functions
Human beings are capable of a wide variety of complex facial expressions. This is most particu-

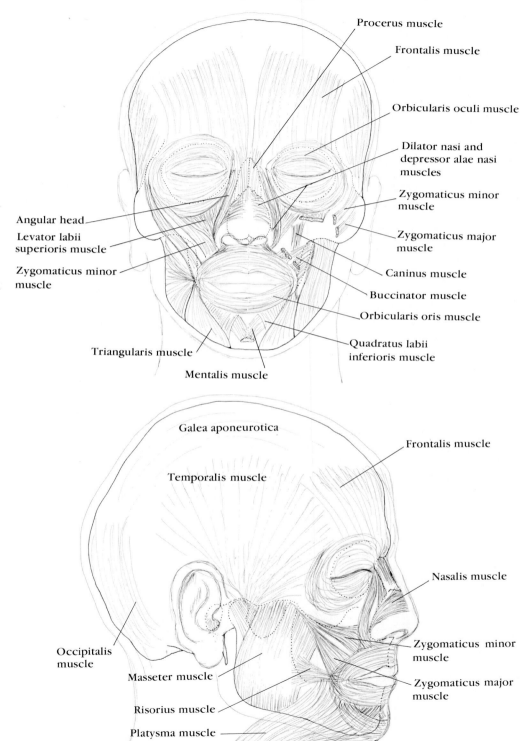

5-67. *Muscles of the face and scalp. A, Anterior view; B, Lateral view.*

Procerus muscle

Frontalis muscle

Orbicularis oculi muscle

Dilator nasi and depressor alae nasi muscles

Zygomaticus minor muscle

Zygomaticus major muscle

Caninus muscle

Buccinator muscle

Orbicularis oris muscle

Quadratus labii inferioris muscle

Quadratus labii superioris muscle

Angular head

Levator labii superioris muscle

Zygomaticus minor muscle

Triangularis muscle

Mentalis muscle

A

Galea aponeurotica

Frontalis muscle

Temporalis muscle

Nasalis muscle

Zygomaticus minor muscle

Zygomaticus major muscle

Occipitalis muscle

Masseter muscle

Risorius muscle

Platysma muscle

B

larly true in the perioral area. The lips can be opened and closed, pursed, extended, and retracted. The corners of the mouth can be drawn medially and laterally with great freedom. In addition, various segments of the lips, including the corners of the mouth, can be drawn in a variety of directions with some independence. Lip motion for speech is of particular concern in the formation of vowels, where such motion controls, in part, the anterior opening of the vocal tract as well as its shape and length.

Muscles

ORBICULARIS ORIS. The orbicularis oris forms the sphincter of the oral opening. It is composed of a deep and a superficial layer. The deep fibers originate from the buccinator muscle and so enter the lips from the sides. The more superficial fibers encircle the lips and are contributed to by fibers entering the lips from the surrounding perioral muscles. Fibers intrinsic to the lips intertwine in a complex manner with some passing between the deep and superficial layers. Some of these fibers attach to adjacent parts of the mandible, maxilla, and perhaps to the anterior part of the nasal septum.

The functional potential of the obicularis oris is sphincteric; that is, to compress the upper and lower lip, to purse and protrude the lips, and to compress the lips against the teeth.

BUCCINATOR. The buccinator is usually considered a muscle of the cheek, but inserts into the lips and therefore could affect their posture. Its origin is at the pterygomandibular raphe and the adjacent surfaces of the alveolar arch of the maxilla and mandible (Figure 5-68). At its origin, the pterygomandibular raphe separates the fibers of the buccinator from those of the posteriorly directed superior constrictor muscle. From its origin, the buccinator is directed anteriorly through the cheek as a relatively broad, thick muscle to the angle of the mouth. Its most superior fibers enter the upper lip. Its middle fibers decussate with the more superior fibers entering the lower lip, and the more inferior fibers entering the upper lip. The most inferior part of the muscle extends into the lower lip.

This muscle would be capable of drawing the angle of the mouth laterally, compressing the cheek against the adjacent teeth, and directing food from the vestibule into the oral cavity proper during mastication.

QUADRATUS LABII SUPERIOR. This muscle is composed of three parts; which have been given separate names. The **infraorbital head** (also called the **levator labii superior**) extends from the lower margin of the orbit to the lateral half of the upper lip. The **zygomatic head** (also called the **zygomatic minor**) extends from the superficial

5-68. *Buccinator muscle.*

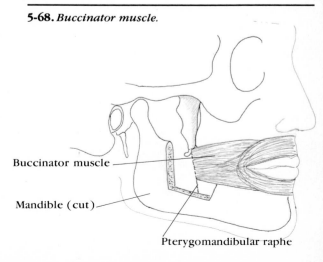

Buccinator muscle

Mandible (cut)

Pterygomandibular raphe

surface of the zygomatic bone to the upper lip in the region of the nasolabial furrow. It is quite variable in form and attachments and may be absent. The **angular head** (also called the **levator labii superior alaeque nasi**) extends from the superior part of the frontal process of the maxilla and inserts into the upper lip. It may also send fibers to the lateral nasal cartilage. The form and extent of this muscle and its parts are quite variable [47]. The functional potential of this muscle is to elevate all or parts of the upper lip and perhaps to dilate the external nares.

CANINUS. The caninus muscle (also called the **levator anguli oris**) extends from its origin at the canine fossa of the maxilla to intermingle with the orbicularis oris muscle at the angle of the mouth. It lies deep to the zygomatic head of the quadratus labii superior. Its function potential is to draw the angle of the mouth superiorly and laterally.

ZYGOMATICUS. The zygomaticus muscle (also called the **zygomaticus major**) lies lateral to the quadratus labii superior. Its origin is from the lateral part of the superficial surface of the zygomatic bone, where it is deep to the orbicularis oculi muscle. It extends inferiorly and medially to insert into the angle of the mouth where it intermingles with fibers of the orbicularis oris. Its functional potential is to move the angle of the mouth superolaterally.

RISORIUS. This small, inconsistent muscle is the most superficial muscle of the cheek lateral to the angle of the mouth. It arises from the fascia superficial to the masseter muscle and courses anteromedially to insert into the angle of the mouth. Its functional potential is to move the angle of the mouth laterally.

QUADRATUS LABII INFERIOR. This thin muscle arises from the oblique line of the mandible lateral to the symphysis and extends to the lower lip from midline to the angle of the mouth. Since its insertion into the lower lip and overlying skin is more superficial than its origin, its functional potential would be to lower and evert the lower lip.

TRIANGULARIS. The triangularis muscle (also called the **depressor anguli oris**) is, as its name implies, a roughly triangular muscle of the lower lip. It takes a broad origin from the oblique line of the mandible superficial and lateral to the quadratus labii inferior. Its fibers converge to insert in the lower lip at the angle of the mouth. Some of its fibers may bypass the angle and extend into the upper lip as a part of the caninus muscle. Its functional potential is to draw the angle of the mouth inferiorly, and perhaps medially.

MENTALIS. The mentalis is a small conical muscle that arises from the incisive fossa of the mandible and courses anteriorly and inferiorly to insert into the skin overlying the chin. Its functional potential is to draw the soft tissue of the chin superiorly and compress the inferior part of the lip against the alveolar arch.

PLATYSMA. The platysma is usually considered a muscle of the neck but may influence the position of the lower lip. Its origin is from the cervical fascia above the clavical immediately deep to the skin. Its fibers course superiorly beneath the skin to insert into the inferior surface of the mandible and into the deep surface of the skin between the masseter muscle and the angle of the mouth (see Figures 5-59, 5-67). This muscle moves the skin of the anterior neck in a superior rather than an inferior direction. Therefore, although its inferior origin would normally suggest influence on lip position, this is doubtful.

OTHER MUSCLES OF THE FACE AND SCALP. Muscles of the nose include the angular head of the quadratus labii superior which has already been described. The **procerus muscle** arises from the superficial surfaces of the lateral nasal cartilage and adjacent nasal bone near midline and extends superiorly to insert into the deep surface of the skin between the eyebrows. It functions to depress the medial end of the eyebrow. The **nasal muscle** arises from the surface of the maxilla superolateral to the incisive fossa and courses toward the midline of the nose below the nasal bones, where it blends with the paired muscle of the other side. Its contraction depresses the lateral nasal cartilage and narrows the aperture into the nasal cavity. The **depressor alae nasi muscle** takes its origin from the area of the incisive fossa of the maxilla and inserts into the ala of the nose and sends some fibers to the nasal septum. It depresses the ala and restricts the nasal opening. The **dilator nasi muscle** (also called the **alar part** of the nasalis muscle) arises with the nasalis muscle and inserts into the wing of the nose. Its contraction dilates the nasal opening.

The large **orbicularis oculi muscle** encircling the eye serves to close the eyelids. Deep to it is the **corrugator muscle,** which originates from the frontal bone superomedial to the orbit and inserts into the skin deep to the eyebrow. Its contraction creates vertical folds in the skin between the brows.

There are two large muscles of the scalp. The **frontalis muscle** is the large vertical muscle of the forehead. It raises the eyebrows and creates horizontal folds in the skin of the forehead. Superiorly this muscle ends in a large flat tendon, the **galea aponeurotica,** which extends over the vault of the skull and gives rise to the **occipitalis muscle** posteriorly. The fibers of the occipitalis continue to their attachment at the superior nuchal line. This muscle is capable of drawing the scalp posteriorly.

INNERVATION. The orbicularis oris, quadratus labii superior, caninus, and zygomaticus muscles are all innervated by the zygomatic branch of cranial nerve VII. The orbicularis oris also receives branches from the cervicofacial branch of cranial nerve VII. All of the other perioral muscles are innervated by the cervicofacial branch of VII. The other muscles of the face and scalp described above are also innervated by various branches of the seventh cranial nerve with one notable exception, the buccinator, which is innervated by cranial nerve V. This exception reflects the fact that the buccinator is a muscle of mastication rather than a muscle of facial expression, even though it is not involved in mandibular motion.

ELECTROMYOGRAPHIC EVIDENCE. With regard to the muscles of the face, electromyographic evidence is less than conclusive owing to the high degree of variability of many of these muscles, especially the muscles of the upper lip. In general, such evidence is consistent with the descriptions of function already presented, however, much of it involves circular reasoning, since electrical activity during specified functions is used as evidence of electrode placement in the specified muscle. Some authors have used dissection techniques on cadaveric material prior to electromyographic studies [52] and recently Kennedy and Abbs [47] analyzed the morphology of the facial muscles in order to establish reliable and valid sites for electrode placement.

REFERENCES

1. Abbs, JH: The influence of the gamma motor system on jaw movements during speech: A theoretical framework and some preliminary observations. *J Speech Hear Res* 16:175, 1973.
2. Abd-El-Malek S: Observations on the morphology of the human tongue. *J Anat* 73:201, 1939.
3. Ahlgren J: Mechanism of mastication. A quantitative cinematographic and electromyographic study of masticatory movements in children, with special reference to the occlusion of the teeth. *Acta Odontol Scand* 24 [Supple 44]:1,1966.
4. Azzam NA, Kuehn DP: The morphology of musculus uvulae. *Cleft Palate J* 14:78, 1977.
5. Barnwell Y: The morphology of musculus styloglossus in the human fifteen-week fetus. University of Pittsburgh, PhD dissertation, 1975.
6. Barnwell YM, Klueber K, Langdon HL: The anatomy of the intrinsic musculature of the tongue in the early human fetus. *Int J Oral Myol* 4:5, 1978.
7. Bell WA: Muscle patterns of the late fetal tongue tip. *Angle Orthod* 40:262, 1970.
8. Bell-Berti F: The velopharyngeal mechanism: An electromyographic study. *Haskins Lab Status Report Speech Res* [Suppl], 1973.
9. Bell-Berti F: An electromyographic study of velopharyngeal function in speech. *J Speech Hear Res* 19:225, 1976.
10. Benson D: Roentgenographic cephalometric study of palatopharyngeal closure of normal adults during vowel phonation. *Cleft Palate J* 9:43, 1972.
11. Bjork L: Velopharyngeal function in connected speech. *Acta Radiol* [Suppl] (Stockh), 202, 1961.
12. Bjork L, Nylen B: The function of the soft palate during connected speech. *Acta Chir Scand* 126:434, 1963.

13. Bjork L, Nylen B: Studies on velopharyngeal closure. *Acta Chir Scand* 131:226, 1966.
14. Blom S, Skoglund S: Some observations on the control of the tongue muscles. *Experientia* 151:12, 1959.
15. Bloomer H: Observations of the palatopharyngeal action with special reference to speech, swallowing and blowing. *Cleft Palate Bull* 2:4, 1952.
16. Bloomer H: Observations on palatopharyngeal movements in speech and deglutition. *J Speech Hear Dis* 18:230, 1953.
17. Bole CT, Lessler MA: Electromyography of the genioglossus muscles in man. *J Appl Physiol* 21:1695, 1966.
18. Bosma JF: A correlated study of the anatomy and motor activity of the upper pharynx by cadaver dissection and cinematic study of patients after maxillofacial surgery. *Ann Otol Rhinol Laryngol* 62:51, 1953.
19. Bryant P, Gale E, Rugh J (Eds): *Oral motor behavior: Impact on oral conditions and dental treatment.* NIH Publication No 79-1845, 1979.
20. Calnan JS: Movements of the soft palate. *Speech (Lond)* 19:14, 1955.
21. Carlsoo S: Nervous coordination and mechanical function of the mandibular elevators. *Acta Odontol Scand* 10 [Suppl 11]:1, 1952.
22. Carlsoo S: An electromyographic study of the activity of certain suprahyoid muscles (mainly the anterior belly of digastric muscle) and of the reciprocal innervation of the elevator and depressor musculature of the mandible. *Acta Anat* 26:81, 1956.
23. Carlsoo S: An electromyographic study of the activity, and an anatomical study of the mechanics of the lateral pterygoid muscle. *Acta Anat* 26:339, 1956.
24. Carlsoo S: Motor units and action potentials in masticatory muscles *Acta Morphol Neerl Scand* 11:13, 1958
25. Carlsoo S, Werner H: Action potentials in the orbicularis oris, temporal and masseter muscles of children and adults. *Acta Odontol Scand* 16:345, 1958.
26. Cooper S: Muscle spindles in the intrinsic muscles of the human tongue. *J Physiol* 122:193, 1953.
27. Croft CB, Shprintzen RJ, Daniller A, Lewin ML: The ocult submucous cleft palate and the musculus uvulae. *Cleft Palate J* 15:150, 1978.
28. Cruveilheir J: *Anatomy of the Human Body.* (Translated by GS Pattison.) New York, Harper and Bros, 1844.
29. Cunningham DP, Basmajian JV: Electromyography of genioglossus and geniohyoid muscles during deglutition. *Anat Rec* 165:401, 1969.
30. Dabelow R: Vorstudien zu einer Betrachtung der Zunge als funktioneller System. *J Morphol Microscop Anat* 91:3, 1951.
31. De Paula Assis JE: Observacios sobre os musculas glosso-palatino e amygdalo-glosso. *Rev Bras Otorinolaryng* 22:39, 1954.
32. Dickson DR: Normal and cleft palate anatomy. *Cleft Palate J* 9:280, 1972.
33. Dickson DR, Dickson WM: Velpharyngeal anatomy. *J. Speech Hear Res* 15:372, 1972.
34. Dickson DR, Grant JCB, Sicher H, Dubrul EL, Paltan J: Status of research in cleft lip and palate: Anatomy and physiology, Part 2. *Cleft Palate J* 12:131, 1975.
35. Doran GA, Baggett H: The genioglossus muscle: A reassessment of its anatomy in some mammals including man. *Acta Anat* 83:403, 1972.
36. Freimann R: Untersuchungen über Zahl und Anordnung der Muskelspindeln in den Kaumuskeln des Menschen. *Anat Anz* 100:258, 1954.
37. Fritzell B: The velopharyngeal muscles in speech. *Acta Otolaryngol* Suppl 250, 1969.
38. Gibbs CH: Electromyographic activity during the motionless period in chewing. *J Pros Dent* 34:34, 1975.
39. Gibbs CH, Messerman T: Jaw motion during speech. In Orofacial function: Clinical Research in dentistry and speech pathology. *ASHA Reports* 7:104, 1972.
40. Greenfield, BE, Wyke BD: Electromyographic studies of some of the muscles of mastication. *Br Dent J* 100:129, 1956.
41. Hesse Fr: Über die Muskeln der Menschlichen Zunge. *Z Anat Entw* 1:80, 1875.
42. Hickey JC, Woelfel JB, Rinear L: The influence of overlapping electrical fields on the interpretation of electromyograms. *J Prosthet Dent* 7:273, 1957.
43. Hilton, Dr. A large bony tumor in the face completely removed by spontaneous separation. *Guy's Hospital Report* 1:493, 1836.
44. Honjo I, Harada H, Kumazawa T: Role of the levator veli palatini muscle in movement of the lateral pharyngeal wall. *Arch Otorhinolaryngol* 212:93, 1976.
45. Hynes DM: A radiological assessment of the oropharynx with special reference to tomography. *Clin Radiol* 21:407, 1970.
46. Junqueira LC, Carneiro J, Contopoulos AN: *Basic Histology.* Los Altos, Calif, Lange Medical Publications, 1977.
47. Kennedy JG III, Abbs JH: Anatomic studies of the perioral motor system: Foundations for studies in speech physiology. *Speech Lang Res* 1:211, 1979.
48. Langdon H, Klueber K, Barnwell Y: The anatomy of m. genioglossus in the 15-week human fetus. *Anat Embryol* (Berl) 155:107, 1978.

49. Latif A: An electromyographic study of the temporalis muscle in normal persons during selected positions and movements of the mandible. *Am J Orthod* 43:577, 1957.

50. Lavorato AS: Normal lateral pharyngeal wall motion during velopharyngeal functioning: A cinefluorographic study. University of Pittsburgh, PhD dissertation, 1975.

51. Lavorato AS, Lindholm CE: Fiberoptic visualization of motion of the eustachian tube. *Trans Amer Acad Ophthalmol Otolaryngol* 84:ORL 534, 1977.

52. Leanderson R: *On the Functional Organization of Facial Muscles in Speech.* Stockholm, Boktryckeri Ab Thule, 1972.

53. Lipke D, Gay T, Gross B, Yaeger J: An electromyographic study of the human lateral pterygoid muscles. *J Dent Res* 66:231, 1977.

54. MacDougall JDB, Andrew BL: Electromyographic study of the temporalis and masseter muscles. *J Anat* 87:37, 1953.

55. MacNeilage PF, Sholes GN: An electromyographic study of the tongue during vowel production. *J Speech Hear Res* 7:209, 1964.

56. Matthews B, Vemm RA: Silent period in the masseter electromyogram following tooth contact in subjects wearing full dentures. *Arch Oral Biol* 15:531, 1970.

57. Maue-Dickson W, Dickson DR: Anatomy and physiology related to cleft palate: Current research and clinical implications. *Plastic Reconstr Surg* 65:83, 1980.

58. McKerns D, Bzoch KR: Variations in velopharyngeal valving: The factor of sex. *Cleft Palate J* 7:652, 1970.

59. McMyn JK: The anatomy of the salpingopharyngeus muscle. *J Laryngol Otol* 55:1, 1940.

60. Minifie, FD, Abbs JH, Tarlow A, Kwaterski M: EMG activity within the pharynx during speech production. *J Speech Hear Res* 17:497, 1974.

61. Minifie, FD, Hixon T, Kelsey C, Woodhouse R: Lateral pharyngeal wall motion during speech production. *J Speech Hear Res* 13:584, 1970.

62. Miyawaki K: A study on the musculature of the human tongue. *Bull Res Inst Logoped Phoniat (Tokyo)* 8:23, 1974.

63. Moller E: The chewing apparatus. An electromyographic study of the action of the muscles of mastication and its correlation to facial morphology. *Acta Physiol Scand* 69 [Suppl. 280]:1, 1966.

64. Moller E: Clinical electromyography in dentistry. *Int Dent J* 19:250, 1969.

65. Moller E: Action of the muscles of mastication. *Front Oral Physiol* 1:121, 1974.

66. Perlman HB: Observations on the eustachian tube. *Arch Otolaryngol* 53:370, 1951.

67. Rakhawy MT: Phosphatases in the nervous tissue. *Acta Anat* 83:356, 1972.

68. Roche AF: Functional anatomy of the muscles of mastication. *J Prosthet Dent* 13:548, 1963.

69. Rosen L: The morphology of the salpingopharyngeus muscle. University of Pittsburgh, MS thesis, 1970.

70. Salter HH: *Todd Cyclopedia of Anatomy and Physiology.* Vol 4. London, Brown, Green, and Longmans. 1852, p 1120.

71. Sauerland EK, Mitchell SP: Electromyographic activity of the human genioglossus muscle in response to respiration and to positional changes of the head. *Bull Los Angeles Neurol Soc* 35:69, 1970.

72. Schaerer P, Stallard RE, Zander HA: Occlusal interferences and mastication: An electromyographic study. *J Prosthet Dent* 17:438, 1967.

73. Shprintzen RJ, Lewin ML, Rakoff SJ, Sidoti SJ, Croft C: Diagnosis of small central gaps in the velopharyngeal sphincter. *Cleft Palate J* 13:415, 1976.

74. Simpson RK, Austin AA: A cephalometric investigation of velar stretch. *Cleft Palate J* 9:341, 1972.

75. Skolnick ML: Video velopharyngography in patients with nasal speech with emphasis on lateral pharyngeal motion in velopharyngeal closure. *Radiology* 93:747, 1969.

76. Sommering ST: Vom Bau des menschlichen Körpers. *Muskellehre* 3:1, 1841.

77. Steiner J, Michman J, Litman L: Time sequences of the activity of the temporal and masseter muscles in healthy young human adults during habitual chewing of different test foods. *Arch Oral Biol* 19:29, 1974.

78. Strong LH: Muscle fibers of the tongue functional in consonant production. *Anat Rec* 126:61, 1956.

79. Sussman HM, MacNeilage PF, Hanson RJ: Labial and mandibular dynamics during the production of bilabial consonants: Preliminary observations. *J Speech Hear Res* 16:397, 1973.

80. Voss H: Zahl und Anordnung der Muskelspindeln in den oberen Zungenbeinmuskeln, im M. Trapezius und M. Latissimus dorsi. *Anat Anz* 103:443, 1956.

The human auditory mechanism serves to translate sound waves striking the ear into neural impulses which, when decoded by the central nervous system, result in the perception of both simple and complex auditory stimuli. The sensory end-organ for hearing is located in the fluid-filled inner ear buried within the petrous portion of the temporal bone. Airborne sound waves reach this fluid-filled mechanism via a membranous "window." Herein a problem arises. Whenever a pressure wave reaches a transition between two media of different densities, the wave may simply be reflected by the interface. For example, most of the energy of an air-borne signal would be reflected by a membrane covering a fluid-filled cavity. Thus, a mechanism is necessary to overcome this loss of energy. That mechanism is contained within the middle ear, the structures of which serve as an impedance-matching transformer between the external space and the inner ear.

The structure of the auditory mechanism may be viewed in two ways. Functionally, it consists of a conduction mechanism and a sensory-neural mechanism. Anatomically, it consists of outer, middle, and inner morphological units with the inner portion linked to the central nervous system via the auditory nerve (Figure 6-1).

EXTERNAL EAR

The external ear is composed of the pinna, the external auditory meatus, and the tympanic membrane. The **pinna** (also called the **auricle**) is the portion of the ear that is visible on the outside of the head. The **external auditory meatus** is the tube-like structure that extends medially from the pinna for about $2\frac{1}{2}$ cm (in the adult) and ends at a thin membrane called the **tympanic membrane** (also called the **eardrum**).

6-1. *The outer, middle, and inner ear.*

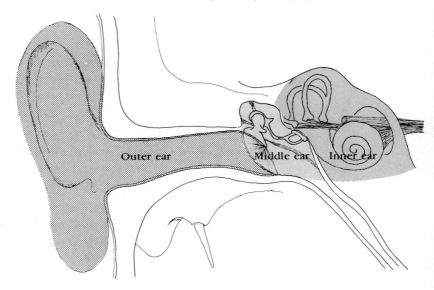

Outer ear   Middle ear   Inner ear

6-2. *The pinna. A, Child; B, Adult.*

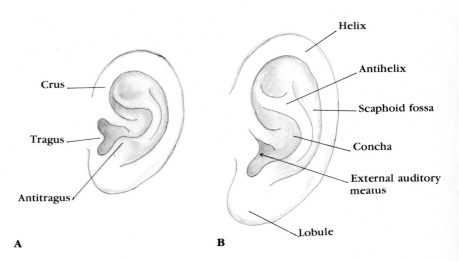

Crus

Tragus

Antitragus

Helix

Antihelix

Scaphoid fossa

Concha

External auditory meatus

Lobule

A   B

Pinna

MORPHOLOGY. The pinna is a cartilaginous structure covered by skin. The various concavities, convexities, and curvatures of the pinna are identified in Figure 6-2. The **helix** is the superior and posterior margin of the pinna. The anterior termination of the helix, which is superior to the entrance into the external auditory meatus, is called the **crus.** The prominent semicircular ridge anterior and inferior to the helix is the **antihelix.** The **scaphoid fossa** is the curved depression separating the helix and antihelix. The bowl-like depression at the entrance into the external auditory meatus is called the **concha.** The flap-like projection at the anterior rim of the concha is the **tragus.**

LIGAMENTS AND MUSCLES. The pinna is attached to the side of the cranium by its continuity with the cartilage of the external auditory meatus and by three ligaments. An **anterior ligament** extends from the pinna to the zygomatic process. A **posterior ligament** extends to the mastoid process. A **superior ligament** attaches to the bony part of the external auditory meatus.

There are also three extrinsic muscles of the pinna: the **anterior, posterior,** and **superior auricular muscles.** They arise from the galea aponeurotica and insert into corresponding parts of the cartilage of the pinna. There are also a number of intrinsic muscles of the pinna. While in lower animals the muscles of the pinna serve to adjust the position of the pinna for localization and reception of acoustic stimuli, they are vestigial in the human form.

FUNCTION. The pinna serves a minor function in directing airborne signals into the external auditory meatus and assists in localizing the source of signals. These functions are muted in the human being by contrast with lower animals.

External Auditory Meatus

MORPHOLOGY. The external auditory meatus is about 2½ cm long and 6 mm in diameter in the adult. It is directed at a slight upward angle from lateral to medial. In young children, before the growth of the face is complete, the external meatus is much smaller and angles downward rather than upward. The external third of the meatus is cartilaginous, while the inner two-thirds is osseous. The skin lining the cartilaginous portion contains sweat glands, sebaceous glands, and hair follicles.

FUNCTION. The products of the sweat glands and sebaceous glands form a waxy substance called **cerumen,** which helps to trap small foreign materials within the external auditory meatus. Ciliary motion of the hairs of the meatus propels the cerumen and any foreign material toward the outside. The external meatus provides for the protected recessed position of the tympanic membrane and provides the membrane with a fairly constant temperature and humidity. The meatus also serves as a resonator for frequencies in the range of 2000 to 5500 Hz [14].

Tympanic Membrane

The tympanic membrane serves as the interface between the external auditory meatus and the middle ear and is frequently classified as a part of both of these structures.

MORPHOLOGY. The membrane (Figure 6-3) is semitransparent, almost oval in shape, and is concave on its external surface. The apex of the concavity of the membrane is called the **umbo.** The membrane is held in position by a circular ligament called the **annular ligament** (also called the **annulus** or **annulus fibrosus**), which attaches the membrane to the tympanic sulcus.

The tympanic membrane is composed of an external, middle, and internal layer. The **external layer** is cutaneous and is continuous with the skin that lines the osseous portion of the external meatus. The **middle layer,** called the **substantia propria,** consists of two layers of connective tissue fibers. Each layer contains both collagenous and scattered elastic fibers. The outer fibers are radial and converge on the umbo. The inner fibers are circular. The **internal layer** of the tympanic membrane is mucosal and is continuous with the mucous membrane that lines the cavity of the middle ear.

One of the three small bones (**ossicles**) of the middle ear, the **malleus,** is embedded in the deep surface of the tympanic membrane. The tip of the **manubrium** (handle) of the malleus corresponds to the umbo. Most of the surface of the tympanic membrane is taut and is, therefore, called the **pars tensa.** Above the malleus, however, the membrane contains only elastic fibers and is flaccid. This part is called the **pars flaccida** (also called **Shrapnell's membrane**). When light is shined into the external meatus, its reflection from the anterior-inferior portion of the cone-shaped tympanic membrane causes a light reflex called the **cone of light.**

FUNCTION. Pressure waves striking the tympanic membrane cause it to vibrate. These vibrations are transferred to the malleus by virtue of its attachment to the membrane. Thus, the function of the membrane is to translate the airborne signal into mechanical motion of the ossicles.

6-3. *The left tympanic membrane as viewed through an otoscope.*

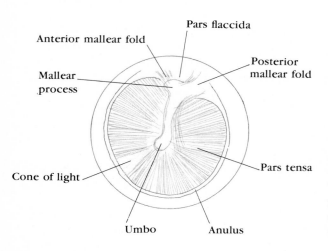

Pars flaccida

Anterior mallear fold

Mallear process

Posterior mallear fold

Cone of light

Pars tensa

Umbo   Anulus

MIDDLE EAR

The **ossicles** form the conduction mechanism between the outer and inner ear; that is, from the tympanic membrane to the oval window. The **oval window** is a membrane-covered opening from the middle into the inner ear. The ossicles are contained within the air-filled middle-ear cavity. In order for the conduction mechanism to function normally, the air within the cavity must be maintained at atmospheric pressure. This is the function of the **auditory tube,** which links the middle-ear cavity (**tympanic cavity**) with the pharyngeal airway.

Tympanic Cavity

For convenience of description the tympanic cavity is divided into the tympanic cavity proper and the epitympanic recess. The **tympanic cavity proper** corresponds to the vertical extent of tympanic membrane. The tympanic cavity superior to the level of the tympanic membrane is called the **epitympanic recess** (Figure 6-4).

The tympanic cavity proper is somewhat cylindrical with convex ends. The lateral convexity is formed by the tympanic membrane. The medial convexity is formed by the lateral wall of the labyrinth of the inner ear. The medial wall of the tympanic cavity proper is marked by the basal turn of the cochlea. This is called the **promontory.** Above the promontory is the **oval window,** one of the two potential openings between the middle and inner ear. The other potential opening, the **round window,** lies below the promontory. The anterior wall of the tympanic cavity proper is a thin plate of bone that separates the cavity from the internal carotid artery and part of the sympathetic plexus. In the upper part of the anterior wall are two small cavities. The more superior cavity forms the entrance into a canal that houses the tensor tympani muscle (to be discussed later). The lower cavity is the entrance into the auditory tube. The posterior wall of the tympanic cavity proper contains the **pyramid,** a small conical projection from which arises the tendon of the stapedius muscle (to be discussed later). The floor of the tympanic cavity lies immediately above the internal jugular vein.

The epitympanic recess is bounded above by the **tegmen tympani,** a thin plate of bone above which are the meninges and the temporal lobe of the brain. The posterior wall of the epitympanic recess contains an irregular opening called the **aditus to the mastoid antrum,** which communicates with the air cells of the mastoid process of the temporal bone.

6-4. *The tympanic cavity. A, Diagrammatic; B, Sectioned to show the medial and lateral walls.*

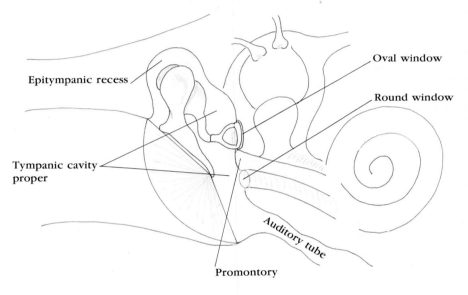

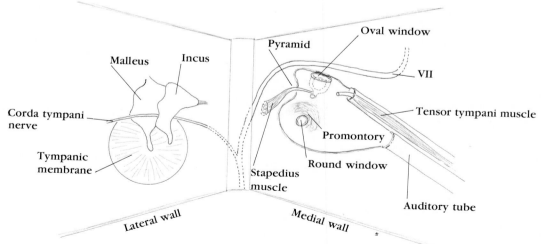

B

Auditory Ossicles

The auditory ossicles are the malleus, incus, and stapes (Figure 6-5). They form a chain with the malleus attached to the tympanic membrane, the stapes attached to the oval window of the inner ear, and the incus intermediate between the other two ossicles.

MALLEUS. The malleus is the largest of the ossicles, weighing approximately 25 mg and measuring about 8 mm in length [12]. It has a club-shaped **head** (also called the **capitulum**) that occupies the epitympanic recess. The head is separated from the **handle** (**manubrium**) of the malleus by the **neck** (**collum**). The handle is a thin, oval rod with a flattened tip. The **lateral process** extends from the lateral side of the superior part of the handle. An **anterior process** extends from the neck of the malleus. The lateral surface of the tip of the handle is covered with cartilage and attaches to the tympanic membrane. The articular surface, which forms part of the joint between the malleus and incus, is on the posterior and medial surfaces of the head and is saddle-shaped.

INCUS. The incus is composed of a rounded **body** with a **short** and a **long process** extending from it. It is slightly heavier than the malleus, weighing approximately 27 mg, and is about 8 mm in length. A saddle-shaped **articular surface** is located on the body of the incus opposite the short process. This surface articulates with the malleus. The tips of both the long and short processes are covered with cartilage. A small **lenticular process** projects from the medial side of the tip of the long process. The lenticular process serves for articulation with the stapes.

STAPES. As its name implies, the stapes is in the form of a stirrup. The **footplate** is oval in shape and fits into the oval window. A **leg** arises from each end of the footplate. These legs converge at the **body** of the stapes. The lateral end of the head articulates with the lenticular process of the incus.

LIGAMENTS AND JOINTS. Three ligaments are associated with the malleus. The **superior malleal** ligament attaches to the superior part of the head of the malleus and extends to the tegmen tympani. The **lateral malleal ligament** attaches to the neck of the malleus and to a small notch at the superior rim of the tympanic annulus. A third ligament, the **anterior malleal ligament,** extends from the neck of the malleus (it also envelops the anterior process of the malleus) and passes through a small **petrotympanic fissure** to attach to the angular spine of the sphenoid bone. Kirikae [12] found that in 42 of his 50 dissections of the ligaments, the anterior ligament consisted of folds in the mucous membrane devoid of ligamentous fibers.

Two ligaments are associated with the incus. The **superior incudal ligament** attaches to the roof of the tympanic cavity and to the superior surface of the body of the incus. The **posterior incudal ligament** attaches to the short process of the incus and extends to the posterior wall of the tympanic cavity.

Folds of mucosa and/or ligamentous fibers are occasionally found attached to the stapes [12]. However, the only consistent ligament is the **annular ligament,** which attaches the rim of the stapedial footplate to the margin of the oval window.

The **incudomallear articulation** forms a synovial saddle joint. However, motion does not occur at this joint over the range of motion associated with usual acoustic stimuli. Only when stimuli reach a degree of loudness associated with pain and tickle does motion occur. Thus, at normal levels of loudness, the malleus and incus move as a single unit. At very high levels of stimulation, motion of the joint tends to limit the conduction of extreme motion to the stapes. The **incudostapedial joint** is formed by the convex extremity of the lenticular process of the incus and the concave surface of the lateral extremity of the stapedial body. This forms a synovial ball and socket joint at which motion is relatively free.

The incudomallear joint rotates in response to vibration of the tympanic membrane around an axis through the anterior malleal ligament [12]. Motion of the stapedial footplate is primarily

6-5. *The ossicles. A, Articulated.* Top, *Medial view;* Bottom, *Superior view. B, Individual ossicles. (Figures A and B reproduced, with permission, from Pernkopf E:* Atlas of Topographical and Applied Human Anatomy *(Vol. 1), 2nd ed. Copyright 1981 by Urban & Schwarzenberg, Baltimore, Maryland.) C, Ligaments of the ossicles.*

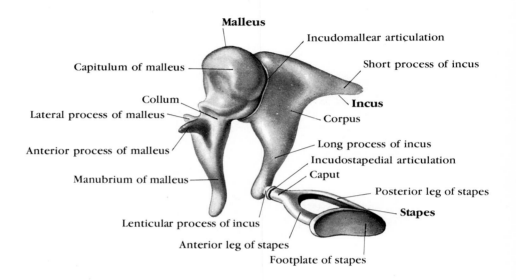

Malleus

Incudomallear articulation

Capitulum of malleus

Short process of incus

Collum

Incus

Lateral process of malleus

Corpus

Anterior process of malleus

Long process of incus

Incudostapedial articulation

Caput

Manubrium of malleus

Posterior leg of stapes

Stapes

Lenticular process of incus

Anterior leg of stapes

Footplate of stapes

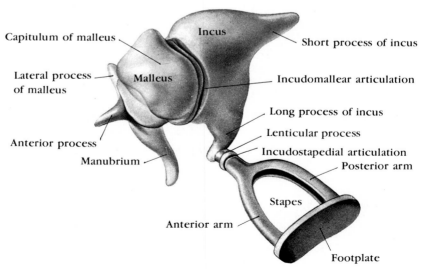

Capitulum of malleus

Incus

Short process of incus

Lateral process of malleus

Malleus

Incudomallear articulation

Anterior process

Long process of incus

Manubrium

Lenticular process

Incudostapedial articulation

Posterior arm

Stapes

Anterior arm

Footplate

A

6-5 (*continued*)

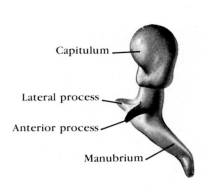

A. Right malleus, anterior view

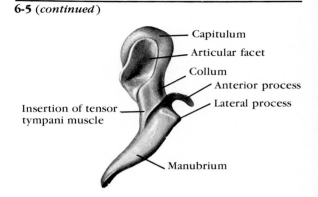

B. Right malleus, posterior view

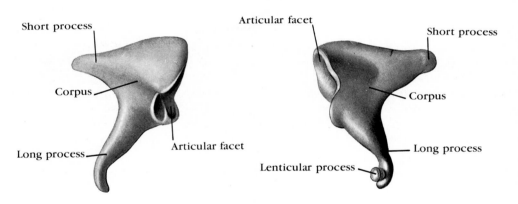

C. Right incus, anterolateral view

D. Right incus, posteromedial view

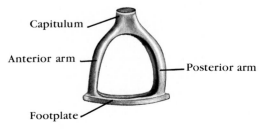

E. Right stapes

B

hinge-like about the lesser diameter of the foot-plate. However, motion around the major axis of the footplate and plunger-like motion also occur.

MUSCLES. There are two muscles of the middle ear. The **tensor tympani muscle** attaches to the malleus. It is a penniform muscle approximately 2 cm in length and arises inferiorly from the tendon of the tensor veli palatini muscle (to be discussed later). The tensor tympani muscle passes through a bony canal in the temporal bone. Its superior tendon emerges into the tympanic cavity, where it passes around a small bony process of the anterior wall of the cavity. This small bony process is called the **cochleariform process.** After rounding the cochleariform process, the tendon inserts into the root of the mallear handle.

The **stapedius muscle** is the smallest striated muscle of the body. It arises within the pyramid and inserts onto the posterior surface of the neck of the stapes.

The innervation of the two muscles is separate. The motor supply to the tensor tympani is from the fifth cranial nerve, while that to the stapedius is from cranial nerve VII.

Auditory Tube

MORPHOLOGY. The first detailed description of the auditory tube was published in 1562 by Bartholomaeus Eustachius [7]; thus, the auditory tube has also been called the **eustachian tube.** Since that time, important refinements in our understanding of its structure and function have been added by numerous investigators [6,15,16].

The adult auditory tube provides a dynamic link between the nasopharynx and the middle ear (Figure 6-6). It is approximately 3.5 cm in length and courses in a lateral, posterior, and superior direction from its pharyngeal orifice to its tympanic orifice. It lies at an angle of approximately 45 degrees to the sagittal plane and 35 to 40 degrees to the horizontal plane. The anteromedial two-thirds of the auditory tube is contained within a cartilaginous semicanal. The posterolateral third lies within a bony semicanal called the **protympanum.** The nasopharyngeal orifice of the tube is a slit approximately 8 mm in height and 1 mm in width. The lumen of the tube decreases in size as it approaches the junction between the cartilaginous and osseous parts. The lumen is narrowest in the cartilaginous portion immediately anteromedial to the beginning of the bony portion. This narrowest

---

6-5 *(continued)*

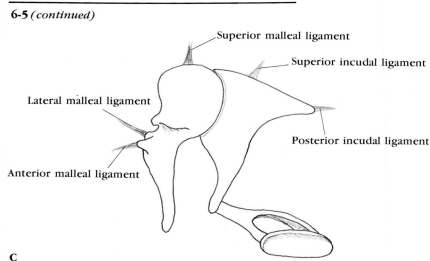

Superior malleal ligament

Superior incudal ligament

Lateral malleal ligament

Posterior incudal ligament

Anterior malleal ligament

C

6-6. *The auditory tube. A, Relationship to the middle ear and nasopharynx (Redrawn, with permission, from Brodel M: Three Unpublished Drawings of the Human Ear. Copyright 1946 by WB Saunders Company, Philadelphia); B, Transverse section of human fetal auditory tube and surrounding structures; C, Longitudinal view with relationships among the lumen, cartilage, and muscles associated with the tube.*

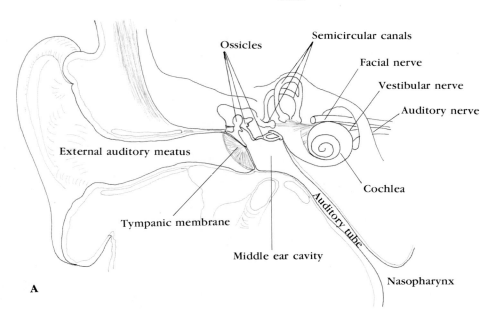

A

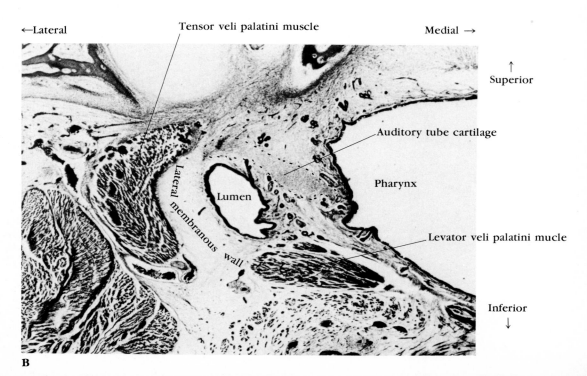

B

part is called the **isthmus.** The lumen then increases in size as it approaches the tympanic orifice. The lumen of the cartilaginous portion of the tube is normally collapsed (that is, closed) at least at the isthmus, while the osseous portion is patent.

The inferolateral lamina of the lumen is lined with pseudostratified ciliated columnar epithelium. The medial lamina and roof of the lumen are lined with simple cuboidal epithelium. Muco-serous glands and goblet cells are present at the pharyngeal orifice and in the midportion of the tube. Lymphoid tissue is present at both orifices but is far less abundant in the midportion of the tube [29].

The cartilage of the auditory tube is composed of a hook-shaped lamina with the major part of the cartilage on the medial side of the lumen and the hook extending over the superior margin of the lumen. The pharyngeal end of the cartilage is enlarged and creates a bulge in the lateral pharyngeal wall medial to the pharyngeal orifice of the tube.

This enlarged end of the cartilage is called the **torus tubarius.**

MUSCLE. The muscle of the auditory tube is the **tensor veli palatini muscle.** It is unfortunate that this muscle was named before its function was understood, since it would more accurately be called the dilator tubae muscle. Its origin is from the anterior velum where it forms the **velar aponeurosis,** which attaches to the entire posterior rim of the hard palate. The fibers of the aponeurosis converge laterally and pass around the hamulus. The tensor veli palatini muscle is bipenniform. Its tendon continues throughout the length of the muscle and, superiorly, becomes the inferior tendon of the tensor tympani muscle [1,4,5,13,20]. As illustrated in Figure 6-7, the fibers of the tensor veli palatini muscle branch from its tendon to two insertions. Laterally, the fibers attach to the scaphoid fossa, sphenoid sulcus, and spine of the sphenoid bone. Medially, the fibers attach to the lateral membranous wall of the audi-

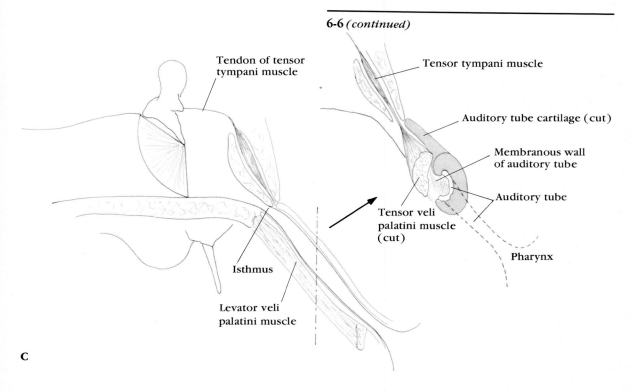

6-6 *(continued)*

Tendon of tensor tympani muscle

Tensor tympani muscle

Auditory tube cartilage (cut)

Membranous wall of auditory tube

Auditory tube

Tensor veli palatini muscle (cut)

Pharynx

Isthmus

Levator veli palatini muscle

C

tory tube. The functional potential of the tensor veli palatini muscle is to open the auditory tube by drawing its membranous wall laterally.

FUNCTION. The two primary functions of the auditory tube are to equalize pressure across the tympanic membrane and to provide an avenue for outflow of fluids from the middle ear. Unfortunately, since its mucosal lining is continuous with that of the pharynx and middle ear, it may also provide a route for the spread of infection from the pharynx to the middle ear and mastoid area.

Functions of the Middle Ear

The tympanic membrane vibrates in response to pressure waves striking it and its action corresponds to the motions of the malleus, that is, it swings inward and outward with the axis of motion at the superior part of the handle of the malleus. The axis of rotation of the ossicles is very

6-7. *Anatomical relationships of the tensor veli palatini and tensor tympani muscles, the auditory tube, and middle ear. (From Maue-Dickson W, Dickson DR. Anatomy and physiology related to the cleft palate: Current research and clinical implications.* J Plast Reconstruct Surg *56:83, 1980. Copyright by Plastic and Reconstructive Surgery, Brookline, Massachusetts.)*

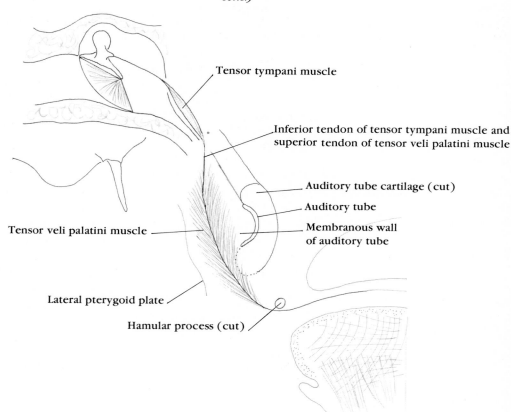

Tensor tympani muscle

Inferior tendon of tensor tympani muscle and superior tendon of tensor veli palatini muscle

Auditory tube cartilage (cut)

Auditory tube

Membranous wall of auditory tube

Tensor veli palatini muscle

Lateral pterygoid plate

Hamular process (cut)

near their center of gravity [12]. Because their inertia is very small, the ossicles are placed into motion easily and cease motion as soon as the stimulus is withdrawn.

Various investigators have studied the amplitude of motion of the umbo of the tympanic membrane and the footplate of the stapes [8,12,17,30]. The motion of the two is very nearly equal, perhaps with a very slight reduction of motion at the footplate. Thus, the lever action of the ossicles can probably be disregarded in determining the transformer function of the middle ear structures (though there is some disagreement on this point). Another important factor is the difference between the area of the tympanic membrane and the oval window. The oval window is much smaller, giving an effective area ratio of about 14 : 1 [30]. However, a 14 : 1 ratio would give a mechanical advantage accounting for only about 23 dB, probably considerably less than the actual advantage provided by the middle ear mechanism [31].

The function of the middle ear muscles has received considerable attention in the research literature. The early concept was that the middle-ear muscles provided protection to the middle ear and cochlea. This was thought to be accomplished by the contraction of the muscles pulling on the malleus and stapes, thereby reducing their response to intense stimuli. This concept has recently been subject to serious dispute. Modern research has demonstrated that while both muscles of the middle ear contract in response to generalized startle, only the stapedius muscle consistently responds to auditory stimuli [24]. Further, contraction of the muscles can account for only a 5 to 10 dB reduction in pressure at the oval window at low frequencies and may actually facilitate transmission of high-frequency energy [3].

A growing body of evidence indicates that the tensor tympani muscle is involved in auditory tube clearance rather than protection of the ear from loud sounds. Greisen and Neergaard [9] demonstrated that the tensor tympani and tensor veli palatini, in response to startle, give rise to small volumes of displacement of air in the middle ear.

Kamerer [11] found that the tensor tympani consistently contracted during swallow and that the two tensor muscles have similar latency response times. A number of studies have confirmed that the tensor veli palatini muscle is an auditory-tube dilator and that the two tensor muscles have common innervation and share a common tendon [18,19,21]. This has led a number of investigators to the hypothesis that the two tensor muscles act together in auditory-tube function. The tensor tympani, by drawing the malleus (and therefore the tympanic membrane) inward, may slightly increase middle-ear and auditory-tube pressure, thereby serving to reflexly stimulate contraction of the tensor veli palatini to open the auditory tube.

The exact mechanism of auditory-tube function is not understood. It is known that the tensor veli palatini opens the tube. However, the stimulus for that action is not clear. Its activity is associated with such events as swallowing and yawning, but evidently a pressure differential across the tympanic membrane is also necessary to stimulate opening of the tube. The opening of the lumen probably also requires the presence of a chemical agent such as surfactant, which lowers the surface tension of the mucous membrane lining of the lumen.

INNER EAR

The inner ear, located within the petrous portion of the temporal bone (Figure 6-8), is composed of the cochlea, the semicircular canals, and a connecting vestibule. The **cochlea** is a snail-shaped, bony spiral canal that lies medial to the middle ear. It contains the sensorineural receptors for audition. The **semicircular canals** are three interconnected bony tubes, each semicircular in shape, that lie in three different planes. The semicircular canals contain the receptors for rotational acceleration of the head. The **vestibule** lies between the semicircular canals and the cochlea. It contains two sensory organs, the **utricle** and the **saccule,** which house receptors sensitive to linear acceleration and position of the head in space. The oval

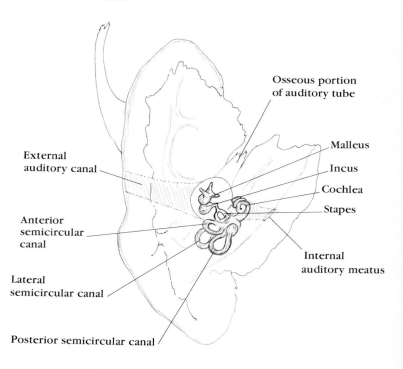

6-8. *The location of the middle and internal ear structures within the left temporal bone, superior view.*

Osseous portion of auditory tube

Malleus

Incus

Cochlea

Stapes

External auditory canal

Anterior semicircular canal

Internal auditory meatus

Lateral semicircular canal

Posterior semicircular canal

6-9. *Relationship between the membranous and osseous labyrinth. (Reproduced, with permission, from Ganong WF:* Review of Medical Physiology, *10th ed. Copyright 1981 by Lange Medical Publications, Los Altos, California.)*

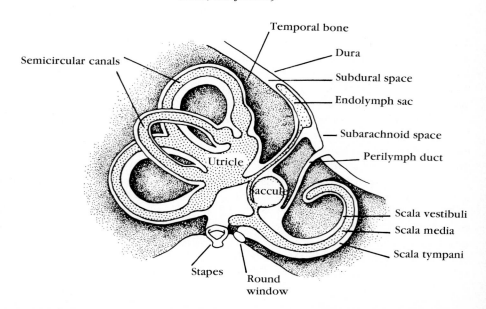

Semicircular canals

Temporal bone

Dura

Subdural space

Endolymph sac

Subarachnoid space

Perilymph duct

Utricle

Saccule

Scala vestibuli

Scala media

Scala tympani

Stapes

Round window

window, which contains the footplate of the stapes, is located in the medial wall of the vestibule. Together, the semicircular canals, utricle, and saccule form the **vestibular apparatus,** which functions to maintain equilibrium. The eighth cranial nerve, called the **vestibulocochlear nerve,** supplies the inner ear structures.

The entire system of bony canals of the inner ear is termed the **osseous labyrinth.** Lying within the osseous labyrinth is a **membranous labyrinth,** which more or less duplicates the shape of the bony canals (Figure 6-9). The interior of the membranous labyrinth is completely closed off from the space between it and the walls of the osseous labyrinth. A clear fluid called **perilymph** fills this space, bathing the inner walls of the osseous labyrinth and the outer walls of the membranous labyrinth. The membranous labyrinth is filled with a more viscous fluid called **endolymph.** The perilymph communicates with cerebrospinal fluid via the **perilymphatic duct,** which extends into the subarachnoid space of the meninges of the brain (see Chap. 7, Nervous System).

Vestibular Apparatus

The three semicircular canals lie at right angles to one another. The membranous canals communicate with the utricle. One end of each semicircular canal, where it joins the utricle, is enlarged. This enlarged end, called the **ampulla,** contains an organ known as the **crista ampullaris** (Figure 6-10). The crista contains **hair cells,** neuroreceptor cells characterized by long hair-like cilia (called **stereocilia** since they are nonmotile) which project from them. The stereocilia of the crista are embedded in a conical gelatinous mass called the **cupula.** The cupula extends across the ampulla and is in contact with the opposite side. Rotational acceleration of the head in any plane causes the endolymph in one or more of the semicircular canals on each side of the head to move relative to the membranous walls of the canals owing to inertia of the fluid. Movement of the endolymph through the ampulla causes the cupula to bend, thus bending the stereocilia of the hair cells. Deformation of the stereocilia in one direc-

tion causes excitation of the sensory cells of the crista. Deformation in the opposite direction causes inhibition (Figure 6-11).

The utricle and saccule are enlargements of the membranous labyrinth in the vestibule of the inner ear. The utricle is the larger of the two and communicates with the semicircular canals. The saccule is thought by some investigators [10] to be vestigial in human beings. The utricle and saccule are interconnected by a Y-shaped ductal part of the membranous labyrinth. The long arm of the Y, called the **endolymphatic duct,** extends through a foramen in the temporal bone and ends in the **endolymphatic sac.** The lining of the endolym-

6-10. *Structure of the crista ampullaris. (Reproduced, with permission, from Wersall J: Studies on the structure and innervation of the sensory epithelium of the cristae ampulares in the guinea pig.* Acta Otolaryngol [Suppl] *126:1, 1956. Copyright by Almqvist Wiksell Periodical Company, Stockholm, Sweden.)*

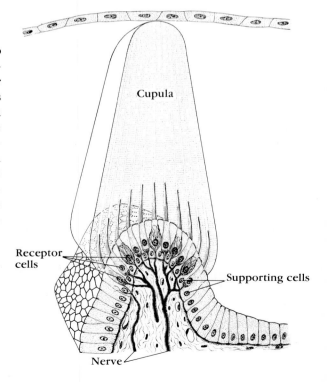

phatic sac is characterized by tall columnar epithelial cells thought to be responsible for absorption of endolymph and digestion of foreign materials within the endolymph.

Within the walls of the utricle and saccule are small specialized organs called **maculae.** The maculae of the utricle and saccule are arranged perpendicular to one another. The structure of the maculae is similar to that of the crista ampullaris. In the maculae, minute calciferous granules called **otoliths** (also called **otoconia**) lie on top of the gelatinous mass (Figure 6-12). The otoliths are denser than the gelatinous mass. Therefore, during linear acceleration or change in head position the otoliths are displaced and place tension on the gelatinous mass and, therefore, on the hair cells. The discharge pattern of the hair cells of the maculae is similar to that of the hair cells of the crista ampullarae.

Cochlea

The part of the membranous labyrinth that lies within the bony cochlea is called the **cochlear duct** (also called the **scala media**). It communicates with the saccule within the vestibule by means of a tiny duct called the **ductus reuniens.**

6-11. *Ampullary responses to rotation. Average time course of impulse discharge from ampulla of two semicircular canals during rotational acceleration, steady rotation, and deceleration. (Reproduced, with permission, from Adrian ED: Discharges from vestibular receptors in the cat.* J Physiol *(Lond.) 101:389, 1943. Copyright by Journal of Physiology (London), Cambridge, England.)*

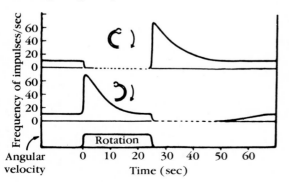

The arrangement of the cochlear duct within the bony cochlea is unique, in that it forms a partition across the bony canal by attaching to opposite sides of it (Figure 6-13). The cochlear duct is triangular in form. The base of the duct is formed by a tough membrane called the **basilar membrane.** The roof of the cochlear duct is formed by a second, extremely delicate membrane called the **vestibular membrane** (also called **Reissner's membrane).** These two membranes are attached to the **spiral lamina,** a bony projection from the central osseous wall of the cochlea. The two membranes diverge as they extend outward from the spiral lamina and attach via a **spiral ligament** to the periosteum of the bony canal. Between their attachments, forming the third side of the triangular cochlear duct, is the **stria vascularis,** which produces endolymph and supplies the cochlear duct with oxygen and other nutrients.

The perilymphatic space adjacent to the vestibular membrane is called the **scala vestibuli** since it communicates with the vestibule. The perilymphatic space adjacent to the basilar membrane is called the **scala tympani** since it communicates with the round window, which is covered by a membrane called the **secondary tympanic membrane.** The cochlear duct ends slightly short of the end of the bony cochlear canal so that the scala vestibuli and scala tympani communicate with one another at the apex of the cochlea. This point of communication is called the **helicotrema.**

ORGAN OF CORTI. The organ of Corti, named for the investigator who provided its first detailed description, is the sensory end-organ for hearing and is located within the cochlear duct. The organ is an aggregate of specialized cells lying on the medial part of the basilar membrane. It extends throughout the length of the cochlear duct and is often called the **spiral organ of Corti,** since it follows the path of the spiraled cochlea. This sensory organ is similar in structure to the cristae and maculae, though more complex. It is composed partly of hair cells, some of whose stereocilia are

6-12. *A, Structure of the maculae; B, Scanning electron micrograph of the surface of a pigeon's macula showing the otoliths. (Reproduced, with permission, from Junqueira LC, Carneiro J:* Basic Histology, *3rd ed. Copyright 1980 by Lange Medical Publications, Los Altos California.)*

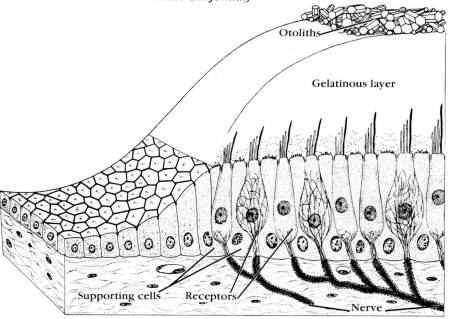

Otoliths

Gelatinous layer

Supporting cells   Receptors

Nerve

A

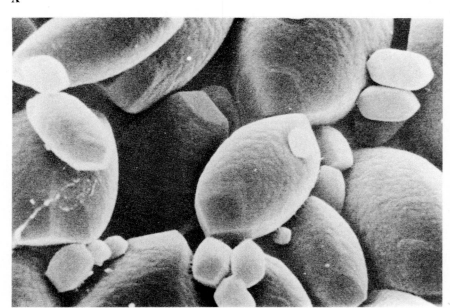

B

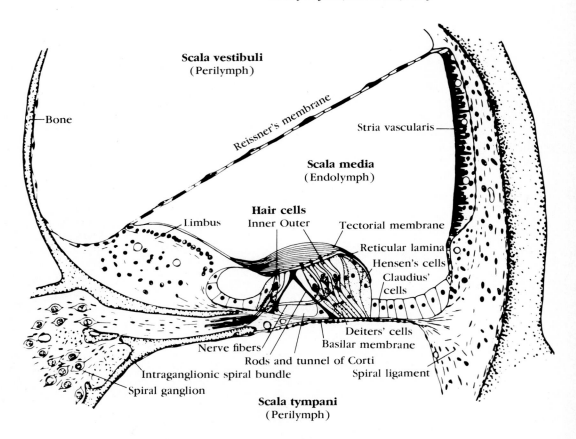

6-13. *Cross-section of the cochlear duct of a guinea pig. (Reproduced, with permission, from Davis H, et al: Acoustic trauma in the guinea pig. J Acoust Soc Am 25:1180, 1953. Copyright by the American Institute of Physics, New York, N.Y.)*

embedded in a gelatinous membrane called the **tectorial membrane.**

The medial part of the organ of Corti is composed of loose connective tissue covered by a layer of epithelial cells extending from the region of the osseous spiral lamina (Figure 6-14). This medial portion is called the **spiral limbus.** The tectorial membrane extends laterally from the superior part of the spiral limbus. The lateral surface of the limbus is concave from superior to inferior. The inferior cells of the limbus, which lie on the basilar membrane, extend laterally and terminate at a single row of hair cells called the **inner hair cells,** since other hair cells lie more laterally on the basilar membrane.

Above the inner hair cells, the enlarged tectorial membrane lies immediately superior to the tips of the stereocilia of the inner hair cells (Figure 6-15). The channel bounded by the spiral limbus medially, the inner hair cells laterally, and the tectorial membrane superiorly is called the **internal spiral tunnel.** Lateral to the internal row of hair cells, separating them from the more laterally placed **outer hair cells,** is a rigid triangular structure composed of supporting cells called **pillar cells** (also called **rods of Corti).** The space between the inner and outer pillar cells is called the **inner tunnel.** Three or four rows of outer hair cells lie lateral to the pillar cells. The longest stereocilia of each of these outer hair cells are embedded in the inferior surface of the tectorial membrane. The outer hair cells are supported by

6-14. *Cross-section of the cochlear partition. CD, cochlear duct; TM, tectorial membrane; OHC, outer hair cell; IHC, inner hair cell; BM, basilar membrane; ST, scala tympani; NF, nerve fibers. (From Ryan A, Dallos P: Physiology of the Inner Ear. In Northern JL (Ed):* Hearing Disorders. *Copyright 1976 by Little, Brown and Company, Boston, Massachusetts.)*

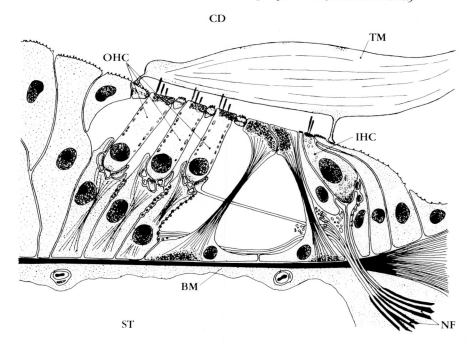

6-15. *Relationship between the supporting cells and hair cells. A, Deiters' cell and associated outer hair cell; B, Schematic representation of the relationship of the outer hair cells to the outer phalangeal cells as revealed on electron micrographs; C, Scanning electron micrograph of supporting cells of Deiters and associated outer hair cells. (From Bloom W, Fawcett DW:* A Textbook of Histology, *10th ed. Philadelphia, WB Saunders, 1975.)*

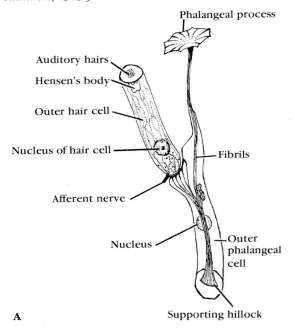

Phalangeal process

Auditory hairs

Hensen's body

Outer hair cell

Nucleus of hair cell

Afferent nerve

Nucleus

Fibrils

Outer phalangeal cell

Supporting hillock

A

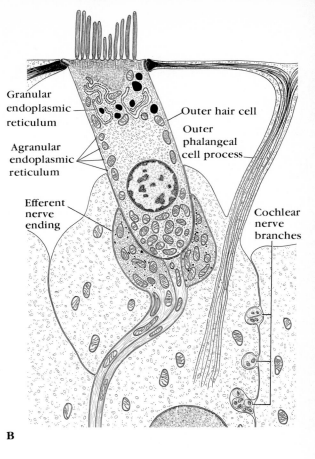

Granular endoplasmic reticulum

Agranular endoplasmic reticulum

Efferent nerve ending

Outer hair cell

Outer phalangeal cell process

Cochlear nerve branches

B

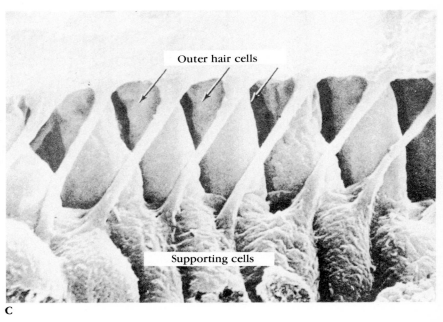

Outer hair cells

Supporting cells

C

cup-shaped cells interposed between the hair cells and the basilar membrane. These supporting cells are called **Deiters' cells.** Each of the Deiters' cells projects finger-like extensions called **phalangeal processes** that pass between adjacent hair cells (Figure 6-16). Each phalangeal process flattens superiorly at the level of the superior surface of the hair cell, providing a rigid separating fibrous support for the hair-bearing end of the hair cells. Lateral to the outer hair cells are additional supporting cells called the **cells of Hensen** and **cells of Claudius.**

The tectorial membrane, which forms the roof of the organ of Corti, also serves to insulate the internal space in which the hair cells reside from the larger space of the surrounding cochlear duct. The tectorial membrane links to the medial supporting cells of the inner hair cells by fibrous projections called **trabeculae,** and, probably in the

same manner, links to the cells of Hensen laterally. The importance of this isolation of the spaces within and around the organ of Corti will become apparent later when we examine the electrical activity of the inner hair cells.

HAIR CELLS. It is important to note that the organ of Corti is very small. The diameter of the entire osseous lumen of the cochlea is on the order of 3 mm. The inner hair cells are about 12 μm in diameter, while the outer hair cells are about 8 μm wide. In all, there are some 3500 inner hair cells and 20,000 outer hair cells within the 35 mm length of the cochlear duct. Each outer hair cell contains approximately 100 stereocilia. Only with the most modern techniques of electron microscopy have many of these details of cochlear structure been discovered [10,23,26] (Figures 6-17 through 6-19).

6-16. *Scanning electron micrograph of guinea pig organ of Corti. (From Bloom W, Fawcett DW:* A Textbook of Histology, *10th ed. Philadelphia, WB Saunders, 1975.)*

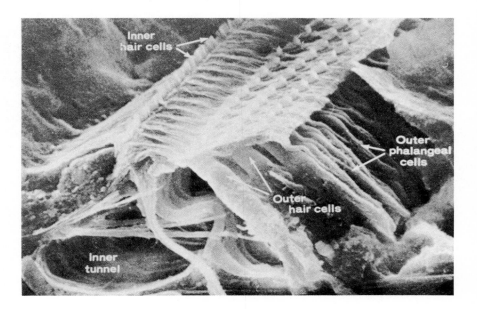

6-17. *Scanning electron micrograph of a surface view of a guinea pig organ of Corti reveals the cilia of the inner hair cells (IH), and the cilia and cell bodies (1,2,3, and A,B,C) of the outer hair cells; Hensen's (H), outer and inner pillar cells (OP,IP) may be observed. An unmyelinated nerve fiber (N) may be seen crossing the tunnel of Corti (Courtesy of Dr. David J. Lim).*

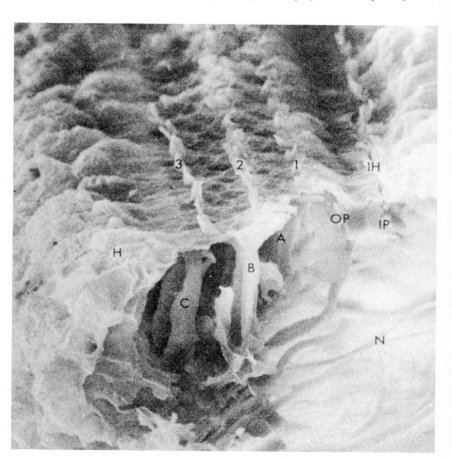

6-18. *Scanning electron micrograph of cellular relationships of a guinea pig organ of Corti. D, Deiters' cell; H, Hensen's cell; IHC, inner hair cell; IS, inner sulcus cell; OHC, outer hair cell; TR, tunnel rod. (Reproduced, with permission, from Smith CA: The Inner Ear: Its Embryological Development and Microstructure. In Tower DB and Eagles EL (Eds):* The Nervous System *(Vol. 3) Copyright 1975 by Raven Press, Publishers, New York, N.Y.)*

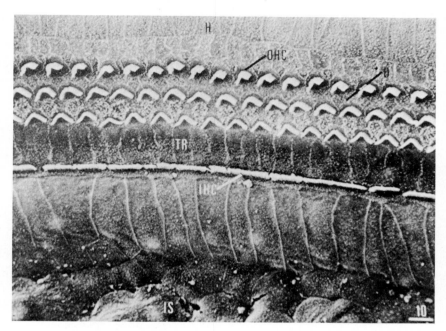

6-19. *Drawing of the cochlear duct, second turn, guinea pig cochlea. Only recent findings are shown in detail. (Reproduced, with permission, from Smith CA: The Inner Ear: Its Embryological Development and Microstructure. In Tower DB, and Eagles, EL (Eds): The Nervous System (Vol. 3) Copyright 1975 by Raven Press, Publishers, New York, NY.)*

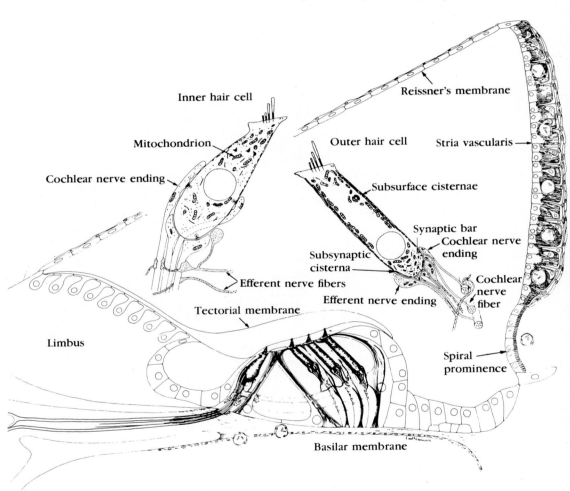

Inner hair cell

Mitochondrion

Cochlear nerve ending

Reissner's membrane

Outer hair cell

Stria vascularis

Subsurface cisternae

Synaptic bar

Cochlear nerve ending

Subsynaptic cisterna

Cochlear nerve fiber

Efferent nerve fibers

Efferent nerve ending

Tectorial membrane

Limbus

Spiral prominence

Basilar membrane

The inner hair cells are goblet-shaped. The inferior end of each cell contains presynaptic structures. Dendritic processes of the **cochlear nerve** (cochlear portion of the vestibulocochlear nerve) synapse with the inner hair cells in a one-to-one relationship and exit from the organ of Corti through small apertures in the lip of the osseous spiral lamina. There are also efferent neurons in the cochlear nerve. Axonal processes of these neurons end on the afferent dendrites in the vicinity of the base of the hair cell (Figure 6-20).

The outer hair cells are cylindrical. They also have presynaptic structures around their bases.

6-20. *Probable pattern of shearing action between the tectorial membrane and the organ of Corti. The hairs of the inner hair cells, which are not attached to the tectorial membrane, are thought to be displaced by fluid movement.* Bottom, *organ at rest;* Top, *during displacement toward the scala vestibuli. (From Ryan A, Dallos P: Physiology of the Inner Ear. In Northern JL (Ed):* Hearing Disorders. *Copyright 1976 by Little, Brown and Company, Boston.)*

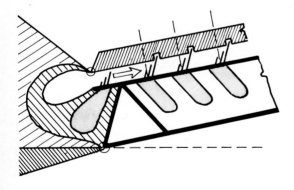

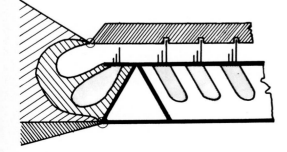

Afferent fibers from the outer hair cells cross the inner and internal tunnels to exit through the osseous spiral lamina. In this case, each afferent fiber synapses with approximately 10 hair cells, and each hair cell synapses with about 10 different afferent neurons [23,28]. Some efferent fibers synapse with afferent fibers of the outer hair cells as well [22,27].

The hair-bearing end of each of the hair cells is composed of a stiff membrane called the **cuticular plate.** Together the cuticular plates, interposed phalangeal processes, and the superior plate of the pillar cells form a fibrous network called the **reticular lamina,** which is thought to hold the superior ends of the hair cells in place. Thus motion between the tectorial membrane and the rest of the organ of Corti would cause the stereocilia of the outer hair cells to bend (Figure 6-21).

There are several differences between the inner and outer hair cells. We have already noted that there are many more outer than inner hair cells. The stereocilia of the outer cells are embedded in the tectorial membrane, while those of the inner cells apparently are not. The inner hair cells have a one-to-one relationship with neurons of the cochlear nerve, while the outer hair cells have multiple relationships. Thus, 95% of the afferent neurons supply the relatively few inner hair cells, while the remaining 5% supply the numerous outer hair cells. The inner and outer hair cells are also different in shape. The possible significance of at least some of these differences will be discussed later in this chapter.

MECHANICS OF HAIR-CELL STIMULATION. We have already seen how sound presented to the ear will result in motion of the footplate of the stapes. As

---

6-21. *Pressure transfer across the cochlear duct.*

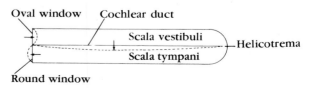

the footplate of the stapes moves inward and outward in the oval window of the vestibule, pressure in the perilymphatic space is alternately increased and decreased. The only mechanism for compensating for this pressure change is by motion of the secondary tympanic membrane in the round window. The pressure differential is introduced by the stapes into the scala vestibuli via the vestibule. The round window is in the basal part of the scala tympani. Since the helicotrema is too small to account for the transfer of pressure between the two scalae, the transfer must occur across the cochlear duct (Figure 6-22). The resulting motion of the cochlear duct, and therefore the organ of Corti, causes a shearing action between the reticular lamina and the tectorial membrane, which results in bending of the stereocilia of the outer hair cells. While the stereocilia of the inner hair cells are not embedded in the tectorial membrane, they also bend, probably in response to motion of the fluid within the organ of Corti during displacement of the cochlear duct [23]. While it is generally ac-

cepted that bending of the stereocilia results in stimulation of the afferent neurons that synapse within the bases of the hair cells, the mechanism of activation within the hair cells is not known.

DISCRIMINATION OF FREQUENCY AND INTENSITY. The exact mechanism by which frequency and intensity information is transformed from mechanical to electrical energy is not known. However, the beginning of this process is fairly well understood as an outgrowth of the monumental work of Georg von Bekesy, begun while he was a communications engineer in Budapest in 1928. The work of von Bekesy demonstrated that motion of the cochlear duct induced by motion of the stapes spreads from the basal portion of the cochlea toward the apex. Further, the amplitude of the displacement increases to a maximum and then diminishes rapidly. The site along the length of the cochlear duct where the maximum displacement occurs varies systematically with the frequency of vibration of the stapes. At low frequencies, the

6-22. *Traveling waves.* Above, *The solid line and short dashes represent the wave at two instants of time. The long dashes show the "envelope" of the wave formed by connecting the wave peaks at successive instants.* Below, *Displacement of the basilar membrane by the waves generated by stapes vibration of the frequencies shown at the top of each curve.* (Reproduced, with permission, from Ganong WF: Review of Medical Physiology, *10th ed. Copyright 1981 by Lange Medical Publications, Los Altos, California.)*

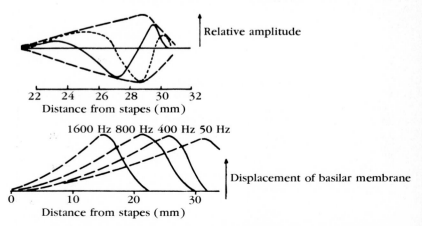

maximum displacement occurs near the apex. As frequency is increased, the site of maximum displacement shifts toward the basal portion of the cochlear duct (Figure 6-23). This pattern of response was first observed by von Bekesy by means of stroboscopic illumination of the basilar membrane of cadavers. Because of the shift in site of maximum response with frequency change, this phenomena was called the **traveling-wave theory.**

The site of maximum response shifts according to stimulating frequency because of variations in the properties of the basilar membrane over its length. The basilar membrane is approximately 0.05 mm wide at its base and approximately 0.5 mm wide at the apex of the cochlea. Concomitantly, the stiffness of the basilar membrane decreases by a factor of 100 from base to apex. Thus while the basal portion of the basilar membrane responds to pressure waves at all frequencies, it is most responsive to high frequencies due to its high degree of stiffness. The apical portion of the membrane, on the other hand, is too compliant to respond to high frequencies. The apparent "travel" of the wave down the cochlear duct from base to

apex is a function of the timing of response of various portions of the basilar membrane as a function of stimulus frequency. The stiffer basal portion of the membrane responds prior to the more compliant apical portion.

Studies of the afferent fibers of the cochlear nerve have demonstrated that individual fibers respond to a limited range of stimulus frequencies (Figure 6-24). The frequency to which an individual fiber will respond is correlated with its cochlear origin. Fibers that respond to high frequencies originate from the basal portion of the cochlea, while those that respond to successively lower frequencies originate from sites in the cochlea closer and closer to the apex. Thus the spatial relationships of site of maximum displacement of the cochlear duct correspond to the frequency responsiveness of the afferent fibers of the cochlear nerve.

6-24. *Comparison of the basilar membrane displacement and cochlear microphonic produced at various frequencies of stimulation and recorded at a cochlear location close to the base. (Reproduced, with permission, from Dallos P, Cheatham MA, and Ferraro J: Cochlear mechanics, nonlinearities and cochlear potentials. J Acoust Soc Am 55:597, 1974. Copyright by the American Institute of Physics, New York, N.Y.)*

6-23. *Guinea pig single auditory nerve fiber responses to tones of given frequencies and intensities. Intensity is in decibels below an arbitrary standard. The dashed line encloses the "response area" of this fiber. (Reproduced, with permission, from Tasaki I: Nerve impulses in individual auditory nerve fibers of guinea pig. J Neurophysiol 17:97, 1954. Copyright by the American Physiological Society, Bethesda, Maryland.)*

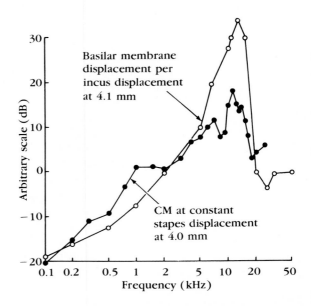

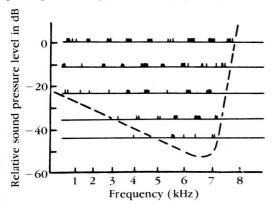

ELECTRICAL ACTIVITY WITHIN THE COCHLEA. The endolymphatic fluid within the cochlear duct is unique electrochemically. Its potassium and sodium concentrations bear a relationship to each other that is closer to that of intracellular than extracellular fluid. In fact, the concentration of sodium is even lower than is typical of intracellular fluid [25]. The values obtained indicate that K^+ must be transported into the endolymph and Na^+ and Cl^- must be transported out of the endolymph [2]. This activity is apparently a function of the stria vascularis, since it is dependent upon the integrity of the stria. The result is a very high **endolymphatic potential (EP),** which is on the order of +80 to +100 mV. By contrast, the intracellular potential of the hair cells is approximately −80 mV. The extracellular fluid within the tunnel of Corti and the tissue of the tectorial membrane are both characterized by a resting potential equivalent to that of the perilymph, about + 2 mV. The result is an exceedingly large potential difference between the endolymph and the hair cells. When a stimulus is delivered to the cochlea, these potentials are disturbed. The resulting changes in potential presumably result in release of transmitter by the hair cells, and thus stimulation of the afferent fibers of the cochlear nerve.

Other components of the complex electrical signal can be recorded from the cochlea. One is the **cochlear microphonic (CM).** The CM is an alternating current that originates in the cochlea and reproduces the time course of a sound wave applied to the ear. It can be picked up in any part of the cochlea even after degeneration of the cochlear nerve (following transection) and for a time even after death. It does not exhibit all-or-none or refractory behavior and is capable of continuous gradation. It is a function of the frequency and intensity of the stimulus sound, and its frequency limits are at least as wide as the audible frequency range. The CM is strongest at the apex for low frequency tones and at the base for high frequency tones. The locus of its greatest intensity corresponds to the peak of the traveling wave along the cochlear duct. The CM has been found to be largely a function of the outer hair cells, since the CM is reduced and altered following their destruction. The remaining CM, thought to be a function of the inner hair cells, is apparently related to the velocity of cochlear duct displacement [23].

Another component of the cochlear potential is the **summation potential (SP).** This is represented by a shift in the baseline voltage and is, therefore, a direct current potential. It, too, is related to the integrity of the outer hair cells, and shifts in the magnitude of the SP correlate with the location of the maxima of the traveling wave.

It is not known whether these electrical events reflect biological events that mediate transmitter release from the hair cells, or are simply a by-product of the events occurring within the cochlea, though the former is more logically appealing. This continues to be a very active area of research. It is tempting to propose a direct relationship between these potentials (CM and SP) and stimulation of the cochlear nerve fibers, given their apparent relationship to the abundant outer hair cells, until one remembers that 95% of the afferent fibers of that nerve arise from the inner hair cells. Some authors have postulated some as yet undefined interaction between the inner and outer hair cells. This might suggest that information is exchanged between the two sets of hair cells [23].

Further consideration of the events that occur within the cochlear nerve and higher centers will be addressed in the following chapter.

REFERENCES

1. Aschan PE, Nylen B: The reconstruction of large defects in the palate or cavity of the mouth using a tubed flap. *Trans Int Soc Plast Surg* 219, 1955.
2. Bosher SK, Warren RL: Observations on the electrochemistry of the cochlear endolymph of the rat. *Proc R Soc Br* 171:227, 1968.
3. Cancura W: Der Einfluss der Binnenohrmuskulatur auf die Schallaubertagung im Mittelohr. *Montssch Ohrenheilk* 1:3, 1970.
4. Dickson DR: Anatomy of the normal velopharyngeal mechanism. *Clin Plast Surg* 2:235, 1975.
5. Dickson DR: Anatomy of the normal and cleft palate eustachian tube. *Ann Otol Rhinol Laryngol* 85 [Suppl 25]:25, 1976.

6. Dickson DR, Grant JCB, Sicher H, DuBrul EL, Paltan J: Status of research in cleft palate anatomy and physiology, July, 1973—Part 1. *Cleft Palate J* 11:471, 1974.

7. Eustachius B: Epistola de auditus organis (Translated by Graves and Galante). *Arch Otolaryngol* 40:123, 1944.

8. Frenckner P: Movements of the tympanic membrane and of the malleus in normal cases and in cases of otosclerosis. *Acta Otolaryngol* 27:707, 1939.

9. Greisen O, Neergaard EB: Middle ear reflex activity in the startle reaction. *Arch Otol* 101:348, 1975.

10. Guyton AC: *Textbook of Medical Physiology*. Philadelphia, WB Saunders, 1971.

11. Kamerer DB: Electromyographic correlation of tensor tympani and tensor veli palatini muscles in man. *Laryngoscope* 88:651, 1978.

12. Kirikae I: *The Structure and Function of the Middle Ear*. Tokyo, University of Tokyo Press, 1960.

13. Lupin A: The relationship of the tensor tympani and tensor palati muscles. *Ann Otol Rhinol Laryngol* 78:792, 1969.

14. Martin FN: *Introduction to Audiology*. Englewood Cliffs, NJ Prentice-Hall, 1975.

15. Maue-Dickson W: Cleft lip and palate research: An update of the art. Section II. Anatomy and physiology. *Cleft Palate J* 14:270, 1977.

16. Maue-Dickson W: The craniofacial complex in cleft lip and palate: An updated review of anatomy and function. *Cleft Palate J* 16:291, 1979.

17. Perlman HB: Some physical properties of the conduction apparatus. *Ann Otol Rhinol Laryngol* 56:334, 1947.

18. Rich AR: A physiological study of the eustachian tube and its related muscles. *Johns Hopkins Hosp Bull* 352:206, 1920.

19. Rich AR: The innervation of the tensor veli palatini and levator veli palatini muscles. *Johns Hopkins Hosp Bull* 355:305, 1920.

20. Rood SR: A functional anatomic study of the muscles related to the eustachian tube. University of Pittsburgh, PhD dissertation, 1972.

21. Rood SR, Doyle WJ: Morphology of tensor veli palatini, tensor tympani, and dilator tubae muscles. *Ann Otol Rhinol Laryngol* 87:202, 1978.

22. Rossi G: The control mechanisms at the hair cell/nerve junction of the central auditory pathways and centers, and the pathways of the cerebral coordination. In Tonndorf J (Ed): *Morphology and Function of Auditory Input Control*. Chicago, Translations of the Beltone Institute for Hearing Research, 1967.

23. Ryan A, Dallos P: Physiology of the inner ear. In Northern JL (Ed): *Hearing Disorders*. Boston, Little, Brown, 1976.

24. Salomon G, Starr A. Electromyography of middle ear muscles in man during motor activities. *Acta Neurol* 39:161, 1963.

25. Smith CA, Lowry OH, Wu ML: The electrolytes of the labyrinthine fluids. *Laryngoscope* 64:141, 1954.

26. Smith CA: The inner ear: Its embryological development and microstructure. In Tower DB, Eagles EL (Eds): *The Nervous System. Volume 3, Human Communication and Its Disorders*. New York, Raven Press, 1975.

27. Spoendlin H: *The Organization of the Cochlear Receptor*. Basel, Karger, 1966.

28. Spoendlin H: The Innervation of the Cochlear Receptor. In Møller A (Ed): *Basic Mechanisms in Hearing*. New York, Academic Press, 1973.

29. Sucheston ME, Canon MS: Eustachian tubes of several mammalian species. *Arch Otolaryngol* 93:58, 1971.

30. Wever EG, Lawrence M: *Physiological Acoustics*. Princeton, Princeton University Press, 1954.

31. Wever EG, Lawrence M, Smith KR: The middle ear in sound conduction. *Arch Otolaryngol* 68:19, 1948.

Nervous System

A chapter on the nervous system is as presumptuous as a chapter on the universe. In many ways, the magnitude of the problems that beset us in our attempts to understand these two topics is similar. In the case of astrophysics, as in the neurosciences, although we can observe some major structures, most are beyond our powers of observation, concealed by distance or, in the latter case, by size. We perceive distant galaxies, which are made up of innumerable stars and planets, as though they were homogeneous units. In the brain we observe clusters of nerve cells and their interconnections in much the same way. We understand principles by which our physical universe operates, such as gravity and relativity, but we have only the vaguest guesses about why the universe behaves the way it does, what it is in the process of becoming, or what it has been. Similarly, we can speak of nerve conduction, synaptic activity, and nerve pathways but have no idea how we remember, form concepts, or process ideas.

In our physical universe we are just now exploring the inner reaches of our own solar system, while events in distant space defy even our imagination. In seeking to understand our own brain, we are just now trying to understand how its parts interrelate, what basic biochemical events occur and what they do, while the interaction between our behavior and its biological basis is largely beyond even the theoretical level.

The behavior that presumably results from activity within the nervous system is itself complex and poorly understood. In addition, it has become clear that the activity of our nervous system is, in part, a function of our behavioral experience. That is, we do not enter this world with an immutable brain, which then acts on its surroundings. Nor is the brain totally plastic and without rules by which it will respond and develop. Thus, when we examine the function of the nervous system and its component parts, we must, in a very real sense, include the world around us as an integral and determinant part of that system. The brain cannot be understood without reference to the world in which it develops and exists. The interaction of the brain and its environment is a determinant of both behavior and brain function.

This chapter will explore some of the basic mechanisms of the nervous system that relate to the perception and production of speech.

CLASSIFICATION AND TERMINOLOGY

There are many ways of subdividing the nervous system in order to make it easier to understand. Such subdivisions can be made along anatomical or functional lines. It should be borne in mind that such subdivisions are for our convenience in study and do not represent real boundaries of neural pathways or functional centers, if such exist. There is still controversy over whether the nervous system, and especially the brain, operates as a series of "centers" or as an indivisible whole.

Anatomical Subdivisions

The most basic anatomical division of the nervous system into parts is between the central nervous system (CNS) and the peripheral nervous system (PNS). The **CNS,** contained within the cranium and the neural canal of the vertebral column, includes the brain and spinal cord. The **PNS** consists of that part of the nervous system external to the CNS.

The CNS is further subdivided into the brain and spinal cord. The junction of the two occurs at the level of the foramen magnum of the occipital bone. The terminology used to describe subdivisions of the brain is complicated by the fact that terms that denote embryological and adult structures are often intermixed. Thus we will examine both briefly (Table 7-1).

By the fourth week of embryonic life, the cephalic portion of the neural tube, which will give rise to the brain, has developed a number of swellings and bends, and anterior, middle, and posterior parts can be identified (Figure 7-1). The anterior part is called the **prosencephalon** (also called the **forebrain).** The middle part is called the **mesencephalon** (also called the **midbrain).** The posterior part is called the **rhombencephalon** (also called the **hindbrain**). By the fifth week, the prosencephalon has formed further and is divided into the **telencephalon** and the **diencephalon.** The mesencephalon undergoes no further subdivision. At the same time, the rhombencephalon has divided into the **metencephalon** and the **myelencephalon.** As can be seen in Table 7-1 and Figure 7-1, the telencephalon gives rise to the adult structures called the cerebrum, corpus callosum, and basal ganglia. The **cerebrum** consists of the two large bilateral masses, each called a **cerebral hemisphere**, which make up most of what can be seen externally as the brain (Figure 7-2). It is the enormous size of the cerebrum that most easily distinguishes the human brain from that of lower animals. It is generally as-

Table 7-1. Embryological Derivations of the Major Parts of the Brain

Embryological Structures		Adult Structures
Prosencephalon	Telencephalon	Cerebrum Corpus collosum Basal ganglia
	Diencephalon	Thalamus "Thalamic" nuclei
Mesencephalon	Mesencephalon	Midbrain
Rhombencephalon	Metencephalon	Pons Cerebellum
	Myelencephalon	Medulla

7-1. *Development of the CNS at approximately 4 weeks (A) and at 6 weeks (B). (Reproduced, with permission, from Moore KM:* The Developing Human, *2nd ed. Copyright 1977 by WB Saunders Company, Philadelphia, Pennsylvania.)*

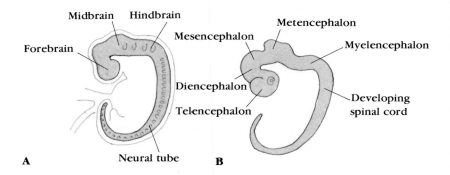

7-2. *The human central nervous system. The higher brain stem, including thalamus, midbrain, and part of the pons are shown within the brain. The lower brain stem, composed of pons and medulla, emerges below with the cerebellum. (From Wilder Penfield and Lamar Roberts,* Speech and Brain-Mechanisms. *Copyright © 1959 by Princeton University Press, Fig. II-1, p. 15. Reprinted by permission of Princeton University Press.)*

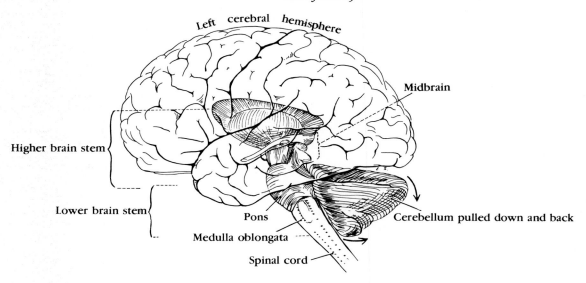

sumed that much of what we think of as "human" brain functions, such as conscious thought, conceptual processing, and abstract problem-solving, are primarily functions of the cerebrum. The **corpus callosum** is a massive pathway of nerve processes that interconnect the two cerebral hemispheres (Figure 7-3). The **basal ganglia** are a group of cell body clusters (more properly called **nuclei;** see Chapter 2, Basic Concepts) that lie on either side of midline between the lower lateral parts of the cerebral hemispheres. The basal ganglia serve as relay stations, primarily within the motor pathways to the muscles of the body.

The diencephalon gives rise to the adult thalamus and the small nuclei around it with names containing the term thalamus. The **thalamus** is the primary relay station between the cerebral cortex and other parts of the brain, especially in the sensory pathways to the cerebrum. The interconnections within the thalamic nuclei, and between those nuclei and other centers are extremely complex, involving many feedback loops in which a part of the brain that receives projections sends projections back to their source.

The mesencephalon gives rise to the adult midbrain. The **midbrain** (Figure 7-4) contains a number of nuclear masses that act as relay stations within the auditory and visual pathways, the nuclei which give rise to some of the cranial nerves, and two large nuclear masses that have recently been included among the basal ganglia because of their functional interconnections with the basal ganglia of the telencephalon. These are the **red nucleus** and the **substantia nigra.**

The metencephalon gives rise to the adult pons and cerebellum (see Figures 7-2 and 7-4). The **pons** contains a number of nuclear masses, some of which give rise to cranial nerves. The anterior surface of the pons is enlarged and contains fiber pathways that course transversely and then posteriorly to enter the cerebellum as the **middle cerebellar peduncles.** The superficial part of the **cerebellum,** like that of the cerebrum, is composed of gray matter, termed the **cortex,** and its inner part is white matter. The cerebellum receives input from all other parts of the central nervous system, including sensory information that arises from the muscles, tendons, and joints of

7-3. *Relationships among the cerebral cortex, corpus callosum, and basal ganglia.*

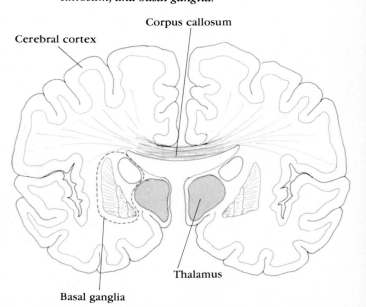

Corpus callosum

Cerebral cortex

Thalamus

Basal ganglia

the body. It apparently also projects fibers to each of the areas of the CNS from which it receives fibers. The cerebellum plays a major role in the modification and control of muscular activity by integration of sensory information coming in from the periphery. It is also a major center for the programming of muscular activity and contains major motor pathways to the cerebral cortex.

The myelencephalon gives rise to the adult **medulla** (also called the **medulla oblongata**) (see Figure 7-4). The anterior surface of the medulla is marked by bilateral longitudinal swellings made up of fibers that form part of the large motor pathway extending from the cerebral cortex to the spinal cord. Within the medulla are nuclei of a number of cranial nerves and other nuclei that are relay stations for sensory fibers projected from the spinal cord. Laterally are the **inferior cerebellar peduncles,** which connect the medulla to the cerebellum. Posterolaterally are bilateral swellings of the **olivary nuclei,** which form relay stations between the spinal cord and brain.

It should be stressed that these divisions of the brain are based on embryological derivations but in no way imply that these parts act independently or constitute anatomical entities. They are all interlaced with ascending and descending pathways and interconnections.

As indicated earlier, the peripheral nervous system consists of all nerves and ganglia external to the brain and spinal cord. This includes all of the nerves to and from all of the structures of the body. The nerves that exit and enter the brain stem are called **cranial nerves;** those that exit and enter the spinal cord are called **spinal nerves.** The cranial nerves supply most structures of the head and neck; internal organs of the body; sensory end-organs for vision, hearing, taste, and smell; and the vascular system. The spinal nerves supply the skeletal muscles of the trunk and limbs and associated tendons, ligaments, and joints. As we will see, this is somewhat oversimplified but will serve for now as an organizing principle.

In general, the cell bodies of peripheral motor nerves are located within the CNS. Those of the cranial nerves lie within nuclei of the brain stem, while those of the spinal nerves lie within the anterior part of the spinal cord. Cell bodies of peripheral sensory nerves are located external to the CNS. They form ganglia that lie next to the brain stem in the case of cranial nerves or next to the spinal cord in the case of spinal nerves.

Other means of subdividing the nervous system have anatomical components but are largely functional divisions and will be described as such.

7-4. *The red nucleus and substantia nigra within the midbrain.*

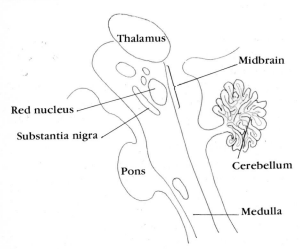

Functional Subdivisions

The nervous system may be subdivided into motor and sensory components. The **motor** components activate peripheral structures such as muscles and glands. The **sensory** components feed information back to the CNS. In the peripheral nervous system, the distinction between motor nerves and sensory nerves is reasonably clear. However, within the CNS such distinctions can become arbitrary. A given neuron that serves to interconnect two parts of the CNS may be classified as sensory or motor depending upon what function it seems to be serving. Frequently we do not know enough to make such distinctions. Also, some neurons interconnect sensory and motor neurons, and others serve such functions as conceptualization and other thought processes in which a sensory-motor classification is clearly not appropriate. Thus, a third category has been added called **internuncial,** meaning to run between.

The term **efferent** is used to refer to motor nerves, while the term **afferent** is used to refer to sensory nerves. However, efferent is also used to refer to nerve processes that conduct signals away from the cell body, nucleus, ganglion, or other center, while the term afferent is used to refer to processes that conduct signals toward the cell body, nucleus, ganglion, or other center. This results in confusion. For example, a sensory neuron can be described, in its entirety, as afferent since it conducts information from a peripheral structure to the CNS. However, the neuronal process of that same neuron that is conducting the signal from the peripheral structure, such as a muscle, toward its own cell body can be described as afferent with reference to the muscle, but as efferent with reference to the cell body. Thus in studying a neurology text, one has to discern how the author is using these terms and hope that they are used consistently. In general, **efferent** is used to mean conduction of a signal toward the periphery (away from the CNS) and **afferent** is used to mean conduction of a signal away from the periphery (toward the CNS).

Peripheral nerves are also classified as somatic or visceral; a distinction based both on the embryological origin of the nerve elements and on the embryological origin of the structures they innervate. Thus, some apparent inconsistencies arise when these terms are applied to adult structures. In general, **somatic** refers to the skeletal muscles, sensory receptors associated with body movement, sensory receptors in the skin, and sensory receptors for hearing and vision. **Visceral** generally refers to those organs and functions of the body that are usually thought not to be under voluntary control, including both motor and sensory nerves that supply the digestive system, cardiovascular system, urogenital system, and other organs such as glands and the iris of the eye. Sensory receptors for taste and smell are also part of the visceral system. There are important exceptions to this general pattern with regard to the skeletal

muscles. Because of their embryological origin, the muscles of the face and larynx and some of the pharyngeal muscles are classed as visceral.

Somatic and visceral nerves are further classified as afferent or efferent and as special or general. The term **special** refers to the "special senses" of vision, hearing, equilibrium (linear and rotational acceleration), taste, and smell and also to the motor innervation of the skeletal muscles included as part of the visceral system. The term **general** refers to everything that is not special. Thus we arrive at classifications that combine somatic-visceral, afferent-efferent, and special-general as in the following examples.

General somatic afferent:	Proprioceptive fibers from muscles of the trunk and limbs
General somatic efferent:	Motor fibers to the muscles of the trunk and limbs
General visceral afferent:	Sensory fibers from the oral and nasal mucosa
General visceral efferent:	Motor nerve supply to smooth muscles
Special somatic afferent:	Optic and vestibulocochlear nerves
Special somatic efferent	None
Special visceral afferent:	Olfactory nerve
Special visceral efferent:	Motor fibers to the muscles of the larynx

The final subclassification of the nervous system that will be considered is the **autonomic nervous system (ANS)**. The term **ANS** is used to describe the motor nerves that supply the "automatic" functions of the body mediated by smooth muscle, cardiac muscle, and the glands of the body. The ANS consists of two subdivisions called the sympathetic system and the parasympathetic system. As a generalization, the **sympathetic** system acts to prepare the body for emergency action, while the **parasympathetic** system is involved in conservative visceral function. Thus the sweating, heart-racing, action-ready state associated with, for example, fear is a function of the sympathetic system. The fibers of the sympathetic system arise from the thoracic and lumbar areas of the spinal cord. The fibers of the parasympathetic system arise from the brain stem and the sacral portion of the spinal cord. Thus the terms **thoracolumbar** and **craniosacral** are often used in place of sympathetic and parasympathetic. Table 7-2 summarizes the classification terms that have been described.

PHYSICAL ENVIRONMENT OF THE BRAIN
Meninges

Within the cranial cavity, the brain is covered by three layers of membrane collectively called the **meninges**, which extend inferiorly to surround the spinal cord. The most superficial layer of membrane is called the **dura mater** (literally, "hard mother"), since it is the toughest and thickest of the membranes. Within the cranium, the dura mater is fused to the periosteum of the deep surface of the cranial bones. Thus, the periosteum is often referred to as the superficial layer of dura mater. In some areas, however, the two layers are separated. Over the posterior cranial fossa, the deep layer extends between the occipital lobes of the cerebrum above and the cerebellum below

(Figure 7-5). This extension of dura is called the **tentorium cerebelli.** In the longitudinal midline, another fold of dura called the **falx cerebri** extends inferiorly between the two cerebral hemispheres.

The middle layer of membrane, called the **arachnoid membrane** (referring to its spider-web appearance), is delicate and is closely applied to the overlying dura. The deepest layer of the meninges, the delicate **pia mater** ("loving mother"), adheres to the surface of the brain and is the only one of the membranes to follow the

7-5. *Extensions of the dura mater.*

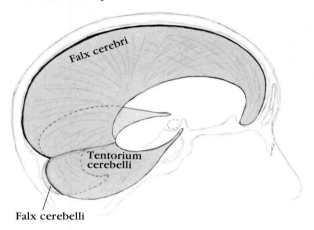

Falx cerebelli

Table 7-2. *Functional Classifications of Components of the Nervous System*

Motor neurons	Activate peripheral structures
Sensory neurons	Send information to the CNS
Internuncial neurons	Interconnecting neurons within the CNS
Efferent neurons	Conduct signals toward the periphery
Afferent neurons	Conduct signals toward the CNS
Somatic system	Includes the skeletal muscles and sensory receptors for body movement, skin sensation, vision, and hearing
Visceral system	Includes the sensory and motor supply to automatic activities of the body
Special	Refers to the senses of vision, hearing, equilibrium, taste and smell, and to the motor innervation to visceral skeletal muscles
General	Everything not listed under Special
Sympathetic system	Includes those parts of the nervous system that ready the body for emergencies
Parasympathetic system	Includes those parts of the nervous system that return the body to its resting functions

cortical convolutions. The space between the arachnoid membrane and the pia mater, termed the **subarachnoid space,** is filled with **cerebrospinal fluid (CSF).**

Delicate interconnections between the arachnoid membrane and the pia mater suspend the brain within the fluid-filled subarachnoid space. The weight of the brain in air is about 1400 g; suspended within the CFS, however, it has a net weight of about 50 g [1]. This buoyancy permits the attachment of the brain via the pia mater to the arachnoid membrane to protect the brain from injury. It takes a fairly substantial blow to the head to drive the brain against the bony wall and produce injury. This motion of the brain may stretch the blood vessels that run between the layers of the meninges, resulting in hemorrhage, usually within the space between the dura and the arachnoid (the **subdural space**). Since this space has no outlet, a bloody mass called a **subdural hematoma** can result and cause pressure on the underlying brain. Prolonged pressure of sufficient degree can cause damage to the brain. Hemorrhage in the subarachnoid space occurs more typically in disease states such as stroke when a weakened portion of a blood vessel ruptures. In this case, blood is released into the CSF, and brain damage is primarily due to failure of oxygen supply to that part of the brain normally supplied by the ruptured vessels.

Ventricles

Embryologically, the CNS develops as a tube with a central cavity. As the brain develops, the central cavity takes on a more and more complex shape. With the early development of the telencephalon, the most cephalic part of the cavity develops bilateral swellings called the **lateral ventricles** (Figure 7-6). Another enlargement of the cavity develops in the area of the diencephalon and is called the **third ventricle** (the lateral ventricles counting as the first and second). A **fourth ventricle**

7-6. *Embryological development of the ventricles. (Redrawn, with permission, from Gardner E:* Fundamentals of Neurology. *Copyright 1963 by WB Saunders Company, Philadelphia, Pennsylvania.)*

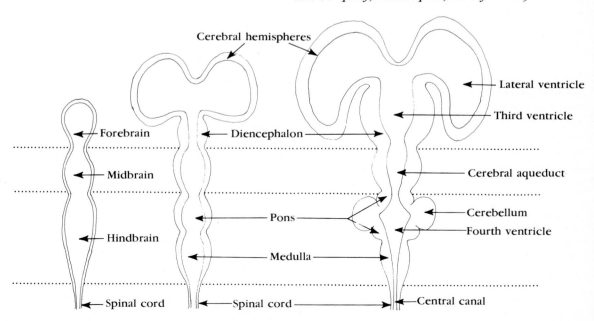

7-7. *The ventricular system of the adult brain. A, Lateral view; B, Anteroposterior view. (Reproduced, with permission, from Curtis BA, Jacobson S, and Marcus EM:* An Introduction to the Neurosciences. *Copyright 1972 by WB Saunders Co., Philadelphia.)*

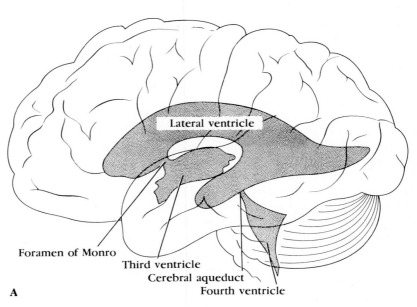

Lateral ventricle

Foramen of Monro

Third ventricle

Cerebral aqueduct

Fourth ventricle

A

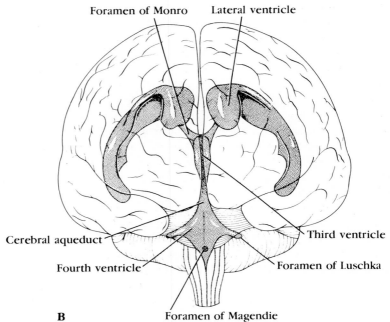

Foramen of Monro   Lateral ventricle

Cerebral aqueduct   Third ventricle

Fourth ventricle   Foramen of Luschka

Foramen of Magendie

B

develops at the level of the rhombencephalon. The communication between the lateral ventricles and from them to the third ventricle is called the **interventricular foramen** (also called the **foramen of Monro**). The passage between the third and fourth ventricles is termed the **cerebral aqueduct** (also called the **aqueduct of Sylvius**). The cerebral aqueduct passes through the mesencephalon. The fourth ventricle opens inferiorly into the central canal of the spinal cord. As the brain assumes a more adult shape, the shapes of the ventricles increase in complexity.

In adult form, the lateral ventricles are by far the largest of these cavities (Figure 7-7). Each is characterized by three projections called **horns**. The **anterior horn** on each side is located near midline and its roof is formed by the corpus callosum. The medial wall is formed by a membrane called the **septum pellucidum,** which extends inferiorly from the corpus callosum. The lateral wall (also called the **floor**) is formed by one of the basal ganglia called the **caudate nucleus.** The inferior horn curves ventrally and rostrally into the temporal lobe. The posterior horn, which is the smallest, extends into the occipital lobe.

The third ventricle is a narrow, vertically oriented cleft interposed between the two thalami. The fourth ventricle is diamond-shaped and lies anterior to the cerebellum and posterior to the pons and medulla. Three openings in the fourth ventricle communicate with the subarachnoid space and thereby permit flow of the CSF. Bilateral openings, located at the termini of the lateral recesses, are called the **lateral apertures** (also called the **foramina of Luschka**). The third opening is through the central portion of the roof and is called the **median aperture** (also called the **foramen of Magendie**).

CSF is produced by the linings of the ventricles and also by special organs called **choroid plexuses** formed by infoldings of the linings of the ventricles. These infoldings are vascularized by a network of blood vessels. About half of the CSF is produced by the choroid plexuses. The importance of CSF production, flow, and uptake to the

protection of the environment of the brain will become evident in the following discussion.

Blood Supply

Four major vessels supply arterial blood to the brain (Figure 7-8). Posteriorly, the two **vertebral arteries** rise toward the brain and join to form the **basilar artery.** Laterally, the two **internal carotid arteries** rise to the brain. The basilar and internal carotid arteries are linked by collaterals at the base of the brain. These vessels and collaterals form a circle called the **circle of Willis,** from which the entire blood supply to the brain arises. Two arteries are given off posteriorly on each side to supply the cerebellum and the posterior part of the cerebrum. These are the **superior cerebellar arteries** and the **posterior cerebral arteries.** The major portion of the internal carotid artery continues superiorly as the **middle cerebral artery. Anterior cerebral arteries** branch from it to supply the anterior part of the cerebrum (Figure 7-9). Each of these large arteries gives off a multitude of branches that penetrate the brain substance to supply all of its parts.

The venous drainage from the brain collects in large vessels called **sinuses**, which are located within the dura mater (Figure 7-10). These subsequently drain into the **internal jugular vein.** Cluster-like projections of dura extend into some of these sinuses. These projections, called **arachnoid villi,** appear at about the age of seven and increase in number until adulthood. Their walls become very thin and permit passage of CSF from the subarachnoid space into the sinuses. Thus the circle of CSF is complete, from the choroid plexuses into the ventricles, from there to the subarachnoid space, and thence to the venous sinuses.

Since the brain lies within a closed bony capsule, any increase in blood pressure produces pressure on the brain which, if prolonged, can result in damage. Since blood pressure does vary somewhat over time, a compensating mechanism is needed. This is provided by the CSF. CSF pro-

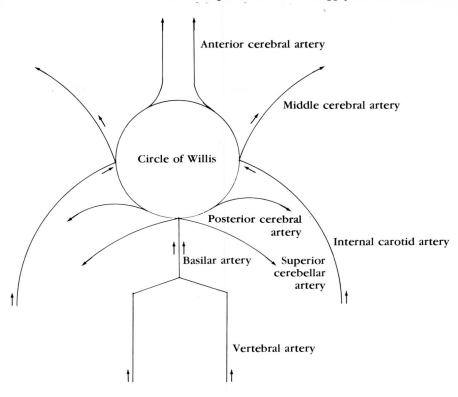

7-8. *Principal arterial blood supply to the brain.*

Anterior cerebral artery

Middle cerebral artery

Circle of Willis

Posterior cerebral artery

Internal carotid artery

Basilar artery

Superior cerebellar artery

Vertebral artery

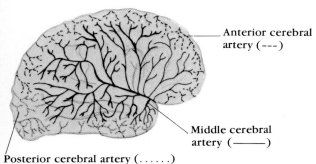

Anterior cerebral artery (- - -)

Middle cerebral artery (———)

Posterior cerebral artery (. . . . .)

7-9. *The cerebral arteries.* Above, *Lateral view;* Below, *Medial view. (Redrawn, with permission, from Ranson SW and Clark SL:* The Anatomy of the Nervous System. *Copyright 1959 by WB Saunders Company, Philadelphia, Pennsylvania.)*

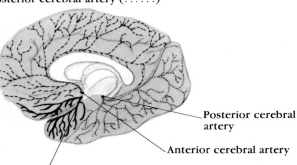

Posterior cerebral artery

Anterior cerebral artery

Middle cerebral artery

duction varies with blood pressure so that under normal circumstances the two are kept in balance.

Since the CSF is normally completely replaced every 12 to 24 hours, blockage of flow can have disastrous consequences in a very short period of time. This can be caused by blockage of the foramina leading out of the fourth ventricle, by obliteration of the subarachnoid space by disease, or by failure of uptake of CSF by the venous system. When this occurs in infancy and goes unchecked, it results in enlargement of the ventricles and consequent destruction of brain tissue, a condition known as **hydrocephalus.** Since it usually occurs before the cranium is completely developed, it also results in massive enlargement of the cranium if untreated.

FUNCTIONAL ANATOMY OF THE NERVOUS SYSTEM
Cerebrum
The cerebrum is composed of two roughly symmetrical bilateral masses termed the **cerebral hemispheres** (see Figure 7-3). Each hemisphere is composed of a superficial layer of gray matter called the **cerebral cortex** and a deep layer of white matter. Together, the cerebral hemispheres form the largest part of the human brain. During fetal development, the cortex becomes folded upon itself so that only about one-third of the surface of the cortex is visible on the surface of the adult brain (see Figure 7-2). The elevations of the folds are called **gyri** (plural of **gyrus,** also called **convolutions**). The depressions that separate the

7-10. *Coronal section through the superior sagittal sinus showing the organization of the meninges (dura, arachnoid, and pia mater), and two of the arachnoid villi.*

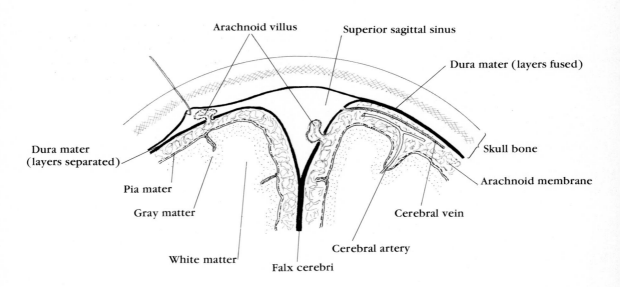

gyri are called **sulci** (plural of **sulcus**) if they are shallow, or **fissures** if they are deep. Some of these sulci and fissures separate areas of the cerebral cortex into **lobes** (Figure 7-11). The most obvious of the fissures is the **lateral fissure,** which separates the **temporal lobe** from the **frontal lobe** anteriorly and from the **parietal lobe** superiorly. The **central sulcus** (sometimes called the **central fissure**), which is the first sulcus to appear in fetal life, is used as a landmark to separate the frontal and parietal lobes. Posteriorly, the parietal lobe is separated from the **occipital lobe** by an imaginary line that connects the **parieto-occipital fissure** on the medial surface of the cerebral cortex to a small notch on the inferior-lateral surface of the cortex called the **preoccipital notch.**

All of these lobes are continuous, and the division into lobes is for convenience of reference. Various of the gyri and sulci are named for their location relative to the fissures, sulci, and lobes already named. Thus, for example, there are superior, middle, and inferior temporal gyri, and a precentral and postcentral sulcus. The specific gyri and sulci on the surface of the brain are subject to individual variation and can be difficult to locate visually on an individual brain. The two cerebral hemispheres are separated from each other at midline by the **longitudinal cerebral fissure.** This fissure extends inferiorly to the corpus callosum.

As with other areas of the human nervous system, much of our information about the function of the cerebrum comes from the study of pathologies. Such studies have led to naming and even numbering of various regions of the cerebrum for reference purposes. Studies of patients whose corpus callosum is absent or has been surgically divided have been of great interest [7]. Division or absence of the corpus callosum essentially isolates the two cerebral hemispheres from each other, so that sensory information provided to one hemisphere is not available to the other hemisphere. (This may not be true for highly emotional stimuli for which there is evidence that acti-

7-11. *Lobes of the cerebral cortex.*

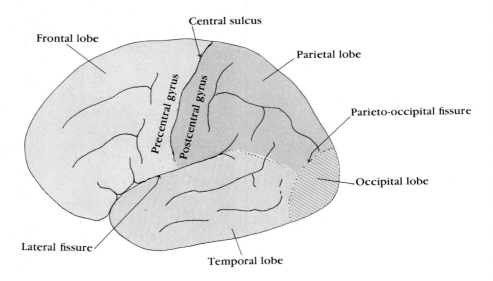

vation of some brain-stem centers gives bilateral stimulation to the cerebrum.) Such studies have shown that each of the two hemispheres is "dominant" for certain kinds of activity. That is, the dominant hemisphere is required for normal function, while the other hemisphere plays a lesser role. Studies of competing messages to the two sides of the brain in normal subjects has added to our understanding of the roles of the two hemispheres. It is of interest that at least some of the functional differences are reflected in anatomical differences between the two hemispheres. However, as pointed out by Milner [3] ". . . one should not be content with delineating the contrasting specializations of the two sides but must also be prepared to tackle the more difficult problem of how they interact in normal behavior."

Our understanding of hemispheric dominance is in its infancy. However, there are general areas in which agreement has been reached by most (but certainly not all) investigators. Current data suggests that the left hemisphere in most persons (probably all right-handed people and the majority of left-handed people) is dominant in activities such as the linguistic aspects of language, including both speech and writing, and for mathematical functions. The right hemisphere seems dominant for nonmathematical and nonlinguistic functions such as melody, including the melodic aspects of speech. In addition, the left hemisphere tends to respond in a holistic manner to perceptual fields, whereas the right hemisphere tends to respond to features that make up the holistic perception.

Damage to the cerebral cortex can result in complex receptive and expressive disabilities depending upon which hemisphere is damaged and the location of the damage. Two of the most clearly delineated areas of the cortex are the precentral gyrus and the postcentral gyrus. The **precentral gyrus,** also called area 4 or the **motor strip,** projects motor fibers to the periphery, while the **precentral gyrus,** also called area 3,1,2 or the **somatic-sensory area,** receives sensory input from the periphery via the thalamus (Figure 7-12). Damage to the precentral gyrus results in flaccid paralysis of the muscles affected, while damage to the postcentral gyrus results in impairment of touch, pressure, and proprioception. Damage to area 6 results in hyperactive reflexes and spasticity. These disabilities will occur on the side of the body opposite to the brain injury, since the fibers that project to and from these areas cross midline before reaching the periphery. Also, damage on the dominant side results in more serious and

7-12. *Areas of the cerebral cortex.*

Precentral gyrus (area 4)

Central sulcus

Postcentral gyrus (areas 3,1,2)

Supramarginal gyrus (area 40)

6

3

4

1

2

40

45

44

22

Broca's area

Wernicke's area

more permanent disability, while damage to the nondominant hemisphere may be transient.

There are a number of areas that, when damaged on the dominant side, produce symptoms that affect the perceptual processes. Damage to area 40 (the **supramarginal gyrus**) may produce tactile and proprioceptive agnosia as well as apraxia. Damage to area 22, called **Wernicke's area,** results in auditory aphasia. Expressive aphasia results from damage to areas 44 and 45, called **Broca's area.** This type of information has led some writers to speculate that specific areas of the brain control specific activities. It is probably more reasonable to assume that the areas mentioned represent areas of convergence of pathways that subserve a complex function or are important relay stations for that function. As an example, if I knock a hole in the wall and the lights go out, I may presume that I have located the "center" that controls the lights. However, I may have damaged any part of the circuitry necessary for their operation including the ground wire, hot wire, switch, fuse, or whatever. Thus, while the functional significance of these centers is important to the understanding of brain function, we must be cautious in interpretation. While the evidence is clear that damage to specific cerebral areas will produce predictable types of symptomatology, it is also true that in most cases of cerebral dysfunction, the area of lesion is unknown. Thus, it is not necessarily true that the site of a lesion can be deduced from behavioral symptoms.

Speech and language perception and production are enormously complex. At this point, both the behavioral aspects and the central processes related to them are almost entirely theoretical. For example, there is still no agreement with regard to the essential components or features of language. Prutting and Elliott (5) take the position that ". . . the traditional definitions of pragmatics, semantics, syntax, and phonology may not, at least on a one-to-one basis, necessarily reflect natural divisions of the language system. Therefore, a question that arises is: What is or are the units of analysis which reflect the synergistic operations?" With regard to brain function, there is evidence

that there are hormonal influences on neuronal and synaptic activity. However, the nature of these influences in what are called "higher mental functions" is largely unknown.

Corpus Callosum

The corpus callosum forms the major portion of the commissural (joining) fibers that interconnect the two cerebral hemispheres (see Figure 7-3). It is massive, containing in excess of 200 million fibers [7]. The fibers generally interconnect analogous sections of the two hemispheres. There are also two smaller bundles of commissural fibers, one anterior to the corpus callosum and one posterior. The anterior bundle, called the **anterior commissure,** interconnects the two olfactory tracts, which conduct stimuli from the olfactory fibers of the nose subserving the sense of smell. The posterior bundle interconnects the hippocampi and is, therefore, called the **hippocampal commissure** (also called the **commissure of the fornix**). The **hippocampus** is a band of cortex in the temporal lobe with functions evidently related to olfaction and also to the development and maintenance of conditioned responses [6].

As indicated previously, the role of these interhemispheric connections in brain function is not well understood. In discussion of patients with callosal ablation, Sperry [7] notes some general tendencies toward reduced perseverance in activities that are "mentally taxing," and some difficulty with the "ability to grasp broad, long-term, or distant implications of a situation," as well as other disabilities. However, he points out that "Most of these symptoms . . . have not yet been subjected to specific study and also most of the patients have substantial extracommissural damage contributing to such effects."

Basal Ganglia

Beneath the mantle of the cortex on either side of midline are concentrations of cell bodies and synapses termed **nuclei**. Many of the clusters have been individually named, as have been groups of these nuclei that are closely related anatomically and/or functionally. **Basal ganglia** is the term used to describe one such collection of nuclei.

Before looking further at the basal ganglia, it will be helpful to examine the entire field of nuclei in the area beneath the cerebrum for purposes of orientation (Figure 7-13). One of the largest struc-

tures in this area is the **thalamus.** The bilateral thalami lie adjacent to midline and form the head of the brain stem. Close to the thalamus and partly wrapped around it are a series of smaller nuclei, including the **caudate, putamen, globus pallidus, subthalamus, substantia nigra,** and **red**

7-13. *Composite of two coronal sections of the brain with the left side of the figure taken more anterior than the right to show the relationships among the thalamus and the basal ganglia. V. 3, third ventricle. (Based on Roberts M and Hanaway J:* Atlas of the Human Brain in Section, *by permission of the publisher. Copyright 1970 by Lea & Febiger, Philadelphia, Pennsylvania.)*

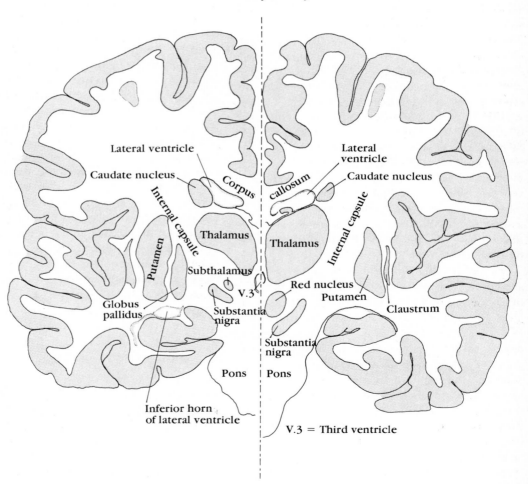

nucleus. All of these have close anatomical and functional relationships. Other nuclei in the area include the **amygdala, claustrum, hypothalamus, epithalamus,** and **interpeduncular nucleus.**

There is not complete agreement as to which of the nuclei should be included in the basal ganglia. Three that are always included are the caudate, putamen, and globus pallidus. Other authors add the major part of the subthalamus, called the **subthalamic nucleus.** A number of recent authors have also included the substantia nigra and sometimes the red nucleus. This is not completely arbitrary; which structures are included depends upon how closely related they seem to be in terms of their interconnections and, therefore, their function. New information is constantly being developed with regard to functional interconnections and the roles of the various nuclei in our behavior. Because the tendency has been to include more and more of the nuclei as a part of the basal ganglia, they will all be considered here.

Table 7-3 presents the terminology used to refer to these nuclei individually and in groups. The **caudate nucleus** is shaped somewhat like the letter *C* with its opening directed inferiorly. The largest part of the caudate, called the **head,** is located on the lateral wall of the anterior horn of the lateral ventricle (Figure 7-14). It is anterior to the thalamus. From there, the caudate curves superolaterally over the thalamus. The tail of the caudate curves downward and then anteriorly posterolateral to the thalamus.

The **putamen** and **globus pallidus** together are called the **lenticular nucleus,** since their shape resembles a biconvex lens. The lenticular nucleus lies immediately anterolateral to the thalamus and within the open arc of the caudate. Massive bundles of fibers interconnect the head of the caudate and the putamen. These fibers are penetrated by a band of white matter called the **internal capsule.** The internal capsule is thus interposed between the lenticular nucleus and the thalamus and the head of the caudate. The internal capsule contains a massive pathway that interconnects the cerebral cortex with structures of the brain stem and spinal cord. The **subthalamic nucleus, red nucleus,** and **substantia nigra** all lie inferior to the thalamus (see Figure 7-13).

One of the important functional roles of the basal ganglia is in the control of skeletal movement. On a simple level, we can consider two major pathways from the motor cortex of the cerebrum to the skeletal muscles. One of these is direct, via the internal capsule to the spinal cord, and is called the **pyramidal tract.** Lesions of this pathway produce spastic paralysis. The other is via the basal ganglia and is called the **extrapyramidal tract** or pathway. Lesions of this pathway interfere with skeletal muscle activity by producing meaningless motions, which are unintentional and unexpected by the individual performing them. It may be helpful to think of the pyramidal system as the main power source for motion, while the extrapyramidal system is necessary for coordinated, skilled activity that involves activation of muscles for motion, supression of other muscles that would interfere with the intended motion and control of sequence, and other factors involved in skilled activity. Two of the primary disabilities that result from basal ganglia damage are parkinsonism and athetosis. The patient with **parkinsonism** exhibits tremor at rest that tends to disappear during purposeful activity, a mask-like face, shuffling gait, and some rigidity. **Athetosis** is characterized by slow writhing movements, especially in the wrists and fingers. More extreme behaviors associated with damage to the basal ganglia include chorea and hemiballismus. **Chorea** is characterized by a sudden dance-like motion of, for example, an arm, which can be brought under

Table 7-3. The Basal Ganglia

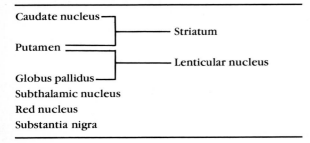

Caudate nucleus ┐
                 ├── Striatum
Putamen ═══╤═══┘
           │
           ├── Lenticular nucleus
Globus pallidus ┘
Subthalamic nucleus
Red nucleus
Substantia nigra

conscious control after the motion starts. Such a patient may be sitting quietly when suddenly his or her arm begins to move in a sweeping type of motion. The patient may then reach for something in order to mask the unwanted motion. **Hemiballismus** is similar, except that the motions involved are violent (hence ballistic) and are, therefore, much harder to control.

Thalamus

The thalamus is composed of a number of nuclear masses that can be differentiated on the basis of projections to and from them. These nuclei are in-

terconnected however. The thalamus serves as the point of convergence of all sensory information from the body which is to be projected to the cerebral cortex and to other parts of the brain. Following the general principle of the organization of the nervous system, the thalamus also receives fibers from the areas of the cortex to which it projects, thus completing feedback circuits. The thalamus thus may provide for integration of sensory information by controlling the relay of sensory information to various parts of the brain. Unfortunately, almost all of our information regarding thalamic projections to the cerebrum comes from

7-14. *Nuclei of the brain stem. A, Horizontal section of the brain shows the relationships among the thalamus and the basal ganglia. B, Basal ganglia and thalamus within the brain. (Adapted from an original painting by Frank H. Netter, M.D., from* The CIBA Collection of Medical Illustrations, *copyright by CIBA Pharmaceutical Company, Division of CIBA-GEIGY Corporation.)*

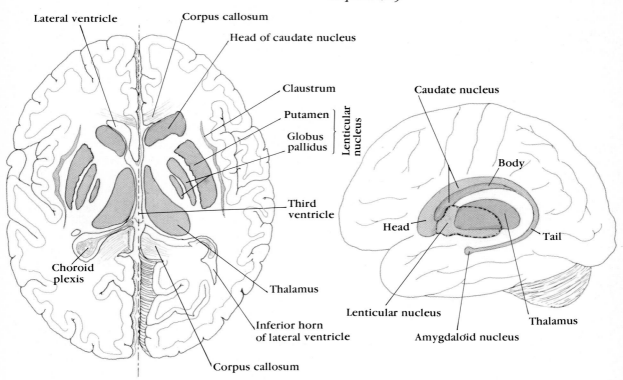

studies of monkeys [4], and so it is possible that descriptions do not completely represent human pathways.

Cerebellum

The surface of the cerebellum contains many sulci and furrows, which give it a laminated appearance (Figure 7-15). It consists of a superficial cortex of gray matter and an internal mass of white matter, which contains a number of nuclei that project fibers to the red nucleus, thalamus, and other brain-stem nuclei. The cerebellum receives great bundles of sensory fibers from throughout the nervous system, including the cerebral cortex, brain stem, and spinal cord, and also has massive projections to the cerebral cortex. It receives input from the proprioceptive and vestibular systems, which led Sherrington to call the cerebellum the head ganglion of the proprioceptive system. The cerebellum governs the synergistic action of all of the skeletal musculature. Both the basal ganglia and the cerebellum send a major portion of their output to the motor cortex of the cerebrum via the thalamus. Thus, in addition to acting to control movement, the cerebellum and the basal ganglia may serve a role in programming complex motion prior to its initiation [2].

Disorders associated with cerebellar dysfunc-

tion include awkwardness, problems in balance, and tremor during purposeful movements, including ataxia, dysmetria, dysdiadochokinesia, and intention tremor. **Ataxia** is characterized by awkwardness of posture and gait, and a tendency to fall. It usually includes some **dysmetria** (overshooting and/or undershooting the goal of motion in reaching) and **dysdiadochokinesia** (failure to perform rapid alternating movements).

Other Nuclei of the Brain Stem

Many other nuclei within the brain stem may be more meaningfully described in the context of the input and output channels of the nervous system of which they form a part. Of special interest will be those that lie in the pathways for proprioception and audition, which will be described in detail. As a first step, we will examine the input and output mechanisms to and from the CNS, that is, the cranial and spinal nerves.

Cranial Nerves

By tradition, there are twelve cranial nerves. However, two of them are actually CNS pathways rather than true cranial nerves. These are the olfactory and visual pathways, which are called the first and second cranial nerves. Table 7-4 presents the cranial nerves, their names and classifications with regard to sensory-motor, somatic-visceral, and special-general functions. As will be seen, three of the nerves are sensory, five are motor, and four contain both sensory and motor components.

The first cranial nerve (**olfactory**) mediates the sensation of smell. The second (**optic**) mediates the sensation of vision. The third (**oculomotor**), fourth (**trochlear**), and sixth (**abducent**) nerves mediate motion of the eyes and constriction of the pupils. The other cranial nerves, which govern functions basic to speech mechanisms, will be considered in more detail.

The fifth cranial nerve (**trigeminal**) has, as its name implies, three major branches, the ophthalmic, maxillary, and mandibular nerves (Figure 7-16). It mediates pain, temperature, touch, and proprioception from various areas of the head and supplies motor nerves to the muscles of the head.

7-15. *Midsaggital section through the cerebellum.*

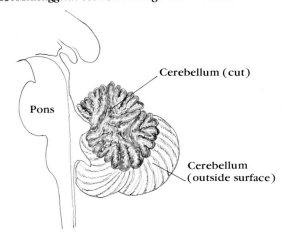

Pons

Cerebellum (cut)

Cerebellum (outside surface)

Table 7-4. The Cranial Nerves and Their Components

No.	Nerve	Classification	Function
I	Olfactory	SVA	Mediates sense of smell
II	Optic	SSA	Mediates vision, including conscious perception, involuntary oculoskeletal reflexes, and simple and consensual light reflexes
III	Oculomotor	GSA GSE GVE	Mediates voluntary eye movements and ipsilateral and consensual light reflexes
IV	Trochlear	GSA GSE	Mediates voluntary eye movement
V	Trigeminal	GSA SVE	Mediates pain, temperature, touch, and proprioception to various areas of the head and voluntary control of various muscles of the face
VI	Abducent	GSA GSE	Mediates voluntary eye movement
VII	Facial	GSA GVA SVA GVE SVE	Proprioception to the face and voluntary control of muscles of the face, suprahyoid area, and stapedius muscle; mediates taste, sensation of oral and nasal cavities, and function of facial and lingual glands
VIII	Vestibulocochlear	SSA	Mediates sense of hearing and balance
IX	Glossopharyngeal	GSA GVA SVA GVE SVE	Motor to stylopharyngeus muscle, sensory to external ear, glands of face, oral cavity, pharynx, velum, auditory tube, carotid sinus; mediates taste
X	Vagus	GSA GVA SVA GVE SVE	Sensory to the cranium, ear, larynx, esophagus, heart, bronchi, abdominal viscera. Mediates many visceral reflexes. Possibly motor to the larynx and velopharyngeal area
XI	Accessory	GSA GVE SVE	Motor and sensory to sternocleidomastoid and trapezius muscles and probably also to intrinsic muscles of larynx and velopharynx
XII	Hypoglossal	GSA GSE	Motor and sensory to muscles of the tongue and extrinsic laryngeal muscles

7-16. *The trigeminal nerve. (Reproduced, with permission, from Chusid JG:* Correlative Neuroanatomy and Functional Neurology, *17th ed. Copyright 1979 by Lange Medical Publications, Los Altos, California.)*

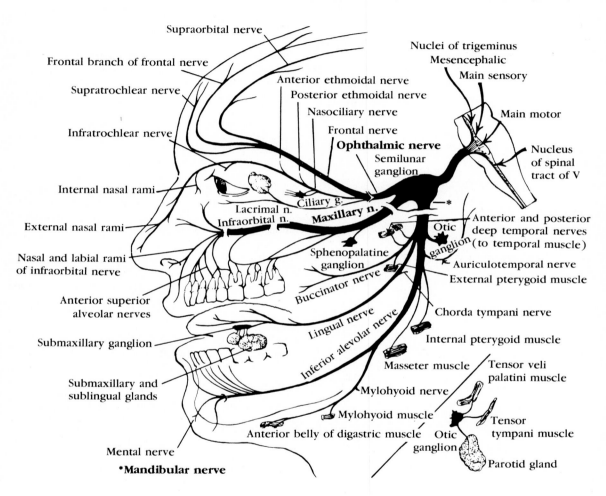

Proprioceptive impulses from and motor supply to the musculature are carried by the third branch, the **mandibular nerve.** It supplies the muscles of mastication (masseter, temporalis, buccinator, medial and lateral pterygoids), and also the tensor tympani and tensor veli palatini muscles, the mylohyoid, and anterior digastric. Tactile sensation from the nasal and oral cavities is also carried by the trigeminal. The proprioceptive fibers go to the mesencephalon (**mesencephalic nucleus**) while the motor fibers arise from the pons.

The seventh cranial nerve (**facial**) is principally motor. It supplies proprioceptive and motor fibers to stapedius, posterior digastric, and stylohyoid muscles as well as to the muscles of facial expression (Figure 7-17). It arises from the pons.

The eighth cranial nerve (**vestibulocochlear**) is sensory from the vestibular and auditory systems (Figure 7-18). As is the case with all peripheral sensory nerves, their cell bodies lie within a sensory ganglion external to the CNS. The fibers of the **vestibular nerve** arise from the semicircular canals, utricle, and saccule. The **vestibular ganglion** lies within the internal auditory

7-17. *The facial nerve. (Reproduced, with permission, from Chusid JG:* Correlative Neuroanatomy and Functional Neurology, *17th ed. Copyright 1979 by Lange Medical Publications, Los Altos, California.)*

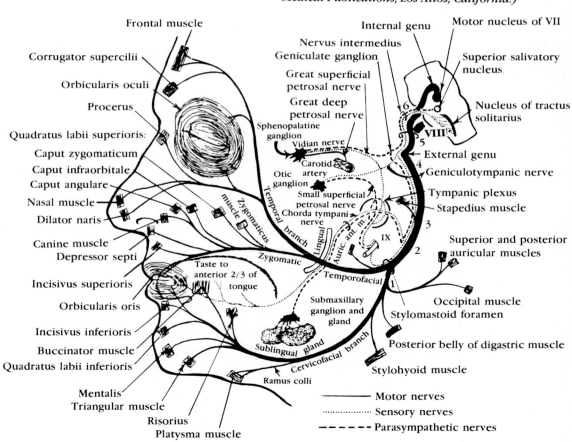

meatus. The vestibular nerve enters the cranium via the internal auditory meatus with the cochlear and facial nerves. Some of the fibers enter the brain stem and pass directly to the cerebellum. The majority are interrupted within the pons and medulla. From there they proceed to the cerebellum, the motor nuclei of the ocular muscles, the motor nuclei of the spinal cord, and perhaps to other locations within the CNS (Figure 7-19). It is interesting that there is no known pathway to the thalamus from the vestibular nucleus [6]. The projections to the cerebellum, ocular muscles, and spinal motor neurons are indicative of the interaction of the visual and balance systems as well as balance, gait, and posture.

The ganglion for the **auditory nerve,** located within the modiolus, is called the **spiral ganglion** owing to the anatomical relationships within the cochlea (see Chap. 6; Audition). Fibers of the cochlear nerve are primarily afferent (that is, project information to the CNS). However, there are also efferent fibers within the auditory nerve that project from the brain stem to the cochlea. These neurons are inhibitory and may be involved in sharpening of responses from the cochlea with regard to specific stimulus features. The following descriptions, except where noted, will concern the afferent pathways.

The cochlear neurons terminate within one of the two brain stem nuclei. These nuclei are the **dorsal** and **ventral cochlear nuclei,** which lie in the lateral part of the medulla (Figure 7-20). The majority of fibers (80% in animals studied) cross midline within the medulla via one of three pathways called the **dorsal, intermediate,** and **ventral acoustic stria.** If one of these pathways is principal, it is the ventral stria (also called the **trapezoid body**). Some of the crossed fibers synapse at the level of the medulla in the superior olive. Fibers from the superior olive rise with uninterrupted fibers from the contralateral cochlear nucleus in a common pathway called the **lateral lemniscus.** Fibers from the cochlear nuclei that do not cross midline synapse within the olivary nucleus of the same side before rising in the ipsilateral lateral lemniscus.

7-18. *The vestibulocochlear nerve. (Reproduced, with permission, from Chusid JG:* Correlative Neuroanatomy and Functional Neurology, *17th ed. Copyright 1979 by Lange Medical Publications, Los Altos, California.)*

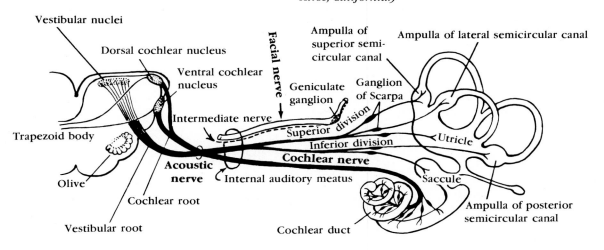

The majority of fibers of the lateral lemniscus rise to the **inferior colliculus,** which is a nucleus within the dorsal part of the midbrain. Some fibers, however, are interrupted in a nucleus located within the lateral lemniscus. From the inferior colliculus, fibers are projected either back across midline to the inferior colliculus of the side of the cochlear origin, or directly to the next relay station, the medial geniculate body. The **medial geniculate body** is a part of the thalamus. From the thalamus, fibers of the auditory pathway are projected to the superior gyrus of the temporal lobe, the **auditory cortex.** Crossing of fibers from one side to the other may also occur at the level of the thalamus and, by means of the corpus callosum, at the level of the cerebral cortex. The probable pathways are illustrated in Figure 7-21.

In Chapter 6 it was pointed out that the peripheral fibers of the auditory nerve are tonotopically related. That is, fibers from the apex of the cochlea are most responsive to low frequency stimuli, while fibers from the basilar portion are most responsive to higher frequency stimuli. This tonotopic relationship is maintained throughout the auditory pathway and is found within the auditory cortex. Damage to the auditory cortex apparently does not prevent perception of frequency or intensity of simple stimuli but does interfere with more complex auditory functions and with localization of the sound source.

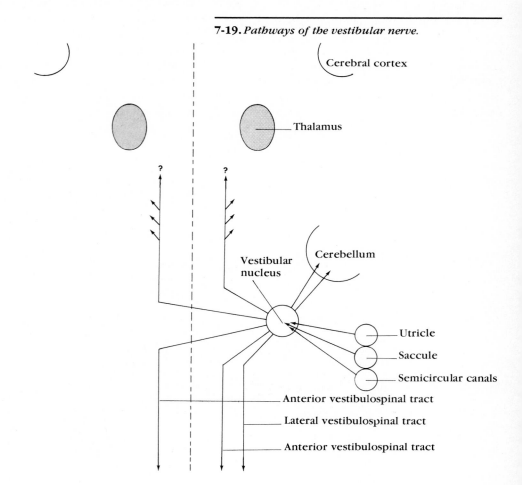

7-19. *Pathways of the vestibular nerve.*

Cerebral cortex

Thalamus

Vestibular nucleus

Cerebellum

Utricle

Saccule

Semicircular canals

Anterior vestibulospinal tract

Lateral vestibulospinal tract

Anterior vestibulospinal tract

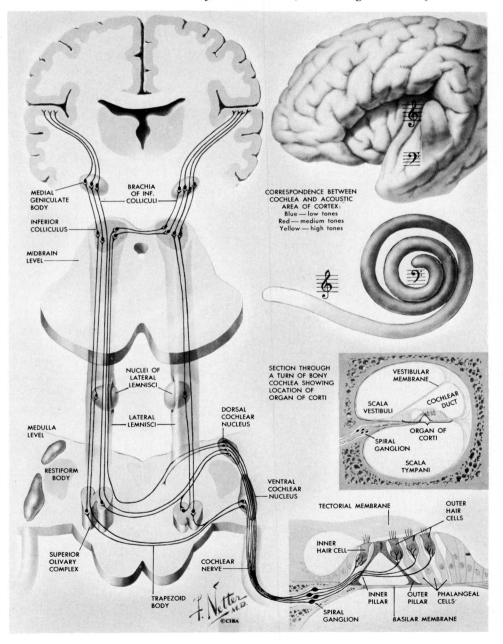

7-21. *Diagram of the auditory pathways from one cochlea.*

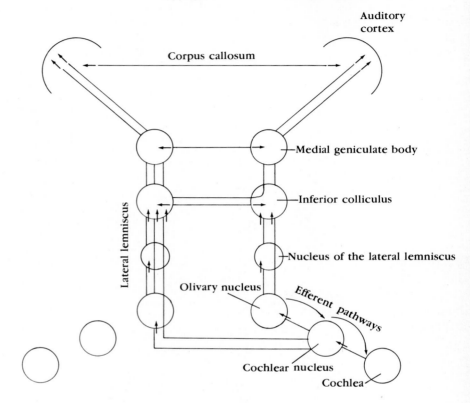

Auditory cortex

Corpus callosum

Medial geniculate body

Inferior colliculus

Nucleus of the lateral lemniscus

Lateral lemniscus

Olivary nucleus

Efferent Pathways

Cochlear nucleus

Cochlea

7-22. *Cranial nerves X and XI and formation of the vagus nerve.*

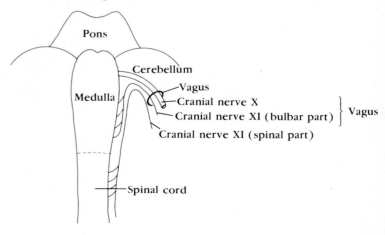

Pons

Cerebellum

Medulla

Vagus

Cranial nerve X

Cranial nerve XI (bulbar part)

Cranial nerve XI (spinal part)

Vagus

Spinal cord

The ninth cranial nerve (**glossopharyngeal**) is primarily a sensory nerve but does supply motor innervation to the stylopharyngeus muscle. It mediates sensation from the external ear, part of the tongue, and the velopharyngeal area. It arises from the medulla.

The tenth cranial nerve (**vagus**) arises from the medulla and joins with part of the eleventh cranial nerve peripherally (Figure 7-22). The vagus consists of both sensory and motor components, which principally supply the visceral components of the body. The nerves supplying the muscles of

7-23. *The hypoglossal nerve. (Reproduced, with permission, from Chusid JG:* Correlative Neuroanatomy and Functional Neurology, *17th ed. Copyright 1979 by Lange Medical Publications, Los Altos, California.)*

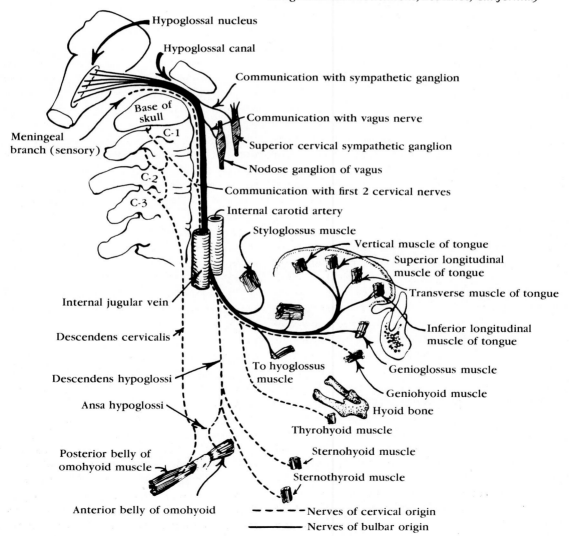

the larynx and the velopharyngeal muscles are usually described as also arising from the vagus; however, this designation is problematic. The peripheral part of the vagus consists of the tenth cranial nerve and also a branch of the eleventh cranial nerve. There is some evidence that the innervation of the laryngeal and velopharyngeal musculature actually derives from the branch of the eleventh cranial nerve rather than from the tenth.

The eleventh cranial nerve (**accessory**) arises from a nucleus within the medulla and also from the upper five or six cervical segments of the spinal cord. The spinal segments give rise to the **external ramus**, which innervates the sternocleidomastoid and trapezius muscles. The **cranial branch** joins the tenth cranial nerve to form the vagus and is probably responsible for innervation of the muscles of the larynx and velopharyngeal complex.

The twelfth cranial nerve (**hypoglossal**) is both sensory and motor. It arises from the medulla and innervates the extrinsic muscles of the larynx and the intrinsic and extrinsic muscles of the tongue (Figure 7-23).

Spinal Nerves

Spinal nerves are associated with each segment of the spinal cord and consist of both motor and sensory components. Some of these are associated with the autonomic system, but we will consider those that are associated with skeletal movement and sensory information related to the control of movement. As a general pattern, the spinal nerves serve areas of the body associated, embryologically, with the particular segment of the spinal cord. This can be most easily seen in the distribution of fibers mediating sensation from the skin (Figure 7-24). Motor and sensory innervation to skeletal muscles of the trunk and limbs follows a similar pattern. Sensory nerves enter the spinal cord from their spinal ganglia to the posterior part of the spinal cord via the dorsal root (Figure 7-25). Motor nerves exit via the ventral root from the anterior spinal cord. The dorsal and ventral roots join lateral to the spinal cord to form the sensory-motor spinal nerve.

Spinal Cord

The spinal cord extends from the medulla oblongata to the level of the first or second lumbar vertebra. A thin filament of pia mater called the **terminal filament** extends from the inferior end of the spinal cord to the posterior surface of the coccyx. In cross-section, the spinal cord is roughly circular, but flattened slightly from anterior to posterior (see Figure 7-25). The surface of the cord is marked by a number of longitudinal furrows. The most prominent of these is the **anterior median fissure**, which is located at the midline anteriorly and extends posteriorly to a depth of about one-third of the spinal cord. A **posterior median sulcus** is found opposite to it. A thin **posterior septum** of pia mater extends from the posterior median sulcus anteriorly to the central canal. The fissure, sulcus, and septum thus described separate the spinal cord into roughly symmetrical left and right halves. Two other furrows on each side of the spinal cord form landmarks for further descriptions of the cord. These are the **anterolateral sulcus**, found in the line of the ventral roots of the spinal nerves, and the **posterolateral sulcus**, located in the line of the dorsal roots of the spinal nerves.

The spinal cord is composed of gray matter and white matter. The gray matter is roughly "H" shaped in the central part of the cord and is surrounded by white matter. The gray matter consists of cell bodies and unmyelinated fibers. Neural fiber pathways coursing longitudinally through the spinal cord are called **fiber tracts.** Fibers serving a particular function, such as proprioception, travel together, Each fiber tract consists of fibers that have the same origin (such as proprioceptive end-organs), the same termination, and the same function. A bundle of fiber tracts located together is called a **funiculus.** Subdivisions of a funiculus, each consisting of a number of tracts, are called **fasciculi.** Terminology of the tracts and fasciculi is not consistent. Fortunately, the historical tendency to name pathways after their discoverer is now out of vogue; instead, pathways are named for their origin and destination (spinocerebellar tract), for their position in the cord (dorsolateral fasciculus), or for their shape (fasciculus gracilis).

7-24. *A typical spinal nerve*

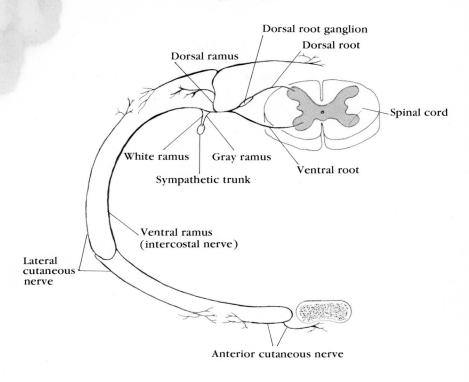

Dorsal root ganglion

Dorsal root

Dorsal ramus

Spinal cord

White ramus

Gray ramus

Ventral root

Sympathetic trunk

Ventral ramus
(intercostal nerve)

Lateral
cutaneous
nerve

Anterior cutaneous nerve

7-25. *Cross-section of the spinal cord.*

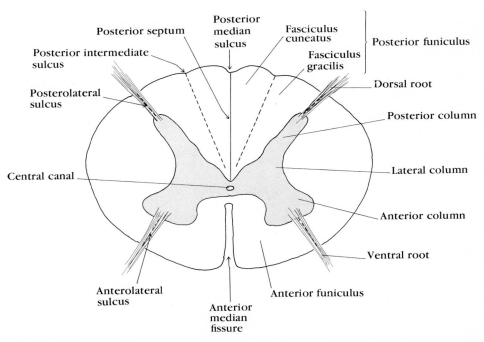

Posterior
median
sulcus

Posterior septum

Fasciculus
cuneatus

Posterior intermediate
sulcus

Posterior funiculus

Fasciculus
gracilis

Posterolateral
sulcus

Dorsal root

Posterior column

Central canal

Lateral column

Anterior column

Ventral root

Anterolateral
sulcus

Anterior funiculus

Anterior
median
fissure

311

Since these tracts, funiculi, and fasciculi course longitudinally within the spinal cord, some of them are also called **columns.** The term **horn** is used to refer to the most anterior and posterior parts of the gray matter, which give rise to the ventral and dorsal spinal roots. This term is descriptive when referring to a cross-section of the cord. However, since the "horns" extend the length of the cord, the horns are also called the **anterior** and **posterior columns.** Thus "anterior horn" and "anterior column" are synonymous. Some of the principal terminology applying to the gray and white portions of the spinal cord is presented in Figure 7-25. It should be noted that some authors

use the term "posterior column" to refer to the posterior funiculi. This is inappropriate and obviously confusing to the unprepared reader.

Sensory Pathways

The pathways of the cranial nerves within the brain stem, cerebrum, and cerebellum beyond those described previously are not known in detail. There is a good deal more information with regard to spinal pathways and their course to and from higher centers. Even here, however, much of our information regarding sensory and motor pathways is based on studies of subhuman animals and clinical studies of human patients. The fol-

7-26. *Pathways for conscious proprioception.*

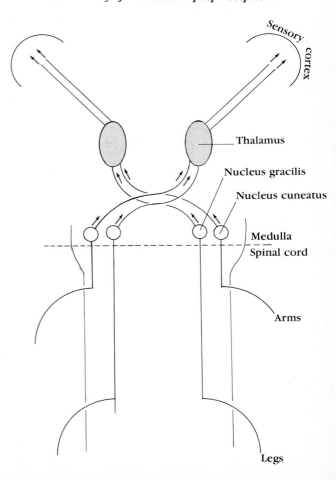

lowing descriptions concern the pathways to and from the spinal nerves.

All sensory input enters the spinal cord via the dorsal spinal roots. Proprioceptive fibers from muscles, tendons, and joints take two routes after entering the cord. One of these is to the thalamus and then to the cerebral cortex and the other is to the cerebellum. It is probable that the pathway to the thalamus subserves conscious proprioception whereas the pathway to the cerebellum subserves unconscious proprioception during already learned motor patterns. The pathway to the thalamus (Figure 7-26) is located in the posterior funiculus. This funiculus is divided into two parts. The more medial of these, the **fasciculus gracilis,** consists of proprioceptive fibers from the lower body and legs. The more lateral part is the **fasciculus cuneatus,** which consists of propriocep-

tive fibers from the upper body and arms. These fibers rise through the spinal cord on the side of origin and terminate in nuclei of the posterior medulla called the **nucleus gracilis** and **nucleus cuneatus.** Here they synpase with fibers that cross midline and rise to the thalamus. Thus damage below the medulla would result in loss of proprioception on the same side as the injury, while damage above that level would result in loss on the opposite side of the body.

The pathway to the cerebellum (Figure 7-27) is called the **spinocerebellar tract** and is located within the lateral funiculus. Fibers of this pathway rise to the cerebellar hemisphere of the same side. Thus, damage to this pathway or its area of projection within the cerebellum results in loss of proprioception to the side of injury.

Fibers subserving the sensations of pain and

7-27. *Pathways for subconscious proprioception.*

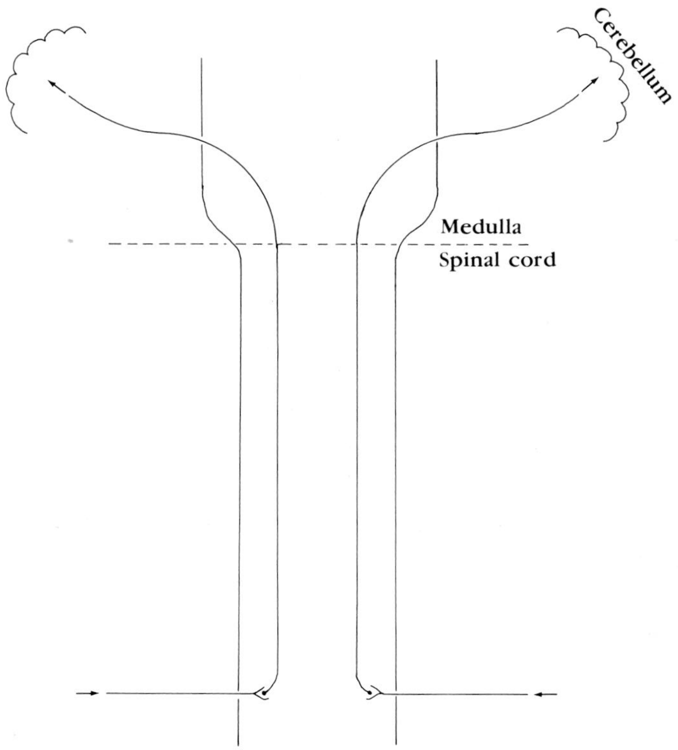

temperature (Figure 7-28) enter the spinal cord and form branches that extend over several segments of the cord within the posterior column. Synapses are formed over several levels of the cord with fibers that then cross midline to the lateral funiculus. Here they form the **lateral spinothalamic tract,** which projects to the thalamus. Damage to this pathway will usually result in loss on the opposite side of the body.

Fibers subserving the sensation of light touch (Figure 7-29) enter the cord and branch over several levels of the spinal cord both above and below the level of entry. Some of these will form synapses on the side of entry and others cross before synapsing. The ipsilateral fibers rise with the pro-

prioceptive fibers in the posterior funiculus and probably aid in sensations relating to shape and stereognosis. The crossed fibers rise in the spinothalamic tract. Because of the extensive branching of the fibers subserving touch, this sensation is unlikely to be abolished by injury to any particular pathway in the cord.

The above descriptions relate to the major pathways for sensation. However, there are innumerable commissural and internuncial fibers within the spinal cord and brain that interconnect the various synaptic pools. Some of the internuncials also interconnect the sensory and motor fibers of the spinal cord and brain stem.

7-28. *Pathways for pain and temperature from one side of the body.*

7-29. *Pathways for touch from one side of the body.*

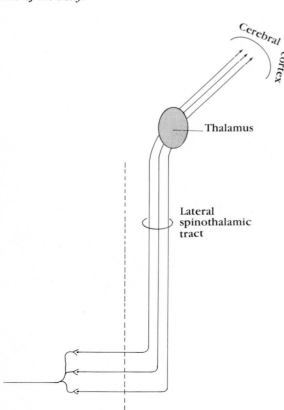

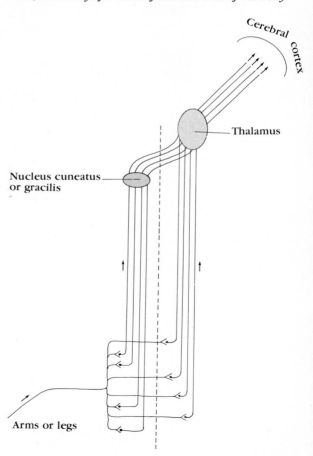

7-30. *Pyramidal tract projections to the anterior horn cells. (© Copyright 1953, 1972, CIBA Pharmaceutical Company, Division of CIBA-GEIGY Corporation. Reprinted with permission from* The CIBA Collection of Medical Illustrations *by Frank H. Netter, M.D. All rights reserved.)*

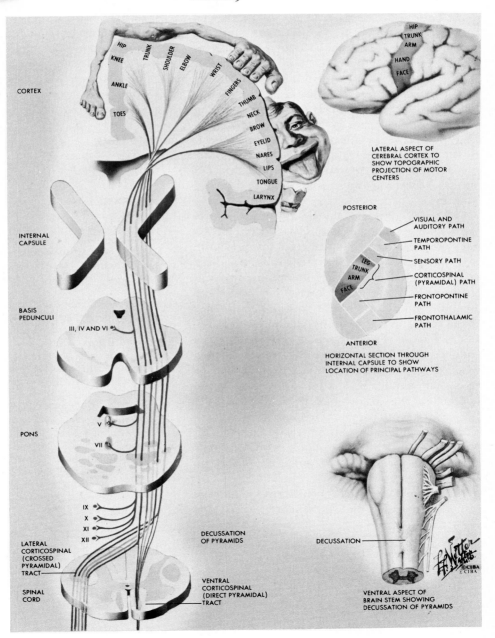

Motor Pathways

For convenience, the motor pathways of the nervous system can be divided into two categories, the lower motor neurons and the upper motor neurons. The **lower motor neurons** have their cell bodies in the anterior columns (horns) of the spinal cord and send their axons to the skeletal muscles. The **upper motor neurons** form the pyramidal and extrapyramidal system and activate the lower motor neurons. The lower motor neurons form the **final common pathway** to the muscle. Thus damage to a lower motor neuron will result in **flaccid paralysis, atrophy** of the muscles supplied, and **hyporeflexia.** Since the upper motor neurons involve pathways connecting the motor cortex, basal ganglia, and other CNS nuclei to the final common pathway, damage to the upper motor neurons results in more complex symptoms.

As previously noted, the upper motor neuron pathways consist of the pyramidal tract and the extrapyramidal tract. Pyramidal tract fibers (Figure 7-30) originate in the motor cortex. From there they pass inferiorly via the internal capsule and **corticospinal tract** to the anterior column, where they form their first synapse with the cell bodies of the lower motor neurons. At the level of the medulla, most of the pyramidal tract fibers cross midline. Thus damage above the medulla results primarily in contralateral symptoms, while damage below the medulla results primarily in ipsilateral symptoms. The majority of those fibers of the pyramidal tract that do not cross at the level of the medulla do so immediately prior to synapsing with the cell bodies of the lower motor neurons at their level of exit from the cord. Some fibers may remain uncrossed.

The extrapyramidal tract consists of a number of pathways through the spinal cord, which are named for their apparent origin. So, for example, there are rubrospinal, olivospinal, vestibulospinal, and other pathways of this system that terminate on the lower motor neurons. Symptoms associated with damage to the various nuclei that make up the basal ganglia have already been described. The term **upper motor neuron lesion** usually refers to damage to the pyramidal tract or to the spinal pathways of the extrapyramidal system. Upper motor neuron lesions are generally described as resulting in **spastic paralysis** and **hyperreflexia.** This would suggest damage to fibers originating in area 6 of the cortex and/or to interference with the inhibitory mechanisms essential to normal motor activity.

REFERENCES

1. Ganong WF: *The Nervous System*. Los Altos, Calif., Lange Medical Publications, 1979.
2. Kornhuber HH: Cerebral cortex, cerebellum, and basal ganglia: An introduction to their motor function. In Schmitt FO, et al (Eds): *The Neurosciences Third Study Program.* Cambridge, Mass.: MIT Press, 1974.
3. Milner B: Introduction to hemispheric specialization and interaction. In Schmitt FO, et al (Eds): *The Neurosciences Third Study Program.* Cambridge, Mass, MIT Press, 1974.
4. Netter FH: *The Ciba Collection of Medical Illustrations: Volume I, Nervous System.* Summit, NJ, Ciba Foundation, 1962.
5. Prutting CA, Elliott JB: Synergy: Toward a model of language. In Lass N (Ed): *Speech and Language: Advances in Basic Research and Practice, Vol 1.* New York, Academic Press, 1979.
6. Ranson SW, Clark SL: *The Anatomy of the Nervous System.* Philadelphia, WB Saunders, 1959.
7. Sperry RW: Lateral specialization in the surgically separated hemispheres. In Schmitt FO, et al (Eds): *The Neurosciences Third Study Program.* Cambridge, Mass, MIT Press, 1974.

Name Index

Subject Index

Pages on which figures or tables appear are given in parentheses. The following abbreviations are used in the text:

A^- = anion
ANS = autonomic nervous system
ATP = adenosine triphosphate
Ca^{++} = calcium cation
Cl^- = chloride anion
cm = centimeter
CM = cochlear microphonic
CNS = central nervous system
CT = computed tomography
EMG = electromyography
EP = endolymphatic potential
EPSP = excitatory postsynaptic membrane potential
Hz = hertz
IPSP = inhibitory postsynaptic membrane potential
K^+ = potassium cation
m = meter
mm = millimeter
μm = micrometer
mV = millivolt
Na^+ = sodium cation
nm = nanometer
PNS = peripheral nervous system
SP = summation potential

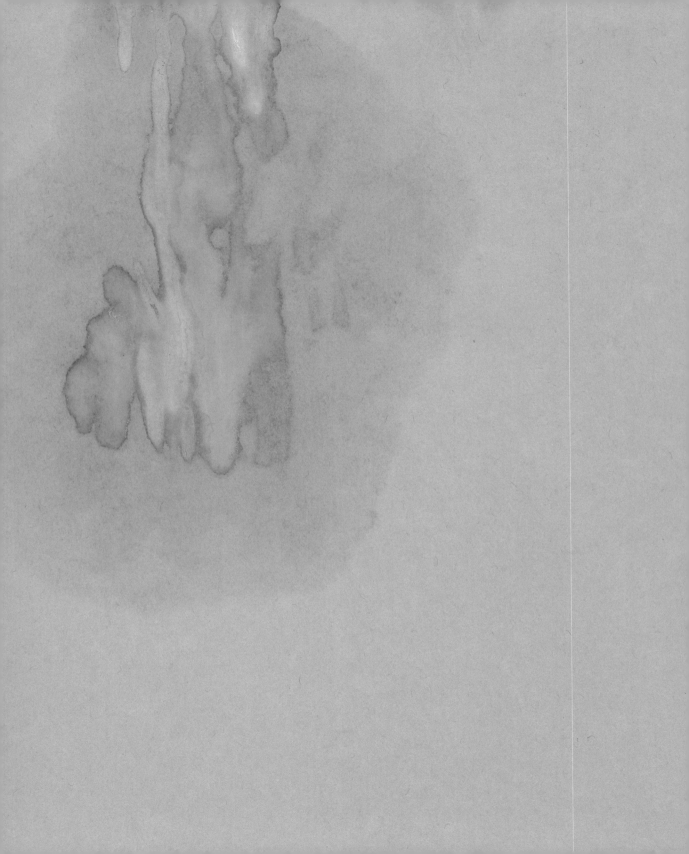

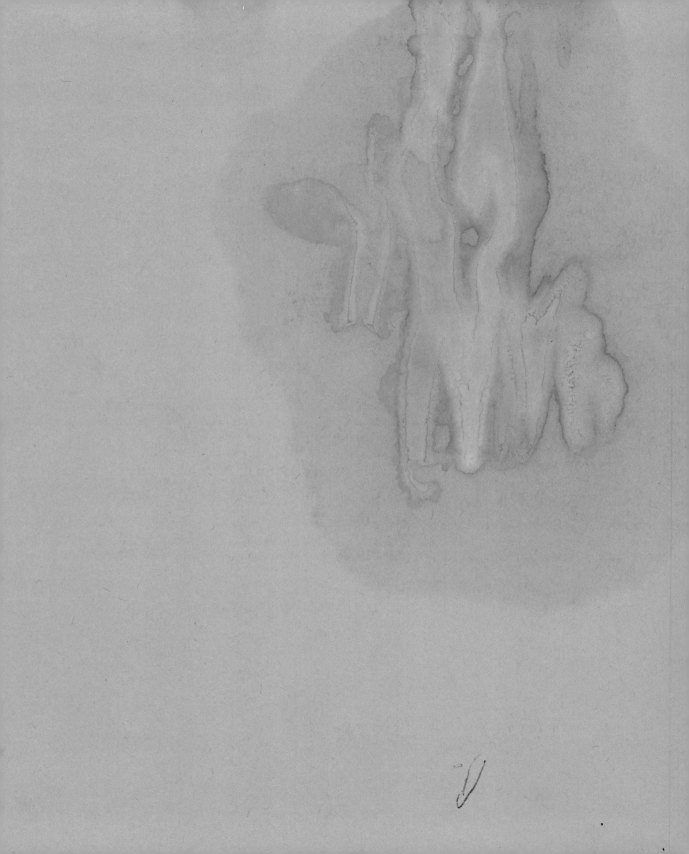